Second Edition

Tutorials in Su[rgery]

Common Surgical Problems

F G Smiddy, MD, ChM, FRCS

Consultant Surgeon to the General Infirmary at Leeds and Clayton Hospital, Wakefield. Member of the Court of Examiners of the Royal College of Surgeons, England. Examiner in Pathology to the College of Surgeons, England.

Pitman

PITMAN BOOKS LIMITED
128 Long Acre, London WC2E 9AN

Associated Companies
Pitman Publishing Pty Ltd, Melbourne
Pitman Publishing New Zealand Ltd, Wellington

First Published 1977
Second Edition 1984

British Library Cataloguing in Publication Data
Smiddy, F.G.
  Tutorials in surgery.—2nd ed.
  1
  1. Surgery
  I. Title
  617   RD 31

ISBN 0-272-79694-8

© F G Smiddy 1977, 1984

All rights reserved. No part of this publication may be reproduced, stored in a retrieval system, or transmitted, in any form or by any means, electronic, mechanical, photocopying, recording and/or otherwise, without the prior written permission of the publishers.

This book may not be lent, resold or hired out or otherwise disposed of by way of trade in any form of binding or cover other than that in which it is published, without the prior consent of the publishers. This book is sold subject to the Standard Conditions of Sale of Net Books and may not be sold in the UK below the net price.

Printed in Great Britain at The Pitman Press, Bath

TO CLARE AND PAUL

Contents

Preface xi

1 Surgical Principles
1.1 Causes and treatment of shock in the surgical patient 1
1.2 Aetiology and treatment of acute renal failure in the surgical patient 11
1.3 Measurements used to monitor cardiovascular function in the severely ill patient 17
1.4 Causes and treatment of fluid and electrolyte imbalance in the surgical patient 22
1.5 Diagnosis and management of pulmonary complications following abdominal surgery 27
1.6 Indications for, and complications of, tracheostomy 35
1.7 Common non-surgical causes of acute abdominal pain 39

2 Endocrine Surgery
2.1 Laboratory diagnosis of primary thyrotoxicosis 45
2.2 Aetiology and treatment of primary thyrotoxicosis 49
2.3 Pathology, diagnosis and treatment of hyperparathyroidism 59
2.4 Diagnosis, investigation and treatment of endocrine-secreting tumours of the adrenal glands 64
2.5 Endocrine-secreting tumours of the gastrointestinal tract 77

3 Surgical Oncology
3.1 Classification, pathology, clinical presentation and treatment of bone tumours 86
3.2 Investigation, pathology and treatment of the thyroid nodule 94
3.3 Common benign swellings of the breast 102
3.4 Different methods of staging breast cancer and factors affecting the prognosis 106
3.5 Tumours of the lymphoreticular tissues with special reference to Hodgkin's disease 114
3.6 Diagnosis and treatment of bladder tumours 121
3.7 Pathology, clinical presentation and treatment of pigmented lesions of the skin 127

4 Orthopaedic Problems
4.1 Causes of an 'irritable' hip in childhood 132
4.2 Pathology, diagnosis and treatment of lumbar disc lesions 141
4.3 Pathology of osteoarthrosis with particular reference to the hip joint 148
4.4 Fractures and the general principles of treatment 153
4.5 Common complications of fractures 158
4.6 Fractures of the cervical spine, their complications and treatment 162

5 Soft Tissue Injury

5.1	Management of head injuries	170
5.2	Diagnosis, complications and treatment of chest injuries	177
5.3	Treatment of blunt injuries to the abdomen	182
5.4	Principles involved in the treatment of nerve and tendon injuries, particularly in the hand and wrist	191
5.5	Aetiology, symptomatology and treatment of tetanus	195
5.6	Aetiology and management of anaerobic infections	199

6 Gastrointestinal Surgery

6.1	Enlargement of the parotid gland: causes and treatment	205
6.2	Causes and treatment of dysphagia	212
6.3	Hiatus hernia: symptoms, treatment and complications	222
6.4	Investigation and treatment of haematemesis, excluding bleeding oesophageal varices	227
6.5	Management of bleeding oesophageal varices	231
6.6	Aetiology of gall-stones	237
6.7	Major complications of gall-stones and their treatment	241
6.8	Causes of jaundice and the evaluation of diagnostic methods	249
6.9	Aetiology, diagnosis, complications and treatment of acute pancreatitis	254
6.10	Diagnosis and management of chronic pancreatitis	263
6.11	Indications for and complications of splenectomy	269
6.12	Classification of intestinal obstruction and the general principles of management	274
6.13	Neonatal intestinal obstruction, excluding anorectal abnormalities	279
6.14	Surgical causes of malabsorption	286
6.15	Aetiology, pathology and management of Crohn's disease	293
6.16	Pathology, clinical course and treatment of ulcerative colitis	298
6.17	Aetiology, pathology, clinical presentation and management of diverticular disease	304
6.18	Pathology and treatment of carcinoma of the rectum	308
6.19	Congenital deformities of the rectum and anal canal	313

7 Urology

7.1	Causes and treatment of urinary tract infections	319
7.2	Diagnosis and treatment of carcinoma of the prostate	323
7.3	Benign prostatic enlargement: pathology, treatment and complications	328
7.4	Pathology, signs, symptoms, treatment and prognosis of renal tumours	334
7.5	Swellings of the scrotum, and the pathology and treatment of testicular tumours	339
7.6	Investigation and surgical management of stones in the renal tract	345
7.7	Causes and treatment of vesicoureteric reflux	351

8 Vascular Diseases

8.1 Anatomy of the sympathetic system, and the place of sympathectomy in surgery — 356
8.2 Embolism and the treatment of arterial embolus — 361
8.3 Pathology, symptoms, signs, and investigations of atherosclerosis in the lower limb — 366
8.4 Arterial reconstruction in the lower limb — 375
8.5 Diagnosis and management of the postphlebitic syndrome — 380

Preface

The genesis of the first edition of *Tutorials in Surgery 1* lay in the needs and aspirations of the many candidates that the author examined during their surgical training.

The necessity for a second edition which has involved the almost complete rewriting of the original text became patently obvious to the author because of the changes which have occurred in surgical practice since the first edition was written in 1977. These changes have sometimes been obvious and sometimes subtle and many examples of both types of change will be found if any reader chooses to compare the first with the second edition. The author is, indeed, reminded of one of the few mistakes made by the father figure of Leeds surgery, Lord Moynihan, when he said that surgery had reached its apogee in the early thirties. Since then advances in diagnostic methods and surgical endeavour have multiplied almost yearly and Lord Moynihan would perforce have to eat his words.

As with the first edition the topics dealt with have been culled from the notes I have made at various courses I have either organized or attended and cover a spectrum that includes many of the subjects universally beloved by examiners.

The practice of surgery consists of two elements; manual dexterity and a basic knowledge of disease processes. In regard to the first of these it is of historical interest that in the past the final fellowship examination of the College of Surgeons of England required the candidate to perform some simple operation on a preserved cadaver but today, of course, it is assumed that technical ability has been mastered in the operating theatre during the course of training and only theoretical knowledge of this subject is required, see *Tutorials 3*.

To some candidates who present themselves for higher examinations in surgery it seems to the author that some find it more difficult to satisfy in the second element and, from the observations I have made over the years, the fault appears to lie not so much in the candidates' lack of knowledge as in their lack of ability to express themselves adequately on paper or in speech when exploring surgical problems. It is to help repair this defect that this book has been written.

Regardless of the type of examination a surgical candidate faces in whatever part of the world he or she lives the requirements of the examiner are much the same—to discover the extent of the candidate's knowledge as he or she reveals it in the written essay, the multiple choice paper or the *viva voce*. The second object of this book, therefore, is to examine the topics enumerated in depth.

I must of necessity express my thanks to several colleagues, to Mr M Flowers who helped in the development of section 5.4, to Mr R Berkin with whom I discussed the various problems associated with fractures and Mr J Beck with whom I discussed the latest development in neonatal surgery.

Finally, as always, Mrs P Docherty struggled with the written word and finally out of chaos came, I hope, order.

F G Smiddy
1983

1 Surgical Principles

1.1 Causes and treatment of shock in the surgical patient
1.2 Aetiology and treatment of acute renal failure in the surgical patient
1.3 Measurements used to monitor cardiovascular function in the severely ill patient
1.4 Causes and treatment of fluid and electrolyte imbalance in the surgical patient
1.5 Diagnosis and management of pulmonary complications following abdominal surgery
1.6 Indications for, and complications of, tracheostomy
1.7 Common non-surgical causes of acute abdominal pain

1.1 Causes and treatment of shock in the surgical patient

Definition. It is difficult to find a definition of shock that meets with the general agreement of both laboratory workers and clinicians.

By clinicians, the term is most commonly used when referring to patients suffering from acute systemic hypotension, a condition usually, but not always, associated with pallor, weakness, sweating and a rapid, thready pulse. Most laboratory investigators, however, feel that this definition is too vague and that, at the very least, the term shock should be qualified by the presumed cause.

Moon, in 1942, found that three general definitions of shock appeared in the literature:

1 those in which the author incorporated a theory of origin;
2 those based purely on clinical signs;
3 those representing a combination of both approaches.

At the present time, most people would accept that 'shock' is a condition in which there is:

1 a persistent deficiency of blood flow through the peripheral vascular bed;
2 inadequate perfusion of vital organs such as the brain, heart and kidneys which, if persistent and severe, will lead to functional failure.

The major causes of shock are:

1 Anaphylactic
2 Cardiogenic

3 Hypovolaemic
4 Bacteriogenic
5 Neurogenic
6 Adrenal insufficiency

Common features observed in the shock syndrome include hypotension, tachycardia, peripheral cyanosis most frequently associated with cold extremities although in some forms of bacteraemic shock the extremities may be warm, increased thirst, oliguria, restlessness and apprehension which may be followed by confusion, unconsciousness, and death.

COMMON PHYSIOLOGICAL DISTURBANCES IN SHOCK

1 *Metabolic acidosis*
This develops because tissue metabolism becomes anaerobic and pyruvic, and lactic acid production increases. With their increasing concentration in the extracellular fluid space metabolic acidosis develops. When the pH falls below 7.2 it may impair myocardial function and interfere with the action of endogenous or exogenous catecholamines. In addition vascular reactivity and permeability is affected and fluid leaks from the circulation into the interstitial space. The continuing loss of plasma gradually increases blood viscosity and hence increases the resistance to flow.

2 *Potassium retention*
This is particularly marked in patients with decreased renal function. Elevation above 7 mmol/l leads to the risk of death due to myocardial poisoning.

3 *Changes in enzyme activity*

4 *Changes in peripheral resistance*
These are in part compensatory but may be due to the immediate cause of the shock syndrome.

5 *Changes in pulmonary function*
The arterial Po_2 frequently falls as low as 50 mmHg (6.7 kPa). The causes of this are discussed under the complications of shock.

6 *Fall in cardiac output*
Cardiac output is a product of stroke volume and heart rate. The former is determined by three variables:

(*a*) ventricular preload, which equates to the ventricular end diastolic volume which in turn is directly proportional to the force of contraction of the heart muscle;
(*b*) myocardial contractility;

(c) ventricular afterload which is an expression of the resistance to ventricular muscle shortening during systole. It can be calculated from the cardiac output and arterial pressure or inferred clinically from the degree of vasoconstriction.

CLINICAL FEATURES ASSOCIATED WITH VARIOUS TYPES OF SHOCK

1 Anaphylactic shock

This type of shock was first described by Richet and Portier in 1902 after they had investigated the severe reactions which occurred in dogs after repeated injections of toxins derived from sea anemones. It occurs in individuals predisposed to develop abnormal amounts of IgE antibody of the reaginic type in response to antigenic stimulation. The first dose of antigen must reach the tissues in an unaltered state and may be injected, inhaled or ingested. Anaphylactic shock follows the administration of a second dose of antigen but only if time is given for the reaginic antibody fixed to the tissue cells to be formed. The second dose of antigen triggers the release of various vasoactive agents of which the most important is histamine. This form of shock is one of the many complications of penicillin and related antibiotics. The World Health Organization estimated the frequency of anaphylactic shock after penicillin injections at between 0.015 and 0.04 per cent of patients treated, with a fatality rate of between 0.0015 and 0.002 per cent. Of those dying, approximately 70 per cent had previously received penicillin and the remainder were suffering from fungal infections, usually of the interdigital clefts of the feet.

In man the effects of anaphylactic shock are acute respiratory distress due to broncho-bronchiolar spasm together with generalized oedema. Itching, urticaria and diffuse erythema of the skin may also occur.

This form of shock is usually treated by the injection of 0.5–1 ml of adrenaline intramuscularly or 0.2 ml well diluted intravenously.

2 Cardiogenic shock

The commonest cause of cardiogenic shock is acute myocardial infarction; less common causes include low cardiac output following cardiac surgery, and massive pulmonary embolus. Infrequent causes include myocarditis, persistent tachycardia, and cardiac tamponade. Clinical manifestations are mainly caused by gross reduction in cardiac output, when the systolic and diastolic pressures fall, the former usually to a greater degree than the latter. Low cardiac output leads to compensatory peripheral vasoconstriction and a cold sweaty skin. There is, usually, but not always, an associated cardiac arrhythmia. Deterioration leads to increasingly inadequate tissue perfusion and increasing metabolic acidosis.

The outlook in cardiogenic shock is dependent on the degree of damage to the myocardium. The treatment of cardiogenic shock consists of potent analgesics to relieve pain and the administration of oxygen together with the use of drugs to improve myocardial contractility. Among the latter are the catecholamines and the digitalis glycosides. Dopamine, which is a catecholamine, has a powerful action on the β-1-adrenergic receptors and is given in a dose of 1–30 µg/kg/min. Digoxin is administered in a dose of 0.5 mg in saline over 30 minutes followed by a further 0.5 mg over 2 hours, after which a maintenance dose is required; its effect should be evident within 10 minutes.

If the cardiac output remains inadequate but the peripheral blood pressure remains high, i.e. above 90 mmHg (12.0 kPa) a reduction in the ventricular afterload may assist the patient and this can be achieved by alpha-adrenergic antagonists such as phentolamine, dose 0.1–0.2 µg/min or salbutamol which is a beta-2-agonist, dose 0.5–1.6 µg/min with haemodynamic monitoring.

3 Hypovolaemic shock

This may be due to loss of whole blood, plasma, or electrolytes and water. In general, the features of hypovolaemic shock can be illustrated by the response to excessive blood loss, which is in three phases.

Phase I. In this phase the venous reservoirs, which normally contain about 70 per cent of the total blood volume, are depleted. These include the large veins, the cutaneous venous plexus, spleen, liver and intestine. The capacity of these areas to contract in volume is shown by lack of response in a healthy individual following the donation of blood. The 500 ml that is lost is immediately compensated for by an appropriate reduction in the capacity of the venous reservoirs, and little, if any, physiological disturbance results.

Phase II. This phase, which is evident from the fall in the systolic arterial blood pressure, usually develops when over 500 ml of blood is rapidly lost from the circulation. If the loss increases to 1000 ml the systolic blood pressure may fall to 90 mmHg. So long as there is no further loss, even if no treatment is given, the blood pressure will return to normal within a matter of hours.

If between 1000 and 2000 ml are lost, the blood pressure falls and usually remains low for some 24–48 hours during which time the secondary effects of 'shock', e.g. renal damage, may develop. During this period of severe hypotension the circulation time through the capillaries decreases, which allows more oxygen to be extracted from the haemoglobin, and as a result there may be peripheral cyanosis. Anyone in this condition is in great danger if there is further bleeding.

Phase III. If there is repeated bleeding or, initially, the volume loss is greater, the compensatory mechanisms are inadequate and death follows. In severe shock the cardiac output is often reduced to the critical level of 2.5 l/min. The final outcome is often determined by the effects of exsanguination on the central nervous system which may lead either to acute respiratory failure or a sudden relaxation of the constricted venous reservoirs.

Treatment of hypovolaemic shock
The treatment of hypovolaemia is by the replacement of the lost fluid by the

fluid which is most appropriate. Although this is accepted as a good general principle, the treatment of both blood and plasma loss can be modified. Thus, high molecular weight dextrans, obtained by the fermentation of sucrose by *Leuconostoc mesenteroides*, can be used as a substitute for plasma. Approximately 60 per cent of an infusion of dextran 70 or 110 is retained in the circulation for two to three days although 40 per cent has already disappeared from the circulating blood volume within 8 hours. If a blood transfusion is required, blood for grouping and cross-matching should be taken prior to the administration of dextran. Large volumes of dextran may prolong the bleeding time. Other substitutes include gelatin solutions, albumin and purified protein fraction; both the latter preparations are extremely costly. When large quantities of blood are given problems may arise as follows.

(a) The first and most obvious is that since blood is stored at 4 °C large volumes may produce hypothermia unless the blood is prewarmed immediately prior to ordering transfusion.
(b) Functioning platelets are absent and the concentration of factors V, VIII and XI are reduced so that when massive transfusions are required these deficiencies must be made good by the administration of fresh frozen plasma and platelet concentrates.
(c) Stored blood contains citrate and in the severely shocked patient citrate toxicity may occur when its concentration exceeds 100 mg/dl, causing muscle tremors and the ECG changes of hypocalcaemia. A warm adult can tolerate 1 unit of blood every 5 minutes but above this level or with associated liver dysfunction as each unit of blood is given it should be followed by 10 ml of 10 per cent calcium gluconate.
(d) Stored blood contains microemboli consisting of platelets, white cells and fibrin. These may contribute to shock lung and renal damage and should be removed by filtration, the pore size being less than 40 μm.

It is interesting that Moyer has shown that in the treatment of 'burn shock' in which the predominant fluid loss is plasma, effective resuscitation can be achieved by the administration of saline and bicarbonate solutions alone, a finding confirmed by the work of the Birmingham Accident Hospital Burns Unit. It has also been appreciated that blood loss can be replaced by electrolyte solutions. It is possible to replace 75 per cent of a whole blood loss by crystalloid solutions so long as large enough quantities are given. Thus, a 1 ml loss of the red cell mass should be replaced by 1 ml of electrolyte solution; 1 ml of plasma loss should be replaced by 3 ml of electrolyte solution. However, if the haematocrit falls below 10 per cent there are simply too few red cells in the circulation to maintain adequate oxygenation, and the red cell mass must be repaired. Using this technique, the volumes of electrolyte solution required may be extremely large. Thus, when a man of 70 kg body weight loses 4000 ml of blood, 12 litres of electrolyte solution are required. The vascular volume returns to normal but the interstitial volume is expanded by approximately 8.1.

In such a patient the haematocrit falls from the normal value of 40 to 10, reaching the critical limit. With smaller losses, e.g. 1500 ml, the volume of Hartmann's solution necessary for adequate replacement would be of the order of 5 litres which would produce a final haematocrit of 30, well in excess of the critical lower limit.

Apart from the replacement of fluid during the period of resuscitation, adequate and repeated observations of the general state and function of specific organs must be made. If necessary a central venous pressure line or even a Swan–Ganz catheter should be established (section 1.3) in order to monitor cardiac function. Pulmonary function must be monitored by repeated blood gas analysis measuring the P_{O_2} and P_{CO_2}. The possible development of metabolic acidosis should be assessed by means of pH determination and bicarbonate. Renal function is measured in terms of volumes, content and osmolality.

'Refractory' shock

If hypovolaemia, from whatever cause, is not adequately corrected, or measures for adequate volume replacement are delayed, the shock state may become 'refractory'. This expression has now replaced the earlier term 'irreversible' which implies that death is inevitable. A variety of physiopathological disturbances may lead to this refractory state:

(a) pooling of blood in the microcirculation. This leads to an increasing reduction in the effective blood volume, increasing capillary permeability, and sludging of the blood;
(b) adrenocortical insufficiency;
(c) superimposed infection;
(d) disseminated intravascular coagulation (DIC);
(e) superimposed cardiogenic shock.

The association between shock and DIC is that both can be initiated by hypoxia, trauma and infection and second, there is a relationship with endothelial cell damage, since the latter results in the liberation of tissue thromboplastins.

Under normal conditions it is thought that the vascular endothelium is being continually damaged by haemodynamic stresses and that the initial reaction to such damage is the deposition of fibrin which is then removed by the fibrinolytic system when the underlying damage is repaired. If the fibrinolytic system fails excessive quantities of fibrin are deposited within the microcirculation.

In DIC rapid fibrin formation occurs when tissue thromboplastins which are probably large lipoprotein complexes are rapidly released into the circulation especially from areas in which they are normally present in high concentration such as the lungs, heart and placenta.

The release of tissue thromboplastin activates clotting factors V and X, the generation of thrombin and the ultimate formation of fibrin. This sequence is accompanied by platelet consumption and enhanced fibrinolysis.

In clinical practice severe infection is a most important cause of DIC in which circumstance the trigger is indirect since the endotoxins activate the intrinsic clotting system or by causing damage to the endothelial cells in the microcirculation activate the extrinsic system.

Clinically DIC is characterized by widespread thrombosis which may affect any or many organs in the body. For example, it is considered that the adult respiratory distress syndrome, i.e. the shock lung, which is particularly associated with massive trauma or severe burns may in part be due to DIC in the pulmonary bed. Similarly, fibrin deposition in the brain produces neurological symptoms and signs whilst impairment of the renal circulation may cause renal failure.

A further feature of DIC is bleeding which may occur alone or in association with consumption coagulopathy. The bleeding tendency may manifest itself as a simple purpura, spontaneous bruising, persistent oozing from wounds and occasionally both genitourinary or gastrointestinal haemorrhage may occur.

The laboratory findings in a typical case of DIC may reveal:

(a) depression of the platelet count;
(b) prolongation of the thrombin, prothrombin and partial thromboplastin times;
(c) specific deficiencies of plasma fibrinogen, prothrombin and clotting factors V and VIII;
(d) the presence of soluble fibrin monomer formed by the action of thrombin on fibrinogen;
(e) distorted and fragmented red blood cells, schistocytes produced by mechanical damage within the microcirculation;

A common concomitant of major trauma, haemorrhagic shock or endotoxic shock is acute respiratory insufficiency, otherwise known as the shock lung.

The development of shock lung is now being more commonly recognized because of the intensive therapy administered to a patient suffering from shock, however caused, which permits the patient to survive long enough to develop this syndrome.

Classically death occurs in the fourth stage of the syndrome's evolution. In stage one the shocked patient is resuscitated and after a latent period of hours or days during which the patient exhibits hyperventilation, respiratory alkalosis and hypoxaemia but no subjective distress, stage two is entered. In this stage marked hypoxaemia, tachypnoea and respiratory distress occur and within 12–24 hours the chest X-ray shows patchy ill-defined densities. In the third stage progressive pulmonary insufficiency occurs and in the fourth and final stage terminal hypoxia and hypercarbia occur which eventually results in hypoxic cardiac arrest.

When the lungs are examined at post mortem the most obvious finding is their great increase in weight which is chiefly due to interstitial oedema although if the patient survives for a sufficient period of time some pulmonary fibrosis also occurs. On microscopic section there is initially widening of the interstitial tissue, vascular congestion and perialveolar haemorrhage. In some areas evidence of disseminated intravascular coagulation will be seen and in the later stages alveolar and interstitial cell proliferation will be found.

Aetiological factors
The precise aetiology of shock lung is a matter for debate, nevertheless a number of factors have been incriminated including:

(a) alteration of pulmonary capillary permeability due to hypoperfusion of the lungs in profound shock;
(b) overtransfusion: the central venous pressure is an inadequate monitoring device in the severely shocked patient undergoing transfusion. A more accurate parameter is the pulmonary capillary wedge pressure which makes it possible to detect left atrial hypertension before the right ventricle fails;
(c) the development of DIC with consequent disruption of the pulmonary microcirculation;
(d) subsidiary factors which may play a part in specific circumstances include the effects of aspiration and/or fat embolism;
(e) oxygen intoxication, the inhalation of oxygen at concentrations over 50 per cent are considered toxic possibly by destroying surfactant.

Treatment

(a) When hypoxaemia arises in the presence of non-ventilated alveoli, action must be directed to reopening the alveoli and preventing further collapse. This can best be achieved at the present time by endotracheal intubation with mechanical ventilation with positive end-expiratory pressure (PEEP). The theory underlying the positive end-expiratory pressure is that this serves to keep open alveoli which have been reflated by the initial application of positive pressure.
(b) Combat infection when present by the appropriate drugs.
(c) Diuretics.
(d) Possibly the administration of steroids although these remain of dubious value.

4 Bacteraemic shock

Bacteraemic shock may be caused by both Gram-positive organisms such as the staphylococci, streptococci and clostridia and by a large number of Gram-negative organisms including *Escherichia coli*, *Klebsiella*, *Proteus*, *Salmonella* and the anaerobic *Bacteroides*.

The chief difference between the two groups of bacteria is in the structure of the wall of the bacterium. In the Gram-positive organisms this is chiefly composed of peptidoglycan and technoic acid and the toxins are within their protoplasm whereas in the Gram-negative organism the outer membrane of the bacterium is composed of lipopolysaccharide, otherwise known as endotoxin which is only liberated upon the death of the organism.

When a bacteraemia occurs, e.g. following instrumentation of the urethra or during an attack of cholangitis, chills, fever or hypothermia and hypotension may occur associated with a warm dry skin indicating a high cardiac output or a cold moist skin indicating a low cardiac output. As shock progresses so marked pallor and cyanosis may develop accompanied by oliguria and anuria and as further progression occurs so the complications of shock develop.

It is usually considered that warm hypotension is a feature of Gram-positive sepsis whereas cold hypotension with peripheral shut down and cold cyanosed extremities indicates a Gram-negative septicaemia.

When a Gram-positive organism such as *Staphylococcus* causes shock the causal factor is chiefly the X toxin which is known to cause:

(*a*) arteriolar vasoconstriction;
(*b*) endothelial damage;
(*c*) increases in cellular membrane permeability;
(*d*) agglutination and lysis of platelets.

When Gram-negative organisms cause shock the offending element is the toxic lipid A which lies within an outer core of hydrophilic polysaccharide between the latter and the peptidoglycan which covers the cell membrane. It is this substance which is detected by the limulus test in which the protein of the white cells of the horseshoe crab *Limulus polyphemus* is coagulated into a gel by even minute amounts of the toxic material.

Gram-negative endotoxaemia is produced whenever Gram-negative organisms disintegrate in the blood stream or alternatively, endotoxin is absorbed from the gastrointestinal tract. Jacob Fine of Boston was the first surgeon to recognize that in severe haemorrhagic shock the end stage was reached when the mucosal resistance of the gut allowed endotoxin to gain entrance from the gut into the blood stream thus greatly aggravating an already serious situation. Normally in the experimental animal sublethal doses of endotoxin although pyrogenic are adequately dealt with by the cells of the mononuclear phagocyte system. If these are overwhelmed death ensues from microvascular breakdown which is directly attributed to the action of endotoxin. In the experimental animal it is possible to enhance the activity of these cells by the repeated injection of sublethal doses of endotoxin and such an animal becomes not only resistant to a supralethal dose of endotoxin but also to severe and prolonged haemorrhagic shock.

The endotoxins have many actions, all of which are potentially damaging to the organism as a whole. These include:

(*a*) non-complement-dependent necrosis of the endothelium of blood vessels;
(*b*) activation and release of complement, kinins, prostaglandins and histamine;
(*c*) depression of cellular respiration by damaging mitochondria;
(*d*) damage to cell-surface phospholipids, notably in the pulmonary alveoli.

Some or all of these effects result in the production of disseminated intravascular coagulation and it is possible since endotoxins are responsible for the Shwartzman reaction that they cause renal cortical necrosis and the shock lung.

The treatment of bacteraemic endotoxaemic shock includes:

(*a*) adequate fluid intake with glucose/insulin infusion in order to achieve an adequate fluid balance;

(b) the infusion of H_2 antagonists in an attempt to avoid stress ulceration of the gastroduodenal mucosa;
(c) large doses of corticosteroids, e.g. 1.5 mg/kg dexamethasone. This should be limited to one or two doses since repeated injection causes depression of the mononuclear phagocytes. The chief reason for the administration of corticosteroids is that they tend to protect the microcirculation by stabilizing various cell mechanisms;
(d) operative removal of the source of toxaemia, e.g. the colon in severe acute proctocolitis, the drainage and lavage of the abdominal cavity following perforation of a colonic diverticulum;
(e) the administration of appropriate antibiotics, e.g. metronidazole combined with an aminoglycoside.

5 Neurogenic shock

The commonest form of neurogenic shock is the vasovagal attack in which a hitherto healthy individual collapses, usually during the course of some minor surgical procedure or at some unpleasant sight. A less common cause is a high spinal injury. In the former, the affected individual faints due to a sudden reduction in peripheral vascular resistance in the splanchnic area, which suddenly diminishes the effective blood volume and, in consequence, brings about a sudden fall in venous return to the heart, the patient becoming cold, clammy and hypotensive, with a feeble slow pulse. Bradycardia is caused by vagal stimulation of the heart, the patient recovering when laid flat with the limbs elevated. The bradycardia can be treated by atropine.

6 Acute adrenal insufficiency

Acute adrenal insufficiency may be the result of:

(a) destruction of the glands by haemorrhage or thrombosis;
(b) stress in a patient in whom adrenal function is already poor;
(c) incomplete replacement therapy in adrenalectomized patients subjected to further trauma.

Acute adrenal insufficiency may occur in patients suffering from severe multiple injuries, or severe infections. The common presenting features are nausea, vomiting, diarrhoea, dehydration and hypotension.

These features may all, however, be caused by the factor or factors which have initiated adrenal destruction and in consequence the diagnosis may be missed unless there is previous evidence of adrenal hypofunction. Furthermore, apart from an estimation of the plasma cortisol level examination of the serum electrolytes is not of great help for the characteristic hyperkalaemia and azotaemia may also be associated with the causative factors.

If the condition is recognized the chief aspects of treatment are:

(a) adequate administration of cortical hormone, e.g. 100 mg hydrocortisone intramuscularly at 4-hourly intervals;

(*b*) control of infection by appropriate antibiotics;
(*c*) support to the cardiovascular system.

1.2 Aetiology and treatment of acute renal failure in the surgical patient

Definition. In absolute terms renal failure can be defined as a situation in which the volume of urine excreted falls below the level required to control the internal environment. In the adult this approximates to between 400 and 600 ml daily.

It is, however, more appropriate to consider renal failure in physiological terms, regarding it as a condition in which the volume of urine excreted is insufficient to prevent nitrogenous end products accumulating in the blood. This definition is better because it recognizes that kidneys damaged by ageing, hypertension or disease, in order to maintain homoeostasis, need to excrete larger volumes of urine than the accepted normal.

In severely ill patients the hourly urinary output is monitored by means of an indwelling catheter, the critical value being, in a normal healthy adult approximately 20 ml/hour. It should be remembered that a catheter is a dangerous instrument. If not aseptically inserted it results in a urinary tract infection and if allowed to drag on the bladder neck or urethra it may well produce an iatrogenic stricture. It is, therefore, important to remove a catheter at the soonest possible moment.

The causes of acute renal failure may be prerenal, renal and post-renal. In the majority of surgical patients oliguria followed by organic changes in the kidney itself are nearly always primarily due to hypovolaemia and hypotension. The causes of hypovolaemia encountered by the surgeon include:

1. blood loss
   (*a*) traumatic
   (*b*) surgical
2. plasma loss
   (*a*) burns
   (*b*) pancreatitis
3. fluid and electrolyte depletion
   (*a*) intestinal obstruction including pyloric stenosis
   (*b*) external fistulae
   (*c*) paralytic ileus
   (*d*) natural diseases such as ulcerative colitis

Physiological effects of hypovolaemia

Nearly 20 per cent of the cardiac output normally flows through the kidneys, 90 per cent passing through the cortical circulation and the remainder through the medulla. In the presence of severe hypovolaemia and the resulting hypotension renal vasoconstriction leads to a marked fall in the renal blood flow with the result that the glomerular filtration rate falls and oliguria develops.

Normally there is an interval of some hours between the onset of hypotension and the development of organic changes in the kidney but once renal vasoconstriction develops it tends to persist so that even though the blood volume may be restored it does not necessarily mean that an immediate increase in renal blood flow will occur with the restoration of normal renal function. In part the persistent low glomerular flow is due to renal renin secretion and swelling of the ischaemic cortical cells.

In many of the conditions listed above additional factors are at work leading from a physiological reduction of renal function to actual organic changes in the kidney. These include:

1 *Haemoglobinuria*
The common causes of haemoglobinuria include:

(*a*) mismatched blood transfusion;
(*b*) plasma hypotonicity after transurethral prostatectomy;
(*c*) thermal burns leading to massive destruction of red cells in the area of burning.

Normally, free haemoglobin in the circulation is bound to a specific binding protein, haptoglobin, and only when the level in the plasma exceeds 100–120 mg/dl does free haemoglobin appear in the urine. However, large amounts of haemoglobin can be intravenously infused into the circulation of an experimental animal without causing adverse effects on the kidney. When a mismatched transfusion is given, it produces a reaction between the patient's antibody and the blood group antigen in the membrane of the donor red cell. The complex thus produced causes intense renal vasoconstriction and, hence, renal ischaemia. Free haemoglobin is also precipitated in the renal tubules because the subsequent renal vasoconstriction causes a reduction of the glomerular filtration rate which depresses urine flow. Another important factor is the increased secretion of antidiuretic hormone which of itself reduces tubular urine flow.

2 *Myoglobinuria*
The common causes of myoglobinuria include:

(*a*) crush injuries of the extremities;
(*b*) sudden arterial occlusion;
(*c*) severe *Clostridium welchii* infections.

Of these conditions the effects of a crush injury are most interesting. The patient may be trapped under debris but, despite suffering severe pain, the general condition remains good until the crushing agent is removed, when, soon after, the affected limb becomes swollen and tense and the blood pressure falls. The haematocrit rises sharply due to a massive extravasation of plasma-like fluid into the damaged limb, and oliguria develops.

3 Jaundice

It has long been recognized that renal failure is relatively common following operations on patients suffering from obstructive jaundice; in some series it was held responsible for 5 per cent of the immediate postoperative deaths.

It had been thought that the important contributory factor was a low blood volume but this has now been disproved. Intensive investigation has shown that risk of renal failure is related to the preoperative level of circulating bilirubin and subsequent investigations suggest that the renal parenchyma is sensitized to changes in blood volume by the presence of high levels of bilirubin glucuronide. The current hypothesis is that bilirubin glucuronide filters through the glomerulus, enters the tubule to form a cast, and exerts a toxic action on the tubular cells.

4 Infection

Infection with Gram-positive or Gram-negative organisms may be associated with the original surgical condition or may follow operation. Both may be nephrotoxic and both may influence the subsequent condition of the patient by converting a normocatabolic into a hypercatabolic state.

5 Hypoxia

The common causes of hypoxia include:

(*a*) road traffic accidents associated with severe chest injuries;
(*b*) abdominal or thoracic operations associated with severe chest complications.

When once there has been a gross disturbance of pulmonary function renal oxygenation may be reduced below tolerable limits.

6 Disseminated intravascular coagulation (see p. 6)

Types of renal dysfunction

Three types of renal disturbance occur:

1 Physiological

This may be temporary and is due to circulatory inadequacy producing a functional change that is not associated with organic disease in the kidney. If, therefore, the aetiological factor, which is usually hypovolaemia, is corrected within a short time of its onset renal function returns to normal.

As a general rule the kidney cannot withstand hypovolaemia that results in a fall in the systolic pressure to the level of the diastolic pressure for longer than 24 hours. However, no specific time limit can be stated because much depends on the condition of the kidney at the time of the 'injury' and the presence or absence of contributory causes.

2 Tubular necrosis

This is an organic condition associated with the following pathological changes in the kidneys: scattered foci of tubular damage in kidneys that may appear macroscopically normal or only slightly paler and more swollen than normal; the basement membrane of the affected tubules fragments and collections of plasma cells, lymphocytes and macrophages surround the affected parts of the tubules; within the tubule there may be haemoglobin, myoglobin or cellular casts.

Because of the association of tubular necrosis with vascular changes in the kidney an alternative terminology, i.e. vasomotor nephropathy, has been proposed. Furthermore, since the changes are normally reparable a further suggestion has been made that the condition should be called acute reversible intrinsic renal failure.

3 *Cortical necrosis*
This is, fortunately, an uncommon irreversible lesion caused by glomerular infarction as well as tubular necrosis. The cut surface of the kidney shows a reddish zone at the corticomedullary junction surrounding which is the paler cortex. Histological examination shows complete necrosis of the glomeruli and the proximal and distal tubules. Fibrin thrombi are present in the glomerular capillaries.

Measures to prevent renal damage

Concerning renal function, particular attention should be paid in the surgical patient to the following aspects of treatment:

1. maintenance of a normal blood pressure, blood volume and cardiac output;
2. prevention of hypoxia;
3. control of infection.

In regard to point 1 above this may require any of the methods described in section 1.1, pages 4–5. Many surgeons would also advise that at least part of the deficit replacement should be made by dextran 40 so that the intravascular 'sludging', commonly seen in the 'shock' syndrome is diminished. In the kidneys this effect is only important in the cortical circulation, for beyond this point red cells are stripped from the renal circulation. The disadvantage of dextran 40 is its tendency to promote bleeding and it is, therefore, contraindicated in patients in whom there has been severe vascular damage.

To prevent hypoxia adequate physiotherapy should be given following surgery and if pre-existing pulmonary disease exists oxygen may need to be administered remembering that concentrations exceeding 50 per cent are toxic and believed to be a causative factor of shock lung.

To prevent infection there is gathering evidence that prophylactic antibiotic therapy will prevent or reduce postoperative sepsis in patients in whom high risk surgery is being performed.

Differentiation of physiological from organic oliguria

Six tests will usually distinguish physiological from organic oliguria:

1 *urine sodium level*. When this remains low it indicates that tubular reabsorption and, therefore, tubular function is intact;
2 *urine urea/plasma urea concentration*. If this ratio remains high it again indicates that tubular function is retained;
3 *specific gravity*. Despite the extreme oliguria that may occur in a physiological disturbance if the specific gravity remains at not less than 1014, it indicates functional activity;
4 *response to volume replacement*. When a physiological renal disturbance only has occurred, the adequate replacement of the blood volume should result in restoration of renal function and an increase in the urine output.
5 *response to mannitol*. This drug, which is an osmotic diuretic, should not be given until the blood volume has been restored. It increases the plasma volume and decreases blood viscosity and renal resistance. Since it is not metabolized the dose, normally 100 ml of a 20 per cent solution administered over 10 minutes intravenously, should not be repeated because over-administration leads to excessive expansion of the extracellular fluid volume and may thus precipitate pulmonary oedema;
6 *response to frusemide*. This is a loop diuretic acting directly on the renal tubules. It is normally given in a dose of 40 mg which may be doubled every 4 hours to a maximum of approximately 3000 mg. When a negative response occurs to the three 'challenges' described it must be assumed that organic renal changes have taken place. As with mannitol the drug should not be administered until the blood volume has been restored.

Biochemistry of renal failure

A patient suffering from renal failure is usually described as normocatabolic or hypercatabolic. In the former, the blood urea rises by 30 mg/dl daily (4.7 mmol/l) and in the latter by 60 mg/dl daily (9.4 mmol/l), or over. In addition to the rising blood urea the plasma concentration of potassium rises. The rate at which hyperkalaemia develops is related to the presence or absence of damaged tissues and the rate of catabolism, the level of 6 mmol/l is regarded as critical since cardiac arrhythmia may then develop followed by peaking of the T waves and later death from cardiac arrest.

Failure to secrete H ions leads to a metabolic acidosis which may initially be controlled by hyperventilation but will later become uncompensated.

Clinical response to acute renal failure

These are all the result of the above biochemical disturbances.

1 Dyspnoea, which may be due to fluid overload causing pulmonary oedema, metabolic acidosis, or pulmonary infection occurring singly or in combination.

2 Cardiac arrhythmias which may be due to hyperkalaemia.
3 Nausea, anorexia and vomiting which may be due to water overload or the result of 'uraemia'.
4 Gastric erosions leading to severe gastrointestinal bleeding.
5 Drowsiness and finally coma.
6 Infection due to damage to phagocytic activity and immunological systems.

PRINCIPLES OF TREATMENT OF ESTABLISHED ORGANIC RENAL FAILURE

The normocatabolic patient

This group of patients can often be treated by a dietary regimen alone. The fluid intake is limited to 400 ml/day with an additional allocation for insensible water loss (particularly significant in a hot environment). To reduce the breakdown of endogenous protein, 1500 non-protein calories are given daily, usually in the form of Hycal which contains 244 kcal/dl. In addition, the daily rise in blood urea of the normocatabolic patient can be further controlled by the use of the anabolic steroid norethandrolone decanoate, dose 50 mg daily by intramuscular injection. The administration of this steroid reduces the rate of protein breakdown by over 40 per cent.

The hypercatabolic patient

This group is not so easily treated and dialysis is usually necessary. In these patients an attempt must be made to control infection either by antibiotics, surgery, or both. If the condition has been caused by a road traffic accident, an associated chest injury followed by hypoxia is often likely. This, again, must be vigorously treated.

Once the blood urea has risen above a concentration of 32 mmol/l, there may be nausea and vomiting which can be controlled by chlorpromazine. Above this level uraemic fits may occur.

If the potentially toxic level of potassium is reached, i.e. above 7 mmol/l, immediate action should be taken to avoid death from cardiac arrest. Emergency treatment consists of the immediate infusion of 100 ml of 50 per cent dextrose together with 10 units of insulin. Once the immediate threat is over, further measures consist of oral administration of ion exchange resins such as sodium polystyrene sulphonate, 15 g three times daily by mouth or, if the patient is vomiting, rectally.

Dialysis

The indications for dialysis vary in different centres but in general when the following parameters are exceeded dialysis should be instituted:

1 a blood urea exceeding 35 mmol/l;

2 a serum creatinine above 900 mmol/l;
3 a serum potassium exceeding 6.5 mmol/l which cannot be reduced by the measures already described.

Dialysis may be performed either by haemo- or peritoneal dialysis. In the former the patient's blood and the dialysing fluid are brought together, separated by a cellophane or cuprophane membrane only, whereas in peritoneal dialysis the peritoneum itself is used as a semipermeable dialysing membrane.

The result of either method depends upon the concentration gradient of solutes existing between the blood and the dialysing fluid. Of the two methods haemodialysis is approximately four times as effective as peritoneal dialysis and, once performed, further dialysis may not be necessary for some 72 hours during which time other aspects of patient care, e.g. the resetting or nailing of fractures, can be accomplished.

The disadvantage of peritoneal dialysis in this type of patient are: first, it is a fairly lengthy procedure; and second, a protein loss of between 20 and 40 g per session may occur. It can only be used if the abdomen is relatively normal; it is, for example, absolutely contraindicated in patients suffering from paralytic ileus. A fluid exchange of 1–2 litres is used, usually at a rate of 2 litres/hour using an approximately isotonic solution with 1.36 per cent glucose.

Natural history of tubular necrosis

The oliguric phase, following tubular necrosis, may last from a few days to a few weeks. It usually ends within three weeks, after which it is followed by the diuretic phase during which large volumes of dilute urine are passed. The renal conservation of sodium and potassium is poor at this time and, despite the polyuria, the blood urea may continue to rise for a few days before gradually declining. Often, many months pass before renal function becomes completely normal. If the oliguric phase persists for longer than three weeks a renal biopsy should be performed because such prolonged absence of function is highly suggestive of cortical necrosis, which is an irreversible condition. Assuming the patient survives, the treatment programme must now include long-term dialysis or renal transplantation.

1.3 Measurements used to monitor cardiovascular function in the severely ill patient

Electrocardiogram

The ECG provides continuous information concerning the heart rate and rhythm and so facilitates the rapid detection and possible correction of various cardiac arrhythmias. It is an essential tool in the monitoring of the severely 'shocked' patient particularly if a history is obtained of previous cardiac disease and it is also routinely used following open heart surgery in which arrhythmias are common in the early postoperative days.

Arterial blood pressure

The level of the peripheral blood pressure is a product of blood flow and resistance. In the severely shocked patient the standard method of measurement using a sphygmomanometer cuff and stethoscope is inadequate and an arterial line should be established which in addition to its use in measuring the blood pressure can be used for the taking of arterial blood samples.

Central venous pressure

Definition. The central venous pressure in precise terms is the venous pressure in the right atrium and assuming the tricuspid valve is functioning normally the CVP equates to the end-diastolic pressure in the right ventricle and is a measure of the preload to this chamber. Assuming that cardiac function is normal the central venous pressure roughly correlates with the blood volume, a high pressure indicating plethora, and a low pressure hypovolaemia. This relationship reflects the fact that as the blood volume falls the vascular compartment shrinks, so decreasing tension, whereas if there is an impediment to blood flow, e.g. left ventricular failure, the pressure rises.

Physiology
In a normal healthy individual, approximately 70 per cent of the effective blood volume lies in the venous side of the circulation. In the absence of compensatory mechanisms a sudden reduction in blood volume would result in a fall in the right atrial pressure (CVP) together with decreased filling of the right ventricle, a fall in the cardiac output and, hence, of the systemic blood pressure.

Fortunately, for the most part these changes are prevented by the vasomotor centres. These exert an ionotropic effect on the heart and produce widespread venous constriction, thus reducing the capacity of the circulation. In this way the CVP tends to remain normal and cardiac output is maintained at normal levels even though the blood volume is much reduced.

Measurement
Central venous pressure is measured by placing a cannula in the right atrium. The precise position of the cannula can be established either by screening, if it is radio-opaque, or by continuously recording the ECG, using a wire down the centre of the cannula as one of the leads. As the cannula enters the atrium the P wave becomes biphasic. The cannula can be inserted, via the median cubital vein, into the subclavian or internal jugular vein.

The ideal place for the tip of the cannula is at the lower border of the superior vena cava or in the upper third of the right atrium. Once it has been inserted, the simplest way of measuring central venous pressure is to use a manometer containing isotonic saline set against a centimetre rule. A reference point is then chosen, and in England this is usually the manubriosternal joint. In a patient reclining in bed supported by five or six pillows the normal pressure measurement from this reference point is between 5 and 10 cm H_2O. In the USA, the central point of the chest is often used and gives lower initial readings than the above. The absolute measurement is, however, not as important as the sequential changes that follow measures designed to improve the patient's clinical state.

Complications
Since this is an invasive technique, complications will inevitably occur. Any method can result in infection, catheter embolus, and sometimes cardiac tamponade due to perforation of the right atrium. However, subclavian puncture is without doubt the most dangerous way of introducing the cannula. The recorded complications resulting from *this* method include pneumothorax, haemothorax, hydrothorax, air embolus, massive subcutaneous emphysema, arteriovenous fistula, and brachial plexus palsy.

Indications

There are several conditions in which measurement of the central venous pressure may be of considerable assistance to the surgeon in the management of the patient, particularly the following:

1 *The severely injured patient*
Even in the absence of an external wound or a soft tissue intra-abdominal injury the blood loss from multiple fractures may be considerable. A fracture of the pelvis may lead to losses in excess of 5 litres, and a fracture of the tibia and fibular losses of up to 3 litres. Such losses are usually associated with systolic arterial pressure of less than 65 mmHg, and if this is not to become irreversible massive transfusions are required. In the aged or patients suffering from cardiac disease, e.g. myocardial ischaemia, the circulatory system is exceedingly 'fragile' and overtransfusion may be as dangerous as undertransfusion. Repeated measurements of the CVP help to avoid cardiac embarrassment and ensure that there is adequate volume replacement. Indeed, the measurement of CVP is, in these circumstances, more accurate than dilution techniques using ^{131}I-labelled plasma albumin because the latter method is limited by the slow and uneven distribution of the indicator in the circulation.

2 *Known or suspected bleeding*
An example of the value of CVP measurements is the patient who has suffered an upper gastrointestinal haemorrhage from any cause. In these circumstances, not only do serial measurements ensure adequate resuscitation without overloading but, in addition, if the CVP falls it indicates that further *bleeding*

has occurred even though the pulse rate and blood pressure have remained constant.

3 Patients in whom oliguria is developing

The volume of urine produced may fall below the 'volume obligatoire' of approximately 400 ml and the blood urea may rise to abnormal levels while the kidneys are still in a stage of functional rather than structural failure. At this stage, organic pathological changes in the kidney, e.g. tubular necrosis, may still be prevented or arrested if the renal blood flow can be restored to normal levels. There is, however, a marked tendency, once the renal blood flow has fallen, for a low level of flow to continue.

Common causes of oliguria in the surgical patient include:

(a) operations accompanied by severe, but possibly unrecognized blood loss, usually greater than 2 litres, lead to persistent hypotension if not replaced;
(b) severe vomiting, diarrhoea or paralytic ileus which results in dehydration;
(c) burns in which hypovolaemic shock due to plasma loss occurs.

All these conditions are associated with a low cardiac output which leads to a reduced renal blood flow. The latter is further diminished by compensatory vasoconstriction. To establish whether the reduced urine flow is due to physiological rather than anatomical causes the response of the circulation to a transfusion of limited volumes of blood or plasma must be noted. The CVP and systemic blood pressure are recorded and an intravenous transfusion of approximately 5 per cent (250–500 ml) of the estimated normal blood volume is then given over a period of 10–15 minutes, after which the pressures are again measured. If little or no change in the CVP occurs and there is only a minimal elevation of the systemic blood pressure, the hypovolaemia has remained uncorrected and further fluid is required.

The clinical history commonly suggests whether the deficit is primarily due to blood, plasma or fluid and electrolyte loss. If the CVP rises by 5–10 cmH_2O without any alteration in the diastolic blood pressure an adequate circulating blood volume for the existing state of cardiac efficiency is suggested.

When there is no change in either the CVP or the systemic blood pressure it can be assumed that the peripheral vascular tone is defective or that there is cardiac insufficiency. These two conditions must then be differentiated one from another so that appropriate treatment can be given.

When the oliguria is due to a reduced blood volume without associated organic changes in the kidney correction of the blood volume can be expected to produce an increased excretion of urine. Following restoration of the blood volume, mannitol may be given; the normal regimen is 100 ml of a 20 per cent solution over a period of 10 minutes. If no increase in urine follows, another 20 g can be given. An alternative regimen is the use of the diuretic frusemide, a first dose of 40 mg is given and doubled every 4 hours. If such treatment fails to produce an increase in fluid and solute output it must be assumed that organic renal changes have taken place and the necessary measures instituted.

4 Pulmonary artery wedge pressure (PAWP)

The pulmonary artery wedge pressure is measured by means of a Swan–Ganz catheter, originally described in 1970. One of its major disadvantages is that of expense, each catheter costing at the present time £90.

The catheter which has a balloon near its tip is introduced via the same routes as a central venous pressure line and the balloon, once the catheter tip has reached a large intrathoracic vein, is inflated after which the catheter is slowly advanced, the blood flow carrying it through the right atrium and right ventricle onwards into a small branch of the pulmonary artery where it becomes wedged. The position of the catheter is monitored throughout its passage by the pressure changes and different wave forms which occur.

In a normal individual the PAWP measured at the end of respiration is from the level of the midaxillary line between 6 and 12 mmHg (0.8 and 1.6 kPa).

Complications. The complications associated with the passage of a Swan–Ganz catheter are those associated with the placing of a central pressure line but an arrhythmia may occur as the catheter passes through the right ventricle and occasionally the catheter may become knotted in the eddying currents it encounters on its passage into the lungs. One complication which may result is a small segmental pulmonary infarct causing a haemoptysis.

Value of PAWP measurement. Whereas measurement of the central venous pressure gives information which can be related to the function of the right side of the heart the PAWP gives a direct measure of the left ventricular filling pressure and left ventricular function, furthermore it can be used to measure the blood volume and Po_2 of mixed venous blood. It is, therefore, particularly valuable in managing patients in whom exact knowledge of left ventricular activity is required. For example, if a high central venous pressure is found in the presence of a low cardiac output it would be appropriate to think in terms of pump failure but if the PAWP is measured and is found to be low the clinical condition may be one of simple hypovolaemia which can be readily corrected. When left-sided failure is not due to low preload the PAWP will be found to be high.

5 Temperature measurement

A simple method of assessing cardiac output is to monitor the difference between the peripheral and the core temperatures. The former is measured from the medial aspect of the big toe and the latter from a monitoring device placed either in the rectum or oesophagus. When the cardiac output is low the difference between the two measurements may even exceed 10 °C, the differential falling as normal output is restored.

1.4 Causes and treatment of fluid and electrolyte imbalance in the surgical patient

Aetiology

A common cause of fluid and electrolyte disturbance in clinical practice is the severe loss of gastrointestinal secretions due to disease or postoperative complications. Loss due to disease may come about through diminished intake, as, for example, when a carcinoma of the oesophagus occludes the lumen of that viscus; excessive vomiting as in pyloric stenosis; or excessive diarrhoea as in ulcerative colitis or the Verner–Morrison syndrome. Some operations, for example, ileostomy, are normally followed by excessive losses in the immediate postoperative period which, under normal circumstances, rapidly revert to normal. The onset of paralytic (adynamic) ileus in the postoperative period may be associated with huge deficits in part due to the excessive quantities of fluid and electrolytes held in the lumen of the distended gut and in part due to the severe vomiting which may ensue. Huge losses may also accompany the development of postoperative fistulae.

Whenever undue gastrointestinal losses are occurring it is essential to compile accurate fluid and electrolyte balance charts comprising an account of all fluid lost including urine volumes and the electrolyte composition of the losses together with an accurate account of all fluids and electrolytes administered.

Although the aetiology of the various depletions is diverse, in general, certain well defined patterns emerge.

1 Hypernatraemia, water depletion

In this condition the serum sodium rises above the normal level of 148 mmol/l (148 mEq/l). The common causes include:

(a) failure to provide sufficient water, usually because the insensible loss has increased beyond the usually accepted level. This could happen in fever, excessive sweating in tropical conditions, hyperventilation with unhumidified air;
(b) patients too ill, too old, or too lethargic to respond naturally to thirst;
(c) lesions of the upper gastrointestinal tract which prevent swallowing;
(d) overenthusiastic administration of osmotic diuretics such as mannitol;
(e) excessive use of hyperosmolar high protein tube feeding.

In the presence of water depletion the volume of urine excreted falls rapidly but a minimum volume is required to excrete the fixed acids formed from protein catabolism. If there is insufficient urine excretion the osmotic pressure of the body fluids increases.

In mild cases of hypernatraemia the extracellular and intracellular compartments contract, and as the condition deteriorates the secretion of aldosterone causes sodium conservation which, in turn, increases the osmolarity of the extracellular compartment, causing a differential intracellular dehydration. In an apathetic patient with a low urine output and a plasma sodium concentration as high as 152 mmol/l (mEq/l) this diagnosis can be assumed. If the condition is allowed to progress, cardiac output falls and may lead, finally, to respiratory failure. Death usually ensues when the total body water has been reduced by approximately 40 per cent, equal to a deficiency of 17 litres in a 70 kg man, a state that, theoretically, could be reached within 13 days.

Treatment
The treatment of water depletion is its replacement, either orally or parenterally. In the conscious patient the relief of thirst indicates improvement. If 5 per cent dextrose solutions are used to replace the water deficit, no more than 20 g of glucose should be administered in every hour, otherwise hyperglycaemia and a solute diuresis may produce a further rise in the serum sodium. Furthermore, too rapid a water transfusion may produce cerebral oedema followed by convulsions.

2 Water intoxication

This is the converse of water depletion and usually comes about in the previously healthy surgical patient because of inadvertent over-administration of too great a volume of fluid. Once the sodium level has fallen to less than 118 mmol/l (118 mEq/l), mental confusion, coma, and finally convulsions develop. If the condition develops insidiously lethargy followed by weakness and disorientation are the common presenting symptoms. High volumes of dilute urine are normally passed.

Treatment
Hypertonic saline, say 300 ml of 5.85 per cent solution, may be given followed by severe restriction in water intake.

3 Sodium depletion

Causation
This condition is usually the result of excessive intestinal losses, e.g. vomiting or diarrhoea, excessive sweating, or excessive infusion of water or diluted salt solutions in patients who are hypovolaemic and suffering from reduced renal efficiency. In the latter type of patient, when the patient is secreting large amounts of antidiuretic hormone the kidneys cannot get rid of the excessive water load and hyponatraemia is inevitable.

Clinical presentation
Clinical symptoms and signs vary with the rapidity of onset and the magnitude of the defect.

Biochemically, the importance of the sodium loss lies in the gradual shrinkage of the extracellular fluid compartment which, after a loss of approximately 30 per cent, leads to hypovolaemic shock.

The clinical diagnosis of sodium depletion rests on the finding of a lowered urine output, loss of skin turgor, and loss of weight. Various compensating mechanisms may maintain the peripheral blood pressure at normal levels, even though the central venous pressure is falling. However, once the fluid debt is of an order of 3.5 litres and the sodium loss between 300 and 500 mmol, hypovolaemic shock is imminent.

Biochemical tests are of limited value because the plasma sodium level does not necessarily indicate the actual sodium mass because of distortion produced by the movement of sodium into the larger intracellular compartment. Once the renal circulation has been affected the blood urea begins to rise.

Treatment

Sodium depletion is treated by saline infusion. If renal function is normal, normal saline, which contains 154 mmol/l of sodium and 154 mmol/l of chloride, can be administered. If renal function is impaired the anion concentration of the replacement fluid should be modified so that each litre contains 100 mmol of chloride and 54 mmol of lactate, and if large quantities of sodium are required it can be administered in the form of a hypertonic (5 per cent) solution, adding 40 ml of molar sodium lactate to each 100 ml.

Once the acute crisis with the threat of hypovolaemic shock and secondary renal failure is over, the problem of continuing therapy remains. Many different intravenous solutions have been described. The solution required is dependent on the source of the loss and if this is taking place from the gastrointestinal tract it should be possible to collect a sample and obtain a relatively accurate analysis.

When the stomach is the major source of the loss a solution of sodium chloride to which potassium chloride has been added may be used, e.g. sodium 63 mmol/l (mEq/l), potassium 17 mmol/l (mEq/l) and ammonium chloride 70 mmol/l (mEq/l) together with 80 mmol/l (mEq/l) of chloride. Adding ammonium chloride produces an excess of chloride ion over sodium ion in the extracellular space and prevents development of a metabolic alkalosis. This is always a possible complication of prolonged gastric aspiration in a normal patient.

If the loss is from lower down the gastrointestinal tract a solution containing sodium, potassium, chloride and lactate is required, an excess of sodium over chloride preventing the development of metabolic acidosis. Darrow's solution which contains 120 mmol/l (mEq/l) of sodium, 36 mmol/l (mEq/l) of potassium, 105 mmol/l (mEq/l) of chloride, and 51 mmol/l (mEq/l) of lactate is a convenient solution.

Potassium

The normal ECF potassium concentration is 3.5–5.5 mmol/l (mEq/l). This compartment contains less than 3 per cent of the total body potassium most of which is within the intracellular compartment, concentration 100 mmol/l. Clinical effects may be the result of either hyper- or hypokalaemia but usually 10 per cent or more of the total body potassium must be lost before definite symptoms and signs develop.

Aetiology of potassium deficiency

A common cause of potassium deficiency is an excessive loss of gastrointestinal secretions, which all contain potassium. When the loss is from the upper gastrointestinal tract, e.g. as in pyloric stenosis, the hypokalaemia is associated with alkalosis because of the accompanying chloride loss. When the loss occurs from the large bowel, e.g. due to a villous tumour of the rectum, a pure potassium loss unassociated with alkalosis may occur.

Clinical presentation

Severe potassium loss is associated with general symptoms, personality changes, drowsiness and, later, coma. There may also be muscle weakness and, in particular, cardiac muscle weakness. The latter produces changes in the ECG but these bear little relationship to the total potassium loss or the fall in plasma potassium. In hypokalaemia the renal blood flow and the glomerular filtration rate are both reduced and there is, therefore, always a risk when correcting a potassium deficiency that the serum potassium will rise above the toxic level of approximately 7 mmol/l.

Treatment

Prior to infusion of potassium solutions it is essential to ascertain that renal function is adequate, after which potassium may be given as a solution of potassium chloride, 60 mmol/l (mEq/l) in a 5 per cent glucose solution. Alternatively, if the condition is not urgent the hypokalaemia can be corrected by giving potassium orally.

Aetiology of hyperkalaemia

Hyperkalaemia is usually seen by the surgeon in patients suffering from renal failure and the danger lies in cardiac arrest in systole. This may be preceded by ECG changes consisting of the shortening of the Q-T interval and peaking of T waves. There may also be bradycardia and hypotension, the latter due to reduction in cardiac output. A patient may complain of paraesthesiae and muscle weakness prior to the cardiac changes.

Treatment

Although the treatment of hyperkalaemia is the treatment of the cause in an emergency during which the plasma potassium is reaching toxic levels, this must be rapidly reduced. It can be accomplished by the rapid infusion of glucose and administration of insulin or its effect countered by administering 10 ml of 10 per cent calcium gluconate.

Less rapid correction can be achieved by giving an ion exchange resin such as calcium polystyrene sulphonate 30 g in a small quantity of water either by nasogastric tube or by retention enema. When the precipitating cause, e.g.

tubular necrosis, requires dialysis for its correction it is performed either by the peritoneal or the systemic route.

DISORDERS OF ACID–BASE BALANCE

The pH of arterial blood lies between 7.33 and 7.45 and accurate diagnosis of disorders of this system requires measurement of arterial pH, the large vessel haematocrit, and the plasma electrolytes.

Acidosis

When the pH falls below the accepted norm acidosis develops. This may be due to the retention of carbon dioxide which, by going into solution and then dissociating, produces an excess of hydrogen ions—respiratory acidosis—or it may be caused by an excessive production of normal or abnormal acidic products in the body—metabolic acidosis. The commonest cause of respiratory acidosis in the surgical patient is carbon dioxide retention due to inadequate pulmonary excretion of carbon dioxide. This is usually the result of alveolar hypoventilation in a patient who has pre-existing chronic pulmonary disease, which is aggravated by abdominal or pulmonary surgery and the postoperative retention of secretions. In this, once the pH has fallen to 7.25, $Paco_2$ probably 60 mmHg (8.0 kPa), the patient develops disordered cerebral function with a tendency to stupor. Because hypercapnia is a potent stimulus to catecholamine release, tachycardia, together with a rise in the systolic and diastolic blood pressure, ensues.

Assuming the cause of the acidosis to be decreased respiratory exchange, endotracheal intubation, possibly with controlled respiration, may be necessary to reverse the condition.

Metabolic acidosis

Metabolic acidosis due to loss of sodium bicarbonate develops in the following:

1. loss of alkaline intestinal juices. This is always a possibility when biliary, pancreatic or high level small bowel fistulae develop as a complication of surgery or disease.
2. diabetic ketoacidosis or lactic acidosis. The former is associated with uncontrolled diabetes and the latter with inadequate tissue perfusion such as occurs in shock.
3. renal failure.

In metabolic acidosis fixed acids of metabolic origin fail to be excreted because of a reduced capacity of the kidney to form ammonia. The falling pH is associated with increasing depth of respiration and air hunger, followed later by mental deterioration, coma, and death. The most important aspect of treatment is to remove the underlying cause, e.g. treatment of the uncontrolled diabetes, but in an emergency, bicarbonate should be given in the form of sodium bicarbonate. This can be administered at a rate of 0.1 mmol/kg/min but not more than 50 ml should be given before re-estimating the Pa_{CO_2} and the pH. If metabolic acidosis has been accompanied by severe hyperkalaemia, as in renal failure, either an ion exchange resin or hypertonic glucose and insulin should be given.

Alkalosis

Metabolic alkalosis, characterized by a high arterial pH and increased plasma bicarbonate level, is usually observed in:

1 patients suffering from high intestinal obstruction, e.g. pyloric stenosis, in which a selective depletion of hydrochloric acid occurs;
2 excessive use of diuretics if supplemental potassium is not administered. Such cases may be complicated by the additional loss of both sodium and potassium so that the simple administration of ammonium chloride is inadequate to correct the metabolic disorder. Severe alkalosis is associated with drowsiness, apathy, confusion and, in addition, tetany may occur due to a fall in the calcium concentration.

Treatment
Treatment should begin with restoration of the sodium and water deficit, the somewhat slower correction of the potassium depletion, which may be as large as 10 mmol/l (mEq/l) per kg of body weight, and administration of extra chloride in the form of either potassium or ammonium chloride.

1.5 Diagnosis and management of pulmonary complications following abdominal surgery

The common pulmonary complications following abdominal surgery are:

1 exacerbation of pre-existing chronic bronchitis;
2 lobular or bronchopneumonia;
3 segmental or massive collapse;
4 pulmonary embolus.

The less common complications include:

1 aspiration pneumonia;
2 lung abscess;
3 pleural effusion followed by empyema;

4 staphylococcal pneumonia;
5 hypostatic pneumonia.

FACTORS INFLUENCING THE FREQUENCY OF PULMONARY COMPLICATIONS

1 Complications associated with infection and collapse

(a) Pre-existing chronic chest disease
The incidence of pulmonary complications following laparotomy rises from approximately 8 per cent in patients with no history or physical signs of chest disease to 26 per cent in those suffering from pre-existing chronic bronchitis.

(b) The incision
Clinically it is well recognized that upper abdominal incisions are associated with a greater number of postoperative chest complications than infraumbilical incisions. This is in keeping with the greater changes in chest physiology that occur after an upper, as opposed to a lower, abdominal incision. Thus, the vital capacity and the maximum inspiratory and expiratory rates are reduced by approximately 60 per cent after an upper as compared to only 40 per cent by a lower abdominal incision.

(c) Sex
The male is more susceptible than the female to postoperative pulmonary complications. This is due in part to the harmful effects of occupation and smoking, both of which may lead to chronic bronchitis. An infective lesion in the respiratory tract before an operation results in a fourfold increase in chest complications.

(d) Postoperative factors

(i) *The position after operation.* The recumbent posture reduces vital capacity by nearly 10 per cent. Elevation of the diaphragm produces pulmonary venous congestion which reduces the elasticity of the lung tissue and, thus, the mechanical efficiency of breathing.
(ii) *Postoperative pain.* At one time, narcotic analgesics were considered harmful because of their depressive action on the respiratory centre and their inhibitory effect on the cough reflex. Evidence recently produced, however, shows that the analgesic effect of the narcotics far outweighs any central effect unless gross inflammatory changes are already present in the lungs. Commonly, the vital capacity of the postoperative patient is actually increased by morphia.
(iii) *Dressing.* The historic many-tailed bandage reduces lung volume by about one-fifth due to the combination of a raised diaphragm and limited chest movement. For these reasons it has, therefore, been abandoned. Never-

theless, the overenthusiastic use of Elastoplast, particularly when used to strap an upper abdominal incision, can be equally harmful.

Frequency of complications resulting from collapse
The frequency of chest complications associated with collapse is difficult to assess. Whereas the incidence certainly differs in different centres and in different parts of the same country a factor of great importance is the diagnostic criteria. This may be either clinical or radiological. Clinical criteria include the development of a productive cough associated with physical signs in the chest not present before operation. Radiological physical signs, used alone, are not easy to interpret with complete accuracy because it is difficult to distinguish purely infective complications from collapse, particularly when the latter is segmental. Using this method, however, some investigators claim that there are pulmonary complications in at least 50 per cent of patients subjected to an upper abdominal laparotomy if no chest physiotherapy is given in the immediate postoperative period. However, if minor radiological signs are ignored the incidence falls to about a quarter.

2 Frequency of venous thrombosis

Assuming that no prophylactic action is taken it has now been established that approximately 30 per cent of all surgical patients will develop a deep venous thrombosis although the incidence varies somewhat according to the type of operation. Thus major surgical operations are followed by a 30 per cent risk of the development of phlebothrombosis whereas the incidence rises to 50 per cent for orthopaedic operations, particularly when these are associated with the hip and lower limb. One of the major problems concerning deep venous thrombosis is that an extensive thrombosis may be present in the absence of either symptoms or signs or conversely in patients in whom classical symptoms and signs are present the deep venous system is found to be normal on phlebography.

Patients particularly at risk of developing phlebothrombosis include patients suffering from cardiac disease, the elderly and obese, the anaemic, the polycythaemic, the debilitated, the hemiplegic, patients suffering from malignant disease and patients in whom splenectomy has been performed and the platelet count has risen to unacceptable levels.

PROPHYLACTIC ACTION

1 Complications due to infection and collapse

At the very least a surgeon should recognize the presence of chronic respiratory disease before operation and then take prophylactic action in both the pre- and postoperative periods. Simple pulmonary function tests can be performed in outpatients or at the bedside. The peak flow, which is easily measured, changes in parallel with the more sophisticated ratio—the forced expiratory volume in one second divided by the forced vital capacity. The FEV_1/FVC is a useful guide to functional impairment. If this test is repeated following the administration of a bronchodilator it may show an improvement, thus differentiating asthma from chronic bronchitis. When this ratio is 80 per cent or above, respiratory function is normal. When the peak flow falls below 350 l/min there is reason to doubt respiratory efficiency. If these relatively simple tests reveal abnormally low values the adequacy of alveolar ventilation should be assessed by measuring the partial pressure of carbon dioxide in the arterial blood.

More sophisticated tests include:

(a) the static lung volume which is measured by rebreathing air containing a known concentration of an inert gas until equilibrium is reached between the gas in the spirometer and that in the lungs;
(b) the transfer factor (TCO) which is a measure of the rate in ml/min per mmHg at which carbon monoxide passes from the atmosphere into the red cells.

When clinical and laboratory tests indicate gross reduction of pulmonary function appropriate steps must be taken both before and after operation. These steps may include preoperative and postoperative physiotherapy, the administration of bronchodilators, the administration of antibiotics and in some patients respiratory support.

2 Prevention of venous thrombosis and its complications

The most important factor in preventing the complications of venous thrombosis is to prevent this complication occurring. It is now recognized that several prophylactic measures are effective in reducing the incidence of postoperative venous thrombosis.

The following have been well documented:

(a) low dose heparin using 5000 units 2 hours preoperatively and then 8-hourly or 12-hourly postoperatively. This regimen is continued until the patient is fully ambulant. Low dose heparin decreases not only the frequency of small ^{125}I-fibrinogen-detectable calf vein thrombi but also major proximal thrombi in the iliofemoral veins. It may also have an indirect beneficial effect when operating on patients suffering from malignant disease in reducing the implantation of micrometastases;
(b) external pneumatic compression (EPC). This method has the advantage of not being associated with bleeding and whilst it is effective following the majority of operations it does not appear to be effective following hip surgery;
(c) dextran 40 or 70 given in volumes of at least 500 ml over a period of 4–6 hours at the time of operation and then daily for 2–5 days. Like heparin the administration of dextran produces a small risk of bleeding and it may in the elderly produce circulatory overload. Unlike EPC it is effective in hip surgery.

Other methods which are being explored at the present time include the use of graduated compression stockings, aspirin and antiplatelet drugs.

Should a deep venous thrombosis be suspected the diagnosis can be confirmed by bipedal phlebography with, on occasion, the addition of pertrochanteric phlebography, to outline the iliac vessels and inferior vena cava. Identification demands anticoagulation but if despite anticoagulation repeated pulmonary emboli occur the loose thrombus can be locked in position by the use of venacaval filter. Thrombolytic therapy using streptokinase may be administered but this drug may give rise to antibodies which preclude any second course of treatment. Immediate allergic reactions and pyrexia can also occur following the administration of this drug.

DIAGNOSIS AND TREATMENT OF SPECIFIC COMPLICATIONS

1 Exacerbation of pre-existing chronic bronchitis and bronchopneumonia

Definition. Chronic bronchitis is defined as a disorder associated with a productive cough that occurs for at least 3 months in 2 successive years. There is nearly always an element of obstructive disease, which produces the second clinical aspect of chronic chest disease in the form of emphysema. In chronic bronchitis, with or without emphysema, the lungs are usually overinflated, which leads to an increase in the residual volume and the functional residual capacity.

Physical types
Two physical types of patient have been described: the 'blue bloater', who is a chronic bronchitic, often short, stocky and commonly cyanosed, and the 'pink puffer', who is purely emphysematous and often asthenic. This patient sits expiring slowly with the lips pursed in order to raise the intrapulmonary pressure and so prevent the collapse of his thin-walled bronchioles. It is these patients who should receive preoperative chest physiotherapy and breathing exercises in order to improve their pulmonary function and mechanics before operation because any interference with pulmonary function, particularly if associated with superadded infection, may tip the patient into respiratory failure.

Postoperative treatment
Immediately the patient has recovered from the anaesthetic, vigorous physiotherapy and postural drainage should begin. Ampicillin should be started and continued until it is clearly recognized that the postoperative course is to be uneventful. If hypoxia develops, continuous oxygen therapy should be administered while still ensuring that administration of the oxygen-enriched gas mixture does not increase the carbon dioxide tension enough to cause a depression of consciousness. If the initial arterial carbon dioxide tension is less than 60 mmHg a 28 per cent oxygen mixture can be given by a mask of the Venturi type.

If infection ensues, bronchopneumonia develops. Increasing respiratory embarrassment follows and the patient brings up large quantities of thick purulent sputum, a specimen of which should immediately be sent for bacteriological examination and to test antibiotic sensitivity.

Chest X-rays at this time show patchy shadows of irregular distribution, usually at the lung bases. These are superimposed on the hypertranslucency of the lung fields in the predominantly emphysematous patient or the more normal chest X-ray of the chronic bronchitic. When the infecting organism is a staphylococcus, the patchy areas of bronchopneumonia are usually 1 cm or less in diameter. Cavitation occurs rapidly and tomography then demonstrates that the abscesses have thick walls.

If the predominant organism is a haemolytic streptococcus a widespread bronchopneumonia with multiple pea-sized areas of consolidation develops.

Any pulmonary infected lesion, particularly if it is near to the pleural surface, may lead to the development of a pleural effusion which may itself become infected (*see* later discussion).

2 Massive collapse

Diagnosis of this condition is usually made some 48 hours after operation when the patient becomes dyspnoeic and, usually, slightly cyanosed. The temperature, pulse, and respiration rate rise, often in an alarming fashion.

Clinical examination is often conclusive, percussion over the affected area revealing dullness, and auscultation absent breath sounds.

The diagnosis may be confirmed by plain radiographs of the chest which may demonstrate:

(*a*) narrowing of the rib spaces over the affected area;
(*b*) deviation of the trachea;
(*c*) elevation of the diaphragm;
(*d*) compensatory emphysema of the unaffected lung tissue;
(*e*) that the affected lobe forms a dense triangular shadow in the paravertebral gutter. On the right side it is clearly visible on the PA film but when collapse occurs on the left side a lateral view is required if the lower lobe is affected.

Treatment

It is necessary to re-expand the affected lung tissue as soon as possible, otherwise subsequent infection may lead to a lung abscess. The principles of treatment include:

(*a*) *frequent active physiotherapy.* To obtain the cooperation of the patient it may be necessary to administer narcotic analgesics before every session or, alternatively, to institute continuous epidural analgesia.
(*b*) *administration of bronchodilators.* Salbutamol given orally or by aerosol spray. Aminophylline administered by slow intravenous injection or as a suppository.

(c) *mucolytic agents*. These drugs are said to lower the surface tension of the viscid sputum but hard evidence to this effect is difficult to obtain.
(d) *antibiotics*. Before obtaining laboratory evidence of bacterial sensitivity, ampicillin is a most suitable agent because it is active against the two most frequently isolated organisms, i.e. *Streptococcus pneumoniae* and *Haemophilus influenzae*.
(e) *aspiration*. If conservative non-invasive physiotherapy fails, the bronchial tree must be aspirated. This can be achieved either by the use of sterile endobronchial catheters, passed without an anaesthetic, or by a bronchoscopy performed after local anaesthesia of the oropharynx, larynx, and trachea.

3 Pulmonary embolus

The various clinical manifestations of a pulmonary embolus include:

(a) in approximately 20 per cent of patients, sudden collapse followed by death, often while straining at stool. A block of at least two-thirds the diameter of the pulmonary artery is probably necessary to produce this condition.
(b) chest pain together with fever, a rise in pulse rate and repeated haemoptysis. If the embolus is small the temperature remains elevated for about 5 days. If a whole lobe is infarcted the temperature may continue for weeks unaffected by antibiotics.

It is also possible for a pulmonary embolus to be completely silent. In practice, only 30 per cent of patients have the classic triad of leg signs, pleural pain, and haemoptysis.

Diagnostic aids
(a) Plain lung films
The classical radiological appearance in the lung field following a pulmonary embolus is a wedge-shaped opacity, but this is rare. More frequently there are changes that resemble the patchy consolidation of bronchopneumonia or pneumonia. Linear opacities, usually basal, pleural effusion, or an elevation of a hemidiaphragm are also seen. A major embolus may produce right ventricular enlargement.

(b) Electrocardiographic changes
Many changes can take place in the ECG appearances but none is specific. Among the changes described are tall P waves in leads 1 and 2, an inverted T wave in lead 3 and, rarely, a partial right bundle branch block.

(c) Pulmonary scanning
Two types of scan are now used and assuming that the lung fields were normal immediately prior to surgery they are extremely reliable diagnostic methods.

Perfusion scanning. In this method isotopically labelled aggregates of capillary size are intravenously injected; either technetium-labelled microspheres or albumin aggregates are normally employed. The particles enter the pulmonary circulation and in normal lungs are evenly distributed thus producing an even density of isotope throughout. Defects in the scan imply a defect in perfusion and the presence of an embolus.

Ventilation scanning. This will differentiate the defects due to obstructive airway disease, e.g. chronic bronchitis and emphysema in both of which the perfusion and ventilation scan will be abnormal. When both the chest radiograph and ventilation scan are normal then defects on the perfusion scan are normally due to a pulmonary embolus.

(d) *Pulmonary angiography*

This invasive technique is now rarely used since the perfection of scanning techniques.

Treatment

Once the diagnosis of pulmonary embolus has been confirmed the patient must be anticoagulated, for repeated emboli are not uncommon and occur in about 30 per cent of untreated patients.

A suitable regimen would be heparin 10 000 units 4-hourly for 24 hours, then 6-hourly. After 48 hours an indirect anticoagulant such as warfarin is given in an initial dose of 30 mg, followed by a continuation dose of between 5 and 10 mg, depending on the prothrombin time.

4 Aspiration pneumonia

As a complication of surgery, aspiration pneumonia is usually seen when a patient, who has not starved before operation or who is suffering from intestinal obstruction, regurgitates at the time of anaesthetic induction before a cuff tube has been introduced. Because the right main bronchus lies more in line with the trachea than the left, aspirated material usually enters the right lung. Changes, therefore, are found with greatest frequency in the axillary segments of the right upper lobe or in the apical segments of the right lower lobe, these being the dependent parts of the lung when the patient is lying on the operating table.

The result of such an accident is a chemical pneumonia that is usually followed by a secondary bacterial infection. The characteristic of the resulting lesion is necrosis of the consolidated areas and, instead of pus, a slimy, smelly fluid that exudes from the necrotic areas.

Treatment

Treatment of this condition consists of bronchial toilet accompanied by lavage, large doses of steroids, and antibiotic therapy.

5 Lung abscess

This may arise as a complication of any of the conditions previously described but the incidence has fallen due to the better care of postoperative chest complications and the introduction of antibiotics.

'Bronchogenic' abscesses are associated with aerobic and anaerobic streptococci, staphylococci, pneumococci, organisms of the Vincent's angina group and, occasionally, *Proteus* and clostridia. A common site is the apical segment of the right lower lobe which is the most dependent part of the lung when the patient is lying on his side or back. The majority of abscesses rupture into a bronchus rather than the pleural space, when the purulent contents are expectorated. Early in the course of their development abscesses appear as a segmental shadow, with the borders blurred and slightly irregular because of oedema in the adjacent segments. Once the abscess has ruptured into a bronchus it appears as a translucent ring containing a fluid level in the middle of the opaque segment. Occasionally, a lung slough is seen as a rounded or oval opacity within the cavity. This usually liquefies and disappears within one or two weeks, thus distinguishing it from a mycetoma in which the 'slough' is permanent.

Treatment
The treatment of lung abscess is essentially conservative. It consists of antibiotics, postural drainage, and percussion by an experienced physiotherapist. Occasionally, lobectomy is required if medical treatment fails, an empyema complicates the condition, or it is thought that the abscess is a cavitated bronchial neoplasm.

1.6 Indications for, and complications of, tracheostomy

INDICATIONS

There are many indications for tracheostomy and they may be classified in a number of different ways. The operation is performed as either a planned or emergency procedure. An example of the former is the formal tracheostomy that accompanies laryngectomy, and of the latter, emergency tracheostomy in severe maxillofacial injury.

The indications can also be grouped under three main headings, but even so these different indications are not mutually exclusive:

1 indications based on respiratory insufficiency;
2 indications in which tracheostomy is necessary before or in the course of treatment;
3 indications based on pharyngolaryngeal dysfunction in which the patient is unable to keep a clear airway.

In clinical practice the indications for immediate tracheostomy are nearly always multiple; for example, a tracheostomy may be indicated in a patient suffering from multiple injuries for the following reasons:

1. the presence of severe maxillofacial injuries may produce airway difficulties;
2. injuries to the chest, if severe, result in the increasing retention of bronchial secretions followed by failure of respiratory function. It is, however, present practice to maintain such a patient by tracheal intubation for at least a week before performing a tracheostomy;
3. respiratory failure following a severe head injury may hasten the onset or worsen cerebral oedema;
4. a tracheostomy may be a necessary part of the treatment of a fractured neck.

Indications based on respiratory insufficiency

This group consists of a large number of different conditions. In many patients respiratory insufficiency is based on airway obstruction the causes of which may be divided into:

(a) infective
   (i) acute epiglottitis
   (ii) acute laryngotracheitis
(b) mechanical
   (i) carcinoma of larynx
   (ii) post-thyroidectomy haemorrhage
   (iii) retention of bronchial secretions
(c) nervous
   bilateral abductor paralysis of the vocal cords.

In other patients respiratory insufficiency may be caused by central factors:

(a) head injury accompanied by brain stem paralysis
(b) severe poisoning
(c) ascending polyneuritis, poliomyelitis and tetanus

Any patient suffering from respiratory insufficiency should have repeated estimations of the blood gases. Whatever the original starting point for the $Pa{co_2}$ this becomes critical at 80 mmHg (11.0 kPa) and at this level, temporary means of improving respiratory function must be instituted.

Measures to deal with temporary respiratory difficulty

When the cause of respiratory difficulty is considered to be temporary the situation may be treated by endotracheal intubation alone.

A modern portex tube can be left *in situ* for about 9 days. The larynx and cords must be carefully inspected at intervals to ensure that oedema and ulceration are not occurring. The advantage of an endotracheal tube over a tracheostomy is that the surgical complications of tracheostomy and the resultant scar are avoided.

Disadvantages of an indwelling tube are as follows:

1. it is less well tolerated than a tracheostomy;
2. it is difficult to fix;
3. it may kink in the pharynx;
4. it may be displaced, usually into the right main bronchus;
5. it increases airway resistance;
6. portex tubes tend to block more readily with inspissated secretions and, therefore, demand excellent humidification for their management;
7. pulmonary infection readily occurs if the tube is improperly managed.

If the glottic anatomy is so distorted that an endotracheal tube is very difficult or impossible to pass, an immediate tracheostomy should be performed because the repeated trauma associated with failure to pass a tube precipitates laryngeal oedema. Endotracheal intubation itself is not without complications but these are most commonly seen in childhood. Complications of intubation include:

1. glottic webs;
2. granulomatous reaction;
3. subglottic stenosis;
4. inexplicable permanent cord paralysis.

In an emergency if the cricothyroid membrane is punctured either by a cricothyrotome or a large bone needle the severe respiratory difficulty may be immediately relieved and the operation can be performed in less difficult circumstances.

A vertical or limited collar incision through the skin can be made. The author would advise the former for the relatively inexperienced operator since it makes the subsequent steps in the operation much easier.

The head should be held in an extended position by an assistant, the trachea being forced into the most superficial position possible. Once the deep cervical fascia is divided, the thyroid isthmus is identified and divided if necessary. The tracheal rings are then identified; the first and second are left undisturbed, after which the third and fourth are divided. An early postoperative complication of tracheostomy is early displacement of the tube. If only an ordinary window has been cut, without any further action the tube is difficult at this stage to reinsert. This difficulty can be overcome by opening the trachea in a T-shaped manner and suturing the angles of the T to the skin of the neck.

Alternatively, an inverted U incision can be made in the trachea, the apex of the U then being sutured to the skin.

Once the trachea is opened either a double lumen silver tracheostomy tube or a plastic cuff tube is inserted and the attached tapes are fastened behind the neck, taking care that they are neither too tight nor too loose. If the tapes are too loose the tube has a tendency to fall out when the neck is flexed.

A tracheostomy reduces the dead space in an adult by approximately 140 ml and also allows freer access to the bronchial tree for removal of secretions. However, the dead space normally warms and humidifies inhaled air and it is important that both functions are replaced by some artificial device otherwise the cilia of the tracheobronchial mucosa lose their mucus covering and become inactive. This leads to the accumulation and inspissation of secretions on the inner wall of the endotracheal tube, the distal trachea, and bronchi.

Once the tracheostomy is in place an air/oxygen mixture is given.

The inspired air oxygen tension should, however, be no greater than that which will maintain the arterial oxygen tension at between 80 and 100 mmHg (10.6–13.3 kPa), because if oxygen is inspired at a Po_2 greater than 300 mmHg (40 kPa) for longer than 36 hours, retrosternal discomfort and cough may occur—the Lorrain Smith effect.

Continuous administration of pure oxygen may eventually lead to bronchopneumonia and death. The mechanism of oxygen poisoning is unknown but it is generally believed that high Fio_2 values interfere with surfactant formation in the alveoli.

Complications of tracheostomy

Complications of tracheostomy are not infrequent. A retrospective study of all tracheostomies performed in the United Oxford Hospitals between 1950 and 1959 showed that some form of complication developed in 252 patients in a total series of 389, and 13 deaths were directly attributed to the operation. The important complications include:

1 *Pulmonary infection*
This is a frequent complication of tracheostomy and special care is needed to avoid it. Sterile plastic endobronchial catheters should be used for bronchial toilet and these should be passed by personnel wearing disposable sterile plastic gloves. Frequent bacteriological examinations of the secretions should be made and intensive physiotherapy, including postural drainage, should always be given to prevent the accumulation of secretions.

2 *Displacement of the tube*
Displacement may be dangerous in the first few days preceding the development of a proper track. Later, angulation of a metal tube may lead to erosion of the trachea and the innominate artery and result in severe haemorrhage followed by death. Alternatively, backward displacement of the tube may lead to oesophageal damage.

3 *Air embolus*
This hazard usually occurs at the time of operation.

4 *Surgical emphysema*
This ensues when the skin around the tracheostomy tube is so tightly sutured that air cannot escape from the neck.

5 *Subglottic stenosis*
This occurs if the first or possibly the second tracheal ring is damaged. If they are divided or eroded chrondritis of the cricoid cartilage may develop which can lead to total collapse of the airway and the need for a permanent tracheostomy.

6 Crusting in the tube and bronchi

Inadequate humidification of the inspired air leads to the accumulation of inspissated secretions which may block the tube.

7 Granulomata of the trachea

These form, proximal to the tracheostomy opening, and cause a ball valve obstruction at the upper lip of the stoma which gives no trouble until the tube is finally removed.

8 Late tracheal stenosis

This is caused by ischaemic necrosis of the tracheal rings by a cuff tube and it can be prevented by releasing the pressure in the cuff every few hours for a few minutes.

9 Pneumothorax

This is due to injury of the dome of the pleura when performing the operation.

1.7 Common non-surgical causes of acute abdominal pain

A discussion on the medical cause of abdominal pain might seem inappropriate to a surgical text but it is essential that a surgeon should be aware of the great many medical causes that may mimic a 'surgical abdomen' if unnecessary laparotomy is to be avoided.

COMMON CAUSES IN CHILDHOOD

1 Mesenteric adenitis

This disease is confined to children and is the commonest cause of misdiagnosis in children suspected of suffering from acute appendicitis. Often, the affected child has suffered from a recent upper respiratory tract infection, signs of which may still be present, particularly in the throat. Abdominal pain may begin in the central abdomen but soon becomes localized to the right iliac fossa. The child is always febrile, in contradistinction to early acute appendicitis, and tender in the lower abdomen. When a laparotomy is performed a mass of enlarged glands are found in the mesentery from which the adenoviruses can be cultured. Later, during convalescence, neutralizing antibodies are found in the serum.

A physical sign said to help in differentiating this condition from appendicitis is the mobility of the point of maximum tenderness. The child is examined supine and the point of maximum tenderness is found by palpation. He is then rolled onto the left side. If the point of tenderness moves medially this is said to favour a diagnosis of mesenteric adenitis rather than appendicitis. This sign should, however, be treated with great caution. The author regards it as useless!

2 Pneumonia

The diagnosis of pneumonia, either bacterial or viral, is often left unconsidered in children but, when it affects the right lower lobe it is a relatively common cause of abdominal pain in childhood. Children under the age of 7 rarely spit and, therefore, the characteristic 'rusty' sputum due to altered blood from areas of red hepatization is not produced. However, in the young child suffering from a pulmonary infection the pulse/respiration ratio, normally about 4:1, decreases and the alar nasae move in the inspiratory phase of respiration. When the cause of the abdominal pain lies below the diaphragm this ratio usually increases and the alar nasae move only when general peritonitis is beginning to restrict diaphragmatic movement. These latter observations are of great importance because the abdominal wall may be rigid in both supra- and infradiaphragmatic conditions.

3 Infestation with worms

Many worm infestations remain symptomless or provoke nutritional changes. Those producing attacks of abdominal plain include:

(a) the whip worm *Trichuris trichura*, which inhabits the large intestine and especially the caecum. When there is a severe infection, pain in the right iliac fossa may mimic acute appendicitis.
(b) the round worm, *Ascaris lumbricoides*, is especially common in tropical countries, and in some parts of Africa is the commonest cause of abdominal pain in childhood when the worms migrate into either the common bile or pancreatic ducts, producing biliary obstruction or acute pancreatitis.
(c) the threadworm, *Enterobius vermicularis*, may well be found within the appendix or even penetrating the wall but it is extremely doubtful whether it is ever responsible for appendicular pain.

4 The exanthemata

In all the exanthemata the prodromal stage may be associated with acute abdominal distress, e.g. scarlet fever, streptococcal sore throat, mumps and measles.

Intermittent abdominal pain of unknown aetiology also occurs in childhood. This type of pain is seen most frequently between the ages of 8 and 10 and the pain may be so severe that the child is not taken to school or, once there, is brought home. Such pain is often in the periumbilical region and may cause the child to vomit for several hours. When the child localizes the pain to the right iliac fossa the parents live in constant fear that each attack may herald acute appendicitis. In these circumstances it is often better to remove the appendix, knowing that it will be normal, after carefully explaining to the parents that the attacks of pain may well continue. Occasionally, investigation of such a child leads to the finding of a previously unsuspected duodenal ulcer, Crohn's disease, or a congenital anomaly of the renal tract.

5 Blood disorders

(a) Henoch Schönlein purpura

Classically, this condition is associated with abdominal pain, a skin rash and joint pains. The diagnosis should go unrecognized only if there is no skin rash. This is usually papular at first and purpuric later. The condition affects children usually 7 to 28 days after an acute respiratory tract infection. The underlying pathological change is in the capillaries which are damaged by an allergic response. As a result, capillary permeability increases and red cells and plasma escape into the surrounding tissues, provoking a perivascular cellular inflammatory reaction. In severe cases a similar lesion in the kidney leads to microscopic haematuria. The abdominal pain is caused by lesions in the bowel. Occasionally, the degree of local irritation is sufficient to induce an intussusception but, more frequently, an ileus develops which leads to repeated vomiting and slowly increasing abdominal distension. Although Henoch's purpura is primarily a medical condition, if an intussusception develops it will require either radiological or surgical reduction.

(b) Sickle cell disease

Sickle cell disease is a common condition in the African negro and descendants from this stock. It is due to the presence of an abnormal haemoglobin in the red cell, known as haemoglobin S. This structural abnormality of the haemoglobin molecule causes it to crystallize into rigid rods when the Pao_2 falls. As a result the red cell twists into the familiar sickle shape.

The effect of this makes the red cells sensitive to trauma and reduces their survival in the circulation and, in addition, the mis-shapen cells tend to migrate to the capillary beds and produce thrombosis. Infarcts occur in the spleen, lungs, and elsewhere and may lead to attacks of abdominal pain, particularly in childhood. The surgeon should be alerted by the skin colour of the patient. A screening test may be positive but this does not necessarily rule out a concomitant surgical emergency.

COMMON CAUSES IN THE ADULT

1 Viral infections

(a) Herpes zoster or shingles

This is a herpetiform eruption affecting sensory nerves and is caused by the same virus as chicken pox. A patient suffering from herpes may transmit chicken pox to a child. Degeneration and demyelination of the posterior horn cells occurs. The first symptom of herpes is usually pain in the cutaneous dermatome of one or more nerve roots. Three to five days later the typical eruption develops. The initial pain of herpes can obviously be mistaken for an acute surgical condition only if the roots between T_7 and L_1 are involved, because these supply the dermatomes with an abdominal distribution. If the T_{10} and T_{11} dermatomes are affected on the right side, the initial pain can easily mimic appendicitis or a twisted ovarian cyst.

(b) Bornholm's disease

This condition caused by the coxsackie B virus, derives its name from the Danish island on which there was an epidemic. It presents with sudden pain, in the lower chest or upper abdomen, which is severe but intermittent, recurring at intervals, usually for about a week. The area of the abdominal wall in which the pain is felt may be tender and rigid. The disease is usually epidemic and affects, in particular, relatively closed communities such as schools, army barracks, and nurses' homes. It is, therefore, common for the first few patients to go undiagnosed. Conversely, the diagnosis is difficult to reach in an isolated case.

2 Pulmonary causes

As in the child, a right-sided diaphragmatic pleurisy may produce severe right upper abdominal pain, thus mimicking acute cholecystitis or perforated duodenal ulcer.

3 Acute coronary occlusion

This condition is usually associated with severe chest pain, radiating to the neck and arms, which may be severe from the onset or build up in crescendo fashion. Weakness, nausea, and even vomiting can occur. Less frequently, the pain and discomfort begin in the epigastrium and are occasionally accompanied by rigidity, suggesting acute cholecystitis, acute pancreatitis, or a perforated peptic ulcer. These different modes of presentation occur regardless of whether the patient is at rest, excessively active, starving or replete, and only rarely does the patient give a history of increasing angina which would assist in the differential diagnosis.

4 Metabolic disease

Diabetes may cause acute abdominal pain during the initial stages of a diabetic crisis as the patient becomes ketotic. The reason is unknown. The severity of the pain appears to be proportional to the ketosis rather than to the level of the blood sugar. Although ketoacidosis may be the first symptom of diabetes, it is more frequently the result of an acute infection in an established diabetic. The classical signs of ketoacidosis are present and include a dry tongue, rapid weak pulse, and hypotension due to sodium depletion and dehydration. The breath smells of acetone and the urine is loaded with ketone bodies and glucose.

The severity of the condition can be assessed by measuring the plasma bicarbonate concentration, a value of less than 10 mmol/l indicating that the patient is severely acidotic. Because such patients are clinically extremely dehydrated, a total body water deficit of 6 litres being common, there is a certain urgency for administering intravenous fluids. Fortunately for the patients, as the dehydration is corrected so the abdominal pain tends to improve, even in the absence of specific measures such as administration of soluble insulin. This has saved many patients from an unnecessary laparotomy.

5 Blood disorders

Porphyria. Acute intermittent porphyria is an autosomal dominant inherited disease, classified into two varieties, the hepatic and erythropoietic. The latter is rare, the first manifestations usually occurring in infancy or childhood. The clinical features associated with hepatic porphyria seldom begin before puberty and consist of episodic attacks of colicky abdominal pain, vomiting, and constipation. Thus, the disease may mimic either small bowel obstruction or acute appendicitis. In keeping with the former diagnosis there may be a number of operation scars. Much less frequently an attack may be associated with lower motor neurone paresis or paralysis, the weakness progressing to a flaccid paraplegia.

The pain of porphyria can be precipitated by many pharmacological agents including oral contraceptives, barbiturates, methyldopa, and alcohol. Since the porphyrins and their precursors are pharmacologically inactive the clinical symptoms are probably due to a neuropathy.

When a patient presents for the first time with this condition, only a high degree of suspicion on the part of the surgeon will lead to the correct diagnosis, unless all patients complaining of acute abdominal pain are routinely screened by the use of Ehrlich's aldehyde reagent (*p*-dimethylaminobenzaldehyde). To 5 ml of this reagent is added 5 ml of urine, after which 10 ml of saturated sodium acetate together with 10 ml of benzylamyl alcohol solution is added. The appearance of an intense red colour indicates the presence of porphyrins. A specimen of urine passed by the patient at the time of admission is normal in colour, and only becomes the classic Burgundy red on standing. This is due to the gradual conversion of colourless prophobilinogen to the red uroporphyrin.

6 Neurological conditions

The gastric crisis of tabes is a cause of abdominal pain. Acute severe intermittent pains are characteristic of tabes dorsalis. Although the pains may affect any part of the body the surgeon's interest is aroused when the pain is abdominal. At this stage in the disease there is symmetrical degeneration of both axons and myelin of the dorsal columns of the spinal cord. Damage to the somatic sensory fibres leads to paroxysmal pain and to impairment of temperature and pain sensation. Damage to the fibres entering the dorsal columns leads to sensory ataxia, and since the afferent arcs of the tendon reflexes are denervated, there is loss of reflexes and hypotonia. The pains do not, in fact, resemble any recognized type of pain produced by the abdominal viscera themselves as they are too severe, too short in duration, and often described as red hot needles. However, they may be associated with vomiting, tenesmus, and strangury. The bizarre description of the pain should alert the surgeon, as should the presence of Argyll Robertson pupils.

7 Psychological pain

A rare cause of abdominal pain in the adult is Munchausen's syndrome. This condition is most commonly seen in females. The patient complains of pain, often colicky in nature, and the presence of abdominal scars suggests a diagnosis of intestinal obstruction. There is usually no associated increase in peristalsis although the patient mimics abdominal rigidity and makes frequent attempts to vomit. Plain X-rays of the abdomen, if obtained, are negative, and sometimes the patient makes certain they are not obtainable, either by fainting on the way to the department or moving as the film is being exposed.

This condition can only be diagnosed if there is a high level of clinical suspicion, which may only be aroused by the multiplicity of abdominal scars. Usually, these patients admit themselves to different hospitals using a variety of aliases to make their movements difficult to trace.

2 Endocrine Surgery

2.1 Laboratory diagnosis of primary thyrotoxicosis
2.2 Aetiology and treatment of primary thyrotoxicosis
2.3 Pathology, diagnosis and treatment of hyperparathyroidism
2.4 Diagnosis, investigation and treatment of endocrine-secreting tumours of the adrenal glands
2.5 Endocrine-secreting tumours of the gastrointestinal tract

2.1 Laboratory diagnosis of primary thyrotoxicosis

Many of the laboratory tests of thyroid function used to diagnose the condition of thyrotoxicosis described in *Tutorials 1*, pages 40–44 are now merely of historic interest and will, therefore, only be briefly reviewed.

The chief clinical conditions from which primary thyrotoxicosis must be distinguished include:

1 an anxiety state;
2 diabetes mellitus;
3 myeloproliferative disorders;
4 phaeochromocytoma;
5 cirrhosis of the liver.

Laboratory tests which are now less commonly used

1 *Protein bound iodine*
This measures the total amount of iodine which can be precipitated with the plasma proteins and is, therefore, an estimate of the total circulating thyroid hormone. This test has now been virtually discarded although when it is accurately performed it remains an excellent reflection of the total amounts of T_3 and T_4 in the plasma.

2 *Tests depending upon the uptake of radioactive iodine*
These tests are also becoming less commonly used and in centres in which isotope uptake is still used as a measure of thyroid function ^{99m}Tc is replacing the iodine isotopes ^{125}I, ^{131}I and ^{132}I. In both children and pregnant females, ^{132}I, with a short half-life of some 2.4 hours, is preferred to ^{131}I with a half-life of 8.1 days, which was once almost universally used. In view of the possible

teratogenic effects of all isotopes it would be regarded as unwise to use any of the materials for diagnostic purposes within the first 3 months of pregnancy.

In the standard tests the isotope is administered orally and the glandular uptake measured by a collimeter. A satisfactory discrimination between the euthyroid and 'toxic' patient can be achieved by measuring ^{132}I at either 4 or 6 hours, the choice depending upon individual laboratories.

The uptake of the isotope by a normally functioning gland at 4 hours varies between 10 and 40 per cent. An uptake in excess of 50 per cent is pathognomonic of thyrotoxicosis although a similar uptake can be observed in endemic iodine deficiency goitres, in gigantism and in acromegaly in which there is increased hormonal activity. The results of uptake studies are invalidated if iodine has been administered to the patient within 2 months of the test, by thiocarbamide therapy and conditions which reduce renal iodide clearance. The last is particularly important since it is assumed that the exogenous iodine is removed from the plasma by either the thyroid or the kidneys. This test has now been abandoned in the majority of centres dealing with thyroid disease because, at best, it is only an indirect measure of thyroid function and the result obtained may not necessarily be related to the level of hormone production.

T_3 *suppression tests.* This test was performed when uptake studies yielded equivocal results. To perform this investigation the uptake of ^{131}I-labelled iodine is measured prior to and 6 days after the continuous administration of 40 μg of T_3 8-hourly. In a normal individual the uptake of ^{131}I is decreased by at least 50 per cent because the production of TSH by the anterior pituitary is suppressed. Similar depression does not take place in primary hyperthyroidism or in toxic thyroid adenomas, because thyroid activity is autonomous rather than controlled by TSH.

3 *Tests based on the peripheral activity of the thyroid hormones*

Basal metabolic rate. This test, the only one available prior to the measurement of protein bound iodine has now been completely discarded since it is not only demanding but also of little use in mild cases of hyperthyroidism in which a high degree of discrimination is required. In order to ensure that the patient is 'basal' prior to the commencement of the test no food must be eaten for at least 12 hours and the patient must remain psychologically and physically at rest for at least 30 minutes before and throughout the duration of the test. The normal scatter of the results about the mean in normal persons is approximately 15 per cent, hence its lack of discriminatory ability.

Duration of the tendon reflex, the photomotogram. The true interval between the start of a muscular contraction and final point of relaxation of a muscle can be measured. Using the Achilles tendon jerk the normal duration of the tendon reflex is about 300 milliseconds. The time interval is diminished in hyperthyroidism although there is a considerable overlap with the normal, making the test as a confirmation of toxicity unreliable. In overt thyroid failure, i.e. severe degrees of myxoedema, the relaxation phase is prolonged but it is not significantly delayed in lesser degrees of thyroid failure.

Tests which are now in common usage

The majority of the tests in use at the present time are designed to establish the circulatory levels of thyroid hormones. Interest is chiefly focused on the levels of T_4 (thyroxine), T_3 (tri-iodothyronine) and TSH. In the common form of thyrotoxicosis the causal agent of the clinical manifestations is an elevation of the thyroxine level but it has now been recognized that in some patients the condition is due to a raised level of T_3. However, it should be appreciated that in the normal course of events an increase in T_4 is always associated with a rise in the circulating level of T_3 but in T_3 toxicosis the magnitude of this discrepancy is greatly exaggerated.

Plasma thyroxine and free thyroxine index

Plasma thyroxine

The commonly used techniques assess the levels of protein bound together with free thyroxine, the normal value lying between 60 and 140 nmol/l (40 and 110 µg/l). Since more than 99 per cent of the thyroxine is bound to a globulin it is predominantly this fraction which is measured. However, in thyrotoxicosis the clinical changes are due to an increase in the free fraction the normal concentration of which is only 26–39 pmol/l (20–30 ng/l). Normal changes in the protein bound and free fractions parallel each other so long as the amount of thyroid binding globulin (TBG) remains constant and for this reason the assay of the plasma thyroxine is a valid measurement of thyroid activity.

If the amount of TBG rises there is no change in the level of free hormone but there is a change in measured T_4. If thyroid activity is normal the proportion of protein saturated with T_4 remains at about 30 per cent whatever the concentration of the TBG. If the amount of TBG in the plasma increases then a proportional increase in both protein bound T_4 and in free binding sites occurs whereas a decrease in the TBG results in both a decrease of T_4 and free binding sites. The former situation could be misinterpreted as thyrotoxicosis and the latter as hypothyroidism if only the T_4 alone is measured and it is, therefore, essential to assess the number of free binding sites available if the correct interpretation is to be put on the assay of the total thyroxine.

In order to achieve the latter an *in vitro* test is used in which more radioactive thyroid hormone (^{125}I–T_3) is added to the patient's plasma than could possibly be bound by the TBG. Obviously the more free sites which are available on TBG the more isotope labelled hormone will be taken up and the less will be left unbound. A resin is added to the mix to bind any free isotopically labelled hormone which has been left unbound, this is separated from the plasma and either the amount of radioactivity on the TBG or on the separated resin is determined. The more left in the plasma, or, the less on the resin, the more free sites there were on the TBG.

Thus in primary thyroid disease the T_4 and free sites vary inversely, i.e. as the T_4 value rises so the free binding sites diminish whereas when the concentration of TBG is altered the T_4 and free binding sites change in the same direction, i.e. as the T_4 value rises so the free binding sites increase.

These results are frequently expressed as the free thyroxine index which is calculated from the following formula:

$$\text{Free } T_4 \text{ index} = \text{Serum } T_4 \times \frac{T_3 \text{ resin uptake of patient}}{T_3 \text{ resin uptake of control}}$$

The normal range of this index is 1.3–3.2.

Abnormal TBG capacity

An increase in TBG capacity is induced by:

1 pregnancy;
2 the administration of oestrogens;
3 the taking of oral contraceptives.

A decrease in TBG is induced by:

1 protein loss caused for example by the nephrotic syndrome;
2 the administration of androgens;
3 severe liver failure;
4 certain drugs which compete from the binding sites. These include the salicylates, dephenylhydantoin and phenylbutazone.

Plasma T_3 concentration

The total T_3 concentration varies between 1.6 and 3.0 nmol/l (0.7 and 20 μg/l). T_3 like T_4 is bound to protein and it may, therefore, be necessary to assess the available binding sites before coming to a definite conclusion. In T_3 toxicity high serum T_3 values are found in association with normal serum T_4. The high T_3 results from the preferential secretion of this hormone by the thyroid, not from peripheral conversion. A biologically inactive form of tri-iodothyronine is also sometimes produced, usually in response to stress, when tetraiodothyronine (thyroxine) is deiodinated in such a manner that iodine atoms are lost from the 5 position of the thyroxine molecule instead of the 5[1] position.

Serum TSH

Assuming that the hypothalamic–pituitary axis is intact, disturbance of thyroid function can be detected by the radioimmunoassay of TSH. In general terms the assay of this hormone is of little use in the diagnosis of hyperthyroidism but a rise in the serum TSH concentration occurs in patients with impaired thyroid function prior to any change in other measurable parameters.

Thyrotrophin releasing hormone (TRH) test

TRH is an easily synthesized tripeptide hormone produced by the hypothalamus which stimulates the release of TSH by the pituitary in a normal person.

200 µg of TRH are rapidly administered by intravenous injection and specimens of blood are taken for TSH assay before, 20 minutes later to detect the peak response, and at 60 minutes to detect delayed response. The response which occurs has been classified as absent, impaired or normal, the latter being a rise in TSH concentration to between 4.2 and 16.1 mu/l in man and 5.9 and 18.20 mu/l in women. Each laboratory must, however, establish its own normal range of response to TRH.

This test is normally used to distinguish between primary and secondary hypothyroidism. In a patient suffering from suspected hyperthyroidism in whom equivocal T_3 and T_4 levels are found a flat response will usually occur. A normal TRH test excludes hyperthyroidism but an absent or impaired response may be seen in some patients who are clinically euthyroid. These patients fall into the following categories:

1. patients with the ophthalmic form of Graves' disease;
2. hyperthyroid patients who have already been treated;
3. patients in whom the cause of hyperthyroidism is an autonomous thyroid nodule which is not under pituitary control.

Because of its convenience the TRH test has superseded the T_3 suppression test.

2.2 Aetiology and treatment of primary thyrotoxicosis

The precise cause of thyrotoxicosis still remains to be established. However, certain features suggest that it is essentially an autoimmune disease probably belonging to the subgroup which includes myasthenia gravis and diabetes mellitus associated with acanthosis nigricans, now labelled the receptor antibody diseases.

The major points in support of the view that primary thyrotoxicosis is an autoimmune disease are:

1. lymphocytic and plasma cell infiltration of the gland are common;
2. patients suffering from thyrotoxicosis may have enlargement of the lymph nodes and spleen;
3. circulating antibodies to various components of the thyroid are frequently found not only in the sufferer but also in the euthyroid relatives;
4. as with all organ specific autoimmune diseases Graves' disease is familial; genetic factors play a part as is indicated by the concordance rates in identical and non-identical twins. The incidence of the disease in monozy-

gotic twins is between 30 and 60 per cent and in dizygotic twins between 3 and 9 per cent;
5 as with all autoimmune disease it is commoner in women than men, the condition being 15 times commoner in the former;
6 antibodies to other structures, e.g. the gastric parietal cell, are found in a large proportion of patients suffering from primary thyrotoxicosis.

With the discovery of TSH it was not unnaturally assumed that this pituitary hormone was the cause of the disease until it was appreciated that in primary thyrotoxicosis the circulatory level of the hormone actually diminishes and that thyrotoxicosis can even develop in hypophysectomized individuals. It is, therefore, now considered that this hormone is only concerned with the normal physiological control of thyroid function.

The first dawning of our understanding of the aetiology of primary thyrotoxicosis was in 1956 when Adams and Purves demonstrated that the serum of many patients suffering from Graves' disease contained two materials capable of stimulating the guinea pig thyroid, a capacity demonstrated by the quantitative release of radioiodine from the thyroids of animals prepared for a normal TSH assay by the administration of exogenous thyroid hormone which suppresses glandular function.

Adams and Purves were astute enough to realize that two responses were occurring. The first, a TSH effect in which a brief but almost immediate release of thyroid hormones occurred was followed later by a delayed but much greater response lasting for several hours. The substance responsible for the second phase was originally known as *abnormal TSH* but this gave way in 1960 to the somewhat non-committal term of long acting thyroid stimulator or LATS which merely reflected the bioassay response.

By 1964 it had been proved that LATS was an immunoglobulin of the IgG class with the result that it is now more properly termed TSI or thyroid stimulating immunoglobulin.

The discovery of a circulating immunoglobulin in at least 50 per cent of patients suffering from primary thyrotoxicosis suggested that Graves' disease was an autoimmune condition. However, one of the difficulties in the immediate acceptance of this hypothesis was the inability of immunologists to demonstrate LATS in 100 per cent of patients suffering from thyrotoxicosis and also that in the serum of patients suffering from even the most florid disease LATS may be absent. However, the standard method for the assay of LATS (the MacKenzie) is relatively crude and insensitive.

The position was resolved when it was demonstrated that the serum of patients suffering from thyrotoxicosis contained another thyroid stimulating immunoglobulin known as LATS-P or long acting thyroid stimulator *protector*. This material is species specific in that whilst LATS itself will stimulate both human and mouse thyroid to produce increasing amounts of thyroid hormone LATS-P is specific for human thyroid only and has, therefore, been named human specific thyroid stimulator or HSTS.

By more advanced and delicate assay procedures it has been established that whilst LATS itself is present in the majority but not all patients suffering from thyrotoxicosis LATS-P, i.e. HSTS, is present in all patients suffering from thyrotoxicosis and *not* in normal individuals. It is, therefore, reasonable to assume that TSIs are an important element in the aetiology of Graves' disease and further evidence of their importance comes from the observation that neonatal thyrotoxicosis can occur in babies born to mothers who are either thyrotoxic or who have been treated for thyrotoxicosis. Such a condition could not arise from the transplacental passage of T_4 or T_3 since these hormones do not pass the placental barrier and it must, therefore, be due to the crossover of TSI, and secondly, from the observation that the injection of plasma or IgG from patients suffering from thyrotoxicosis into normal human volunteers increases their thyroid activity.

Whether the TSIs, i.e. LATS and LATS-P, are autoantibodies depends finally on identifying an antigen. At present it is considered most likely that the determinant is associated with the TSH receptor on the thyroid follicular cell membrane.

How then does primary thyrotoxicosis arise? The following hypothesis has been put forward:

1. Possibly triggered by some unrecognized viral infection or by non-specific stress an abnormal clone of T-lymphocytes directed against the thyroid follicle cell may arise.

   Normally such a clone would be destroyed by suppressor T-lymphocytes exercising their normal surveillance over the immunological system but in this group of individuals perhaps lacking some genetically determined controlling mechanism the forbidden clone proliferates to interact with their complementary antigen, presumably on the thyroid cell membrane setting up a localized cell-mediated (CMI) response.
2. Subsequently the activated helper T-lymphocytes programme normally functioning B-lymphocytes to produce humoral antibodies. These take the form in PT of the thyroid stimulating immunoglobulins already described which appear to be antibodies directed against the TSH receptor on the follicular cell. Interacting with the TSH receptor in the thyroid cell membrane they appear to stimulate the follicular cells in a manner indistinguishable from normal TSH.

Further evidence that the immunoglobulins found in Graves' disease are antibodies to the TSH receptor is supplied by the following observations:

1. these immunoglobulins activate adenylate cyclase;
2. there is good correlation between the degree of displacement of TSH and ^{131}I uptake.

From this hypothesis it will be appreciated that TSI is an antireceptor antibody even though it provokes a thyroid stimulating effect. This is not a unique biological situation as has already been stated.

An alternative theory is that an abnormal stimulus produces receptors which are hived off in such quantities that they stimulate B-lymphocytes directly.

The following steps, therefore, may explain the development of primary thyrotoxicosis:

1. Genetically predisposed individual.

2 Exposed to stress or ? viral infection.
3 Development of abnormal T-cell clone which responds to receptor site on the follicular cell.
4 T-cell plus B-cell cooperation follows leading to the production of B-cells responsive to the antigenic properties of the TSH receptor on follicular cell.
5 Antireceptor antibody produced = LATS-P or HTSI which is an immunoglobulin of the IgG class.
6 This inhibits binding of TSH to thyroid membrane but activates receptor thus producing a TSH-like action and hence thyrotoxicosis.

TREATMENT OF PRIMARY THYROTOXICOSIS

It is now generally accepted that in areas of the world in which close supervision of the patient can be achieved the primary treatment of Graves' disease is medical. Only if relapse occurs is surgery considered in the highly developed countries of the West and in patients over the age of 40 radioactive 'iodine' may be used if some contraindication to surgery exists.

Antithyroid drugs

1 *The iodides*
These are classically administered in the form of Lugol's iodine which consists of iodine 5 g, potassium iodide 10 g, water to 100 ml. The dose is 1 ml in divided doses. Whereas the various antithyroid drugs described below take several days, usually between 10 and 14, before there is any observable effect, iodine exerts its effect within 24 hours by preventing the release of hormone which is already formed from the thyroid gland. It is, however, unsuitable for long term treatment of thyrotoxicosis because an 'escape' from its effect occurs after approximately 2 weeks.

Until recently it was customary to replace the antithyroid drugs described below with iodine for a period of 10–14 days in the belief that this would lead to a reduction in the vascularity of the diseased glands. Experiments using labelled xenon injected into the parenchyma of the gland lead the author to doubt that this effect occurs and as a result he has abandoned this phase of preoperative treatment.

2 *The thiocarbamides*
Included in this group of drugs are the thiouracils and the imidazoles. The most frequently used, carbimazole, belongs to the latter group. The drugs were introduced following the observation that thiourea resulted in the development of a goitre in normal experimental animals. They exert their therapeutic effect by blocking the incorporation of iodine into the tyrosyl residues to form mono- and di-iodotyrosine.

3 Potassium perchlorate

This compound which is only used when the thiocarbamides produce toxic effects achieves its therapeutic effect by blocking the uptake of iodide by the gland by competitive inhibition.

Other valuable drugs

Although the above are specifically 'antithyroid' drugs the β-adrenergic blocking agent, propranolol, can be used alone for the preoperative preparation of a patient, since many of the symptoms exhibited by the thyrotoxic patient are due to the direct action of T_3 and T_4 on the sympathetic end organs. Propranolol can be given orally when a dose of 0.25–1 mg/kg in divided doses can be administered for 3 days prior to surgery, the last dose being twice the normal and given 2 hours prior to surgery. The drug is then continued in the same dose for at least 3 days postoperatively giving the drug intravenously during the first 12 hours maintaining the pulse rate below 80/min. The only contraindication to the use of β-blockers is the presence of asthma, chronic pulmonary disease, heart block or in patients receiving monoamine oxidase inhibitors.

In addition to these agents the use of psychotropic drugs will often frequently help the severely agitated patient.

Therapeutic use and complications

Carbimazole

This drug can be administered orally in doses of up to 20 mg 6-hourly. Following ingestion it is rapidly metabolized to its active metabolite, methimazole. After about 10–14 days the patient is able to appreciate an improvement in well being even though no objective signs are apparent. Shortly after, however, the pulse rate begins to fall and the weight to rise. Serial measurements of the now abandoned basal metabolic rate have shown that it falls by about 2 per cent a day. Therefore the time taken for normality to be achieved is roughly proportional to the size of the overactive gland which, in turn, roughly parallels the amount of hormone which must be metabolized. In addition to its effects on the synthesis of thyroxine it has recently been demonstrated that carbimazole can influence the autoimmune processes involved in thyrotoxicosis by inhibiting autoantibody production probably by acting on the lymphocytes within the gland. This action appears to be specific since whilst the thyroxine stimulating hormone receptor antibody is decreased following the administration of the drug, gastric parietal cell antibody activity shows no significant alteration.

The continued use of large doses of carbimazole may rapidly lead to hypothyroidism and overt myxoedema. This complication can be avoided by the simultaneous administration of tri-iodothyronine. One theoretical advantage of this combination is that it remains possible to measure thyroid uptake and, therefore, to assess whether thyroid suppression has occurred. Alternatively by careful clinical observation the dose can be reduced once the patient has become euthyroid to a maintenance dose of between 5 and 15 mg daily.

The toxic effects of the thiocarbamides include:

1. macular or papular skin rashes. These are seen in approximately 1:20 patients. They are usually controlled by the administration of antihistamines but if this fails the drug must be abandoned and perchlorate commenced.
2. agranulocytosis. This is rare, affecting not more than 1 in 200 patients. However, all patients taking thiocarbamides should be warned to stop taking the drug should they develop a sore throat.
3. comparatively rare complications of the thiocarbamides include fever associated with lymphadenopathy, arthralgia, polyarteritis, polyneuritis and prothrombin deficiency.

Potassium perchlorate

The normal dose of perchlorate is between 300 and 800 mg daily, orally, in divided doses.

The drug has fewer toxic effects than the thiocarbamides but nausea and vomiting may occur requiring the administration of an antacid. Hypersensitivity reactions such as maculopapular rashes and lymphadenopathies may also occur but are rare if the dose is kept below 1 g daily. No drug containing iodine should be given at the same time because it may reduce the efficacy of the perchlorate. If this drug is given over a long period thyroid function may be depressed for some time following the cessation of its administration.

Prognosis

Whichever drug is used it now is customary to continue its administration for 18–24 months after which the drug is withheld and the patient observed for signs of relapse.

Whichever series of patients is examined it has been clearly shown that 50 per cent will relapse and that approximately 60 per cent of the relapses occur within the first 3 months, after which the risk becomes increasingly less. Clinical observation suggests that patients with severe disease or with a large goitre are more liable to relapse than those patients with mild disease and small goitres.

Predictive tests

It is obvious that if a predictive test of high discriminatory value existed it would be possible to select those patients in whom surgery or radioactive iodine was the only satisfactory method of treatment at a much earlier date.

One predictive test was described by Alexander and Harden in 1967. The basic principles of this test are as follows: the 20 minute uptake of ^{132}I is measured prior to the commencement of therapy after which the patient is treated with adequate doses of carbimazole and tri-iodothyronine. After 6 months the ^{132}I uptake is remeasured. In some patients it will be found that there is little reduction in the uptake of the isotope whereas in others a profound depression occurs. Such results indicate that relapse is much more likely to occur in the former group. These workers interpreted suppression as indicating that the thyroid was once again under the control of TSH rather than LATS.

This test has unfortunately a large overlap relapse occurring in many patients in whom suppressibility has been demonstrated and vice versa.

Measurement of thyroglobulin. When methods are available to measure the level of circulatory thyroglobulin it has been shown that the patient in whom the circulating level of thyroglobulin level is high prior to and during treatment is liable to relapse.

Measurement of receptor antibodies. If the receptor antibody is high prior to and following treatment this group of patients is particularly liable to relapse.

HLA typing. In 1980 it was shown that Graves' disease is associated with the HLA type DRW3 and nearly all these patients are liable to relapse following the cessation of medical treatment. If HLA typing is combined with receptor antibody measurements the occurrence of remission or relapse can be predicted in the vast majority of patients.

Surgical treatment

The surgical treatment of primary thyrotoxicosis is subtotal thyroidectomy. The technical details of this operation are described in *Tutorials 3*, 1.6, 13. This operation is remarkably safe so long as the patient is euthyroid or controlled by propranolol at the time of the operation and that great care is taken with haemostasis.

Object
The object of subtotal thyroidectomy is to reduce the mass of the gland sufficiently to cure hyperthyroidism but to leave sufficient to avoid the development of hypothyroidism. The optimum size of the remnant is difficult to determine and within broad limits is probably relatively unimportant. The author, for example, attempts to reduce the bulk of the thyroid remnant on each side of the neck to the size of the terminal digit of the first finger, i.e. the thumb, since this represents the approximate bulk of the normal thyroid lobes. However, the residual secretory activity is determined by other factors including damage to the blood supply, the degree of lymphocytic infiltration, the extent of thyroid regeneration and alterations in the immunological status.

Following operation, thyroid regeneration occurs; this is reflected in the TSH levels. The TSH level rises following operation, falls gradually for several months and then becomes stable. The thyroid stimulating immunoglobulin (LATS-P) (p. 50), also falls after subtotal thyroidectomy thus indicating that surgery alters the immunological disturbance.

The complications may be divided into immediate, intermediate and late.

Immediate complications
1   *Respiratory obstruction.* This complication is nearly always the result of uncontrolled bleeding from the cut surface of the thyroid lobes. Bleeding occurs within the confines of the deep cervical fascia which is normally sutured

at the termination of the operation and which is indistensible. Occasionally bleeding deep to the skin flaps may also cause difficulty.

Once the tension within the neck has risen pressure on the deep veins of the neck is produced which is rapidly followed by laryngeal oedema and asphyxia.

The condition is recognized by the development of increasing stridor in the immediate postoperative period.

Treatment consists of passing an endotracheal tube using local anaesthesia prior to administering relaxant drugs. If the latter are administered prior to passing the tube the oedema rapidly increases and the passage of the tube becomes increasingly difficult, if not impossible.

When any difficulty at all is encountered the surgeon should not hesitate to open the wound and perform an immediate tracheostomy after which the bleeding can be controlled. In the author's experience it is exceedingly rare to find a specific bleeding point and if doubt still exists in the surgeon's mind two packs should be placed in the wound, one on each side of the neck. These will control bleeding and can be removed after 48 hours.

2 *Division of the recurrent laryngeal nerves.* Damage to the recurrent laryngeal nerves leads to a variety of symptoms. If only one nerve is divided vocal weakness follows which may last for several months and if, by chance, the patient is a singer previous performance will never be attained. When both cords are divided the patient develops an inspiratory stridor which becomes rapidly worse during exertion so that the patient must be subjected either to a tracheostomy or bilateral fixation of the cords.

The incidence of this complication varies in different series but there is little doubt that its frequency is reduced if the nerve is identified and it can be almost abolished by not only identifying the nerve but by tracing the course of the nerve from its emergence from the root of the neck to its disappearance beneath the lower border of the cricopharyngeus muscle to enter the larynx. Normally as the thyroid lobe is pulled forwards the nerve is also displaced forwards usually angulating sharply backwards at the level of the inferior thyroid artery.

3 *Thyroid crisis.* Apart from bleeding this complication was once the primary cause of death following subtotal thyroidectomy. The condition normally occurs within 48 hours of surgery, the patient becoming agitated and finally stuporose. At the same time fever, tachycardia, tachypnoea and finally cardiac failure develop. This complication should never be seen if the toxic state has been completely brought under control prior to surgery. The mechanisms underlying this complication are incompletely understood.

Treatment consists of:

(a) the rapid infusion of large doses of iodine in the form of sodium iodide, 1–2 g in order to curb the release of thyroid hormone;
(b) the slow infusion of propranolol at a dose sufficient to control the tachycardia;
(c) cortisol (hydrocortisone) 100 mg hourly;
(d) intravenous fluids to prevent dehydration;
(e) large doses of diazepam in order to achieve adequate sedation.

Intermediate complications

The major intermediate complication of subtotal thyroidectomy is hypoparathyroidism. This may be associated with hypocalcaemia without overt evidence of tetany or in a smaller percentage of patients the latter develops commonly between the fourth and sixth postoperative days.

The condition may arise from either actual excision of the glands or, more commonly, damage to the blood supply to the glands causes their infarction. An alternative theory to explain the transient hypocalcaemia after thyroidectomy is that it follows the retention of calcium by the bones.

At first sensory symptoms such as paraesthesia and numbness develop, usually in the fingers and toes, followed by motor symptoms the chief manifestations of which are due to increased neuromuscular excitability. Muscle twitching, muscle cramps, carpopedal spasm, laryngeal stridor and even convulsions may occur. The classic physical signs of overt tetany are eponymously known as Chvostek and Trousseau's sign. In general the earlier the symptoms following operation the more severe the injury. The diagnosis is confirmed by measurement of the serum calcium.

Treatment of the overt condition consists of the immediate infusion of 20 ml of 10 per cent calcium gluconate which can be repeated if necessary. Additional calcium can be administered orally in the form of milk supplemented by calcium gluconate or lactate 6 g three times a day. To ensure the absorption of calcium, calciferol (vitamin D) or cholecalciferol (vitamin D_3) should be given, 1.5–5 mg daily. Spontaneous improvement tends to occur with the passage of time but during treatment repeated estimations of the serum calcium are required.

Late complications

1 *Myxoedema.* The incidence of this complication varies with the series examined; incidences between 3 per cent and 35 per cent have been reported. The probable norm is within the region of 5 per cent and in the majority of cases the maximum incidence occurs within 1 year of surgery. Many factors are involved one of the most obvious being the amount of thyroid tissue removed at the time of operation but in some patients there are more subtle reasons for the development of this complication. It has been shown that in many patients suffering from thyrotoxicosis circulating thyroid cytoplasmic antibodies are present in the plasma, a serological finding which is reflected in an abnormal infiltration of the toxic gland with focal deposits of lymphocytes. Investigations have shown that the greater the initial focal lymphocytic infiltration the more probable is the late development of myxoedema. Treatment consists of the administration of 0.1 mg L-thyroxine twice or three times daily.

2 *Recurrent thyrotoxicosis.* The incidence of recurrent thyrotoxicosis has been variously reported in different series as between 1.2 and 28 per cent but a more realistic figure is of the order of 5 per cent. Recurrence normally occurs within the first 4 years following operation. The condition can be treated by antithyroid drugs, radioactive iodine or further surgery. The decision to perform further surgery depends on the technical difficulties encountered at the first operation and the presence or absence of a recurrent laryngeal palsy

following the first operation. If a nerve has been divided at the first operation any subsequent surgical interference should be approached with caution.

Furthermore, recurrent toxicity is more commonly seen in patients suffering from severe Graves' disease often with obvious extrathyroidal manifestations of the disease and in this group further surgery is frequently followed by yet another recurrence.

3   *Advancing exophthalmos.* It is imperative that patients in whom exophthalmos and ophthalmoplegia are present should be warned that the effects of surgery are completely unpredictable. If the exophthalmos progresses following surgery to the point at which corneal ulceration threatens a lateral tarsorrhaphy may be required or very occasionally an orbital decompression either by the frontal or lateral approach.

The place of radioactive iodine in the treatment of primary thyrotoxicosis

The treatment of hyperthyroidism by means of ^{131}I was first introduced in 1942. There is no evidence that such treatment is followed by an increased frequency of thyroid carcinoma, leukaemia or congenital abnormalities in the children of previously treated women.

The accepted indications, however, for this mode of treatment remain:

1   a patient over the age of 45 years;
2   a general contraindication to surgical intervention is present;
3   the patient has relapsed following surgical treatment and there has been recurrent laryngeal nerve or parathyroid damage.

Dose and mode of action of ^{131}I

It should not be given during pregnancy or to children in whom there may be a risk of developing thyroid carcinoma. ^{131}I destroys both the thyroid cell and its nucleus by β-irradiation. The dose required is difficult to assess because it is affected by a number of factors including:

1   percentage uptake of the isotope by the gland, this can be assessed by preliminary tracer studies;
2   the size of the gland;
3   nodularity of the gland, i.e. the gland geometry;
4   the sensitivity of the thyroid cells to ionizing irradiation.

The normal mode of administration of radioactive iodine is to administer an empirical dose of between 5 and 12 mCi (111–296 mBq) depending on the size of the gland. A further dose should not be given until 12 months have elapsed.

Because the ^{131}I becomes incorporated in the thyroid cell it continues to have a direct radiation effect for about 70 days. However, the physiological reflections of cell death and, hence, of overactivity are not controlled immediately and 2–3 months elapse before the patient becomes euthyroid so that the disease continues to require control by β-blocking agents throughout this period.

Complications of treatment by radioactive iodine

The chief complication of this form of treatment is the development of hypothyroidism. Approximately 10 per cent of patients develop hypothyroidism within a year of treatment after which a further 2–3 per cent become hypothyroid annually thereafter. The rapid development of hypothyroidism is believed to be due to damage to the thyroid cells and thereafter to damage to the nucleus of the thyroid cell.

2.3 Pathology, diagnosis and treatment of hyperparathyroidism

Hyperparathyroidism due to an increased secretion of parathyroid hormone is a rare disease. It is classified as follows:

1 *primary*: due to adenoma, hyperplasia or malignant tumours of the parathyroids. The latter are extremely rare.
2 *secondary*: in which hyperplasia and overactivity of the parathyroids is secondary to a peripheral cause; e.g. chronic renal failure, malabsorption or vitamin D deficiency.
3 *tertiary*: in which parathyroid secretion becomes autonomous. This always follows secondary hyperplasia.

Pathology

Parathyroid adenomas, which are purplish in colour, well defined and encapsulated, consist of chief cells arranged in sheets, clusters, and occasional acini. Pleomorphism of both nucleus and cell are frequent. Local areas of degeneration, sometimes with cyst formation, fibrosis or calcification are met with. Solitary adenomas account for 80 per cent of cases of primary hyperparathyroidism; multiple adenomas 6 per cent.

Hyperplastic glands vary both in size and weight. The common form of hyperplastic gland is composed of water-clear cells, which may be four times the usual size with a highly vacuolated cytoplasm, but general hyperplasia of the chief cells can also exist.

Carcinoma of the parathyroids, usually, but not always, produces a non-functioning tumour. The cells and nuclei are usually uniform, with the cells arranged in trabeculae. Mitotic figures may be present. Lymphatic and blood stream metastases are found, together with invasion of the surrounding tissues.

Pathological changes produced by parathyroid overactivity are as follows:

1 *Skeletal changes*
These fall into four different categories:

(*a*) osteitis fibrosa cystica

(b) cyst formation
(c) giant cell tumours
(d) osteomalacia

The fundamental bony change in hyperparathyroidism is resorption of both cortical and cancellous bone and its replacement by vascular connective tissue in which abortive bone formation (calcium-free osteoid) takes place. The bones most commonly involved are the spine and pelvis, the skull and face, and the long bones.

Cysts may be single or multiple, small or large, unilocular or multilocular. They are lined by connective tissue and contain a brownish fluid. Giant-cell tumours are reddish in colour and closely mimic osteoclastoma. Histologically they are composed of osteoclasts set in a cellular stroma. In the jaw they expand the cortex and form a variety of epulis. Elsewhere they may form tumours of a considerable size.

2 *Renal lesions*

Two lesions are commonly met with in the renal tract: stone formation and nephrocalcinosis. Severe hyperparathyroidism leads to stone formation in 60 per cent of patients and so the pathological changes in the kidneys may be confusing because the changes associated with the endocrine disorder may eventually be masked by those secondary to the presence of calculi.

One major factor concerned in stone formation is the excessive urinary excretion of calcium. Two other factors may also be important: first, the hypersecretion of protein, which may form matrix, and second, the calcific deposits in the calyces which produce the nuclei for the further deposition of calcium. The stones of hyperparathyroidism are composed of calcium oxalate or mixed calcium phosphate/oxalate. Nephrocalcinosis is also common. This consists of focal deposits of calcium large enough to be seen radiologically throughout the cortex and medulla and involving both the glomeruli and the tubules. Microdissection of the kidney shows that the portions of the individual nephron most commonly involved are the distal convoluted tubule, the ascending loops of Henle, and the collecting tubules. Fibrosis and tubular distortion follow the deposition of calcium and, finally, the degree of renal damage may be severe enough to produce renal failure.

Nephrocalcinosis may result from many other conditions, including renal tubular acidosis, pyelonephritis, and medullary sponge kidney, but in many cases the aetiology is unknown.

Physiopathology

The adenomatous or hyperplastic gland secretes an excess of parathyroid hormone and the serum calcium rises above the normal level of 2.5–2.6 mmol/l.

The biological effects of excessive secretion of parathyroid hormone are:

1 an increased production of $125(OH)_2$ vitamin D_3, which is the biologically active form of vitamin D;

2 an increased absorption of calcium from the bowel, probably due to the production of vitamin D;
3 direct action on the bones, increasing resorption;
4 decrease in the tubular resorption of phosphate;
5 an increased tubular reabsorption of calcium.

Nephrocalcinosis and (or) stone formation eventually decrease renal function. This is always greater when there is nephrocalcinosis which, because it results in permanent renal damage, may lead to death from renal failure or hypertension. With lesser damage, particularly when renal stone formation is met with in the absence of nephrocalcinosis, the loss of tubular concentrating power undergoes reversal after parathyroidectomy. Some patients without a gross pathological lesion of the kidneys secrete large volumes of a low specific gravity urine.

Clinical presentation

Hyperparathyroidism can exist at any age and is more common in females. Pyrah stated that the disease presents a great array of symptoms deployed in depth. The symptoms are protean and may vary from minimal to severe. In addition to organic symptoms affecting the skeletal, renal and abdominal systems, severe psychological disturbance may occur.

Hypercalcaemia, from any cause, may produce anorexia, nausea, vomiting, constipation, thirst, muscular weakness, fatigue, and drowsiness. Skeletal symptoms include vague non-specific aching in the back, hips and shoulders. The bones become painful and tender to pressure and swellings appear if cyst formation develops. Pathological fractures are not uncommon.

Renal symptoms are related to:

(a) stone formation, which may result in renal pain, haematuria, renal colic or infection;
(b) nephrocalcinosis which, when advanced, produces hypertension and renal failure; and
(c) polyuria and polydipsia may occur in the absence of any demonstrable organic lesion.

Abdominal manifestations of hyperparathyroidism include constipation, nausea and vomiting, but the condition is also specifically associated with peptic ulceration and the development of pancreatitis. The duration of symptoms prior to diagnosis has decreased, especially in patients presenting with renal calculi because of routine estimations of serum calcium in this group. In the absence of such specific symptoms, however, the history may stretch over many decades. Apart from the chronic form of the disease, the symptoms of which have already been described, there is an acute variety that may be rapidly fatal. Usually, the patient has a long history, then transient attacks of unconsciousness and mental confusion occur. Finally, the patient passes into a coma associated with hypotension and circulatory collapse. This condition is associated with extremely high levels of serum calcium.

Emergency treatment of the acute condition consists of infusion of large volumes of saline by the intravenous route and the concomitant administration of a diuretic such as frusemide. The emergency usually arises because of decreased renal function. Alternative treatments of this condition are administration of disodium hydrogen phosphate or calcitonin.

Diagnosis

The diagnosis of hyperparathyroidism is usually made by a combination of tests. Important among these, and the simplest screening test, is repeated estimation of the serum calcium. The normal value is 2.5–2.6 mmol/l. However, a raised serum calcium may be due to many other causes such as excessive milk intake, vitamin D poisoning, sarcoidosis, thyrotoxicosis, immobilization, multiple myelomatosis, and secondary deposits in bone. All these must be considered and excluded. In addition to raised serum calcium urine calcium excretion is increased. The normal 24-hour calcium excretion in adults varies from 100 to 300 mg (2.5 to 7.5 mmol) with a mean value of approximately 180 mg (4.5 mmol). All the causes of hypercalcaemia enumerated above produce a hypercalciuria and, in addition, a small number of apparently healthy people suffer from idiopathic hypercalciuria and regularly excrete more than 300 mg (7.5 mmol) of calcium a day. In parathyroid disease approximately 50 per cent of patients suffer from hypercalciuria.

The serum phosphate is usually below the normal level of 0.8 mmol/l but, again, low levels also exist in idiopathic hypercalciuria and renal calculi not associated with hyperparathyroidism.

Other biochemical tests of value are calcium perfusion tests, phosphate clearance, and phosphate deprivation. At the present time an elevation of the serum calcium and a raised parathyroid hormone level detected by immunoassay are regarded as the most specific tests. Occasionally, the tumour can be localized by selective venous catheterization, which permits selective measurement of the effluent hormone levels from the various glands. In addition to the biochemical changes, characteristic radiological changes are met in various systems.

In the skeleton subperiosteal bone reabsorption is particularly likely in the middle phalanges of the hands. The X-ray shows a spiculated pattern beneath the periosteum, giving the outer cortical bone a ragged appearance resembling a rotten-wood gatepost. These changes may be accompanied by rarefaction of the cortex or whole bone. The bony tufts disappear from the distal phalanges. These changes are reversible following removal of the pathological gland or glands. The generalized demineralization of the skeleton is also reversible after parathyroidectomy. In the central parts of the shafts of the long bones, metacarpals, ribs, and pelvis, bone cysts may develop. Occasionally, the patient complains of sudden pain in a limb, when a pathological fracture is observed.

A plain radiograph of the neck may very occasionally reveal a calcified tumour.

Renal radiography may show either renal, ureteric calculi or nephrocalcinosis in approximately 60 per cent of patients.

Eye changes are found in approximately one-quarter of the affected patients, slit lamp examination showing calcification in either the cornea or, more rarely, the conjunctivae.

With the increasing use of multichannel biochemical screening a proportion of patients in whom asymptomatic primary hyperparathyroidism is present are being identified.

The criteria on which such a diagnosis can be made according to the Mayo Clinic group is as follows:

1. mean serum calcium $\leqslant 2.8$ mmol/l;
2. creatinine clearance $\geqslant 60$ ml/min;
3. no radiological evidence of bone disease;
4. no evidence of nephrocalcinosis or renal calculi;
5. no history of duodenal ulceration or pancreatitis.

Nevertheless such patients have asymptomatic accelerated bone turnover, as manifest by an elevated strontium space, alkaline phosphatase activity and urinary hydroxyproline, which is only slightly less than in symptomatic patients and many are in negative calcium balance under test conditions.

Furthermore, when compared to matched controls it can be shown that the bone mineral content is reduced in asymptomatic patients and it has also been shown that the incidence of osteoporosis is greatly increased in postmenopausal females suffering from primary hyperparathyroidism, the mechanism suggested for this phenomenon being that parathyroid hormone plays a permissive role in the osteoporosis of euparathyroid patients.

Treatment

In the absence of absolute contraindications the accepted treatment of hyperparathyroidism is surgical although this need never be regarded as an acute procedure. Operative removal of the pathological gland or glands reverses the skeletal changes and halts the renal pathology. In the early postoperative period the commonest cause of death is renal failure which is particularly likely in patients suffering from an advanced renal lesion.

In asymptomatic hyperparathyroidism it is also considered that exploration of the neck should be performed since evidence has been produced showing that the disturbed parameters of bone metabolism already described return to normal after the removal of the offending adenoma.

The basic principle of the operation is that all the parathyroids should be identified. The upper glands are situated on the posterior surface of the thyroid dorsal to both the inferior thyroid artery and recurrent laryngeal nerve, when the thyroid is folded medially, and the inferior glands, when situated beside the lower pole of the thyroid gland, are ventral to both the inferior thyroid artery and recurrent laryngeal nerve.

Adenomata are met with somewhat more frequently in the inferior glands and may, occasionally, be found in the substance of the thyroid gland itself. Any tissue removed should be immediately examined histologically by frozen section techniques. Strict haemostasis during the operation helps to identify parathyroid tissue by maintaining the usual colour contrasts between thyroid and parathyroid tissues.

The size of the adenoma is roughly proportional to the elevated serum calcium and the level of the parathyroid hormone in the plasma; the presence of a single adenoma often leads to atrophy of the remaining glands, making identification difficult.

Causes of surgical failure include:

1 inadequate anatomical knowledge;
2 inadequate surgical technique;
3 unusual situation of the parathyroids.

In the great majority of patients sternotomy is rarely necessary if complete exploration of the neck includes cervical thymectomy. In approximately 50 per cent of patients subjected to re-exploration the abnormal gland will be found to be in a perfectly normal position.

Within 24–48 hours after operation the serum calcium falls to normal or subnormal levels. The rapid fall may precipitate tetany which can be treated by an infusion of calcium gluconate and vitamin D. The fall in serum calcium is usually aggravated by the functional deficiency of the remaining parathyroids. If the anticipated fall does not take place and the diagnosis is not in doubt the operation is a failure and a further exploration may be necessary.

2.4 Diagnosis, investigation and treatment of endocrine-secreting tumours of the adrenal glands

The adrenal gland is composed of two elements, the cortex and medulla which differ in development, structure, function and pathology.

Development of the cortex and medulla

The primitive adrenal cortex arises from the coelonic mesothelium whereas the medulla is derived from the neuroectoderm of the corresponding side of the body, its chromaffin cells representing postganglionic sympathetic neurones of which only the cell body has developed.

Whereas in man the adrenal cortical tissue is restricted to the adrenal gland itself the adrenal medullary tissue is more widely dispersed and tumours of the extra-adrenal chromaffin tissue may produce the same syndromes as are produced by medullary tumours themselves.

In the fetus the chromaffin tissue forms spherical bodies, the chromaffin bodies, which reach a diameter of about 2 mm. These are found in all parts of the sympathetic chain, plexuses and splanchnic nerves. Of these bodies the best known are the para-aortic bodies, the organs of Zuckerkandl, which lie on either side of the aorta in the region of the origin of the inferior mesenteric artery. Elsewhere chromaffin bodies are found within or abutting on the ganglia of the sympathetic trunks in which site they are known as chromaffin paraganglia to distinguish them from the non-chromaffin paraganglia which are the chemoreceptors.

Structure of the adrenal cortex and medulla

1 *The cortex*
This is composed of three zones, the outer zona glomerulosa which merges with the intermediate zona fasciculata and a distinct inner layer of compact cells containing much less lipid known as the zona reticularis. In both males and females the weight of the adrenal glands as a whole rapidly increases both relatively and absolutely from childhood to early adult life and then slowly falls. The relationship between these various histologically recognizable zones and the specific secretion of the various hormones produced by the cortex remains to be fully elucidated.

2 *The medulla*
In the adult the medulla forms only between a tenth and a twentieth of the total substance of each gland. It is composed of cords and nests of cells, each cell containing basophile granules which give a characteristic staining reaction when the tissue is freshly fixed in a solution of potassium dichromate, the granules then appearing brown in colour. This staining reaction indicates that the granules are composed of catecholamines although it is non-specific and a more accurate means of identifying these substances now exists, chiefly formaldehyde-induced fluorescence.

Secretions of the adrenal cortex

The secretions of the adrenal cortex are essential for normal existence; their sudden destruction as in the Friderichsen–Waterhouse syndrome is rapidly fatal and its slow destruction leads to Addison's disease.

The chief steroid hormones which can be isolated from the venous blood draining from the glands are:

1 the glucocorticoids, the primary effect of which is to promote gluconeogenesis but which are also catabolic on protein metabolism. These are the $C_{(21)}$-steroids, cortisol and corticosterone;
2 the mineralocorticoid, aldosterone, the primary effect of which is to promote sodium resorption by the distal renal tubules and diminish sodium secretion by the gastric, sweat and salivary glands;
3 the androgenic $C_{(19)}$-17-oxosteroids, dehydroepiandrosterone and androstenedione, which not only produce an androgenic effect but are also anabolic;

4 the $C_{(18)}$-oestrogen, oestrone, which pursues a role in feminization.

Under normal conditions there is a marked diurnal variation in the secretory activity of the cortex. The high level of cortical activity on awakening gradually falling to a low level by early evening.

Secretions of the adrenal medulla

The phaeochromocytes secrete the catecholamines, dopamine, noradrenaline and adrenaline. These compounds are basically derived from phenylalanine, in turn converted to L-tyrosine which is oxidized to L-dopa which is then decarboxylated by means of decarboxylase to dopamine. This produces a variety of physiological effects on the splanchnic and renal blood flow. Dopamine is then oxidized to noradrenaline and finally it is converted by methyltransferase into adrenaline which constitutes about 80 per cent of the total catecholamine content of the adult adrenal medulla. Noradrenaline is the chief neurohumoral transmitter agent of the adrenergic fibres of the autonomic nervous system.

Plasma levels of the adrenal hormones

1 *Adrenal cortex*
The plasma concentration of the chief hormone of the adrenal medulla, cortisol, can be measured in a variety of ways. The normal level is between 110 and 525 nmol/l, 10 and 25μg/dl, a level which can be greatly increased when the adrenal reserve is normal by the infusion of ACTH.

Normally the adrenocortical production of androgens and oestrogens is trivial in comparison to their production by the gonads.

The aldosterone concentration can also be measured although it is much lower than that of cortisol, the normal level being of the order of 10 ng/dl. In practice it is much more valuable to measure the aldosterone concentration in the venous blood draining directly from the adrenal veins if the facilities for this exist.

2 *Adrenal medulla*
The plasma concentration of dopamine, adrenaline and noradrenaline can be measured by radioenzymatic methods, the normal resting values being 0.7, 0.5, and 4.0 nmol/l respectively.

Degradation products of the adrenal hormones found in the urine

1 *Degradation products of cortical hormones*
The excretion products of the steroid hormones are composed of the 17-oxosteroids (ketosteroids) and the 17-oxogenic steroids; the latter are so-called because they yield 17-oxosteroids on oxidation. In the male, 17-oxosteroids are also produced from the testicular androgens.

The urinary excretion of the 17-oxosteroids, formerly known as the 17-ketosteroids in the normal individual, varies with age but in the adult the range is between 20 and 60 μmol/24 hours in men and in women. These degradation products are derived from androstenedione in addition to cortisol, and are markedly elevated in females showing a marked degree of mascularization in addition to Cushinoid signs.

The urinary excretion of the 17-oxogenic steroids in the normal individual also varies with age but ranges from 30 to 75 μmol/24 hours in adult females. These products are derived principally from corticosterone, cortisol and aldosterone but a variety of intermediate compounds also make some contribution to the total.

The urinary secretion of aldosterone can also be measured, approximately 10 per cent of the hormone being excreted as a water-soluble glucuronide, the normal value being 2–10 μg/24 hours.

2 Adrenal medulla

The chief degradation product of the catecholamines which can be readily measured in the urine is vanillylmandelic acid, the normal value is below 35 μmol/24 hours (7 μg/24 hours) but in the presence of an active tumour this value may rise several-fold. An elevation of VMA occurs in 90 per cent of all patients suffering from a tumour of the medullary cells, i.e. a phaeochromocytoma. The concentration of catecholamines, normally 1.5–4.5 nmol/l, can also be measured.

SYNDROMES PRODUCED BY CORTICAL HYPERPLASIA, ADENOMATA AND CARCINOMA

1 Overproduction of androgens

In infants and young children a congenital form of adrenal cortical hyperplasia causes sexual precocity in boys and pseudohermaphroditism in girls. This form of hyperplasia is associated with a lack of specific enzymes in the cortex leading to abnormally small amounts of cortisol being produced. This, in turn, by feedback mechanisms leads to the oversecretion of ACTH by the anterior lobe of the pituitary and consequently stimulation of the adrenal cortex which leads to hyperplasia. In addition to the two major elements of sexual precocity and virilism, salt loss and/or hypertension may also occur. In boys adrenal hyperplasia leads to the infant Hercules and in girls some degree of labial fusion occurs together with clitoral enlargement. In girls the condition is distinguished from pseudohermaphroditism not of adrenal origin by the finding of excessively high levels of 17-oxosteroids in the urine.

2 Overproduction of oestrogens

This is a rare condition which is usually associated with cortical carcinoma. It is associated with sexual precocity in girls and feminization in the male with loss of libido and gynaecomastia. The urinary output of oestrogens, 17-hydroxycorticosteroids and 17-oxosteroids is abnormally high.

3 Overproduction of mineralocorticoids: primary aldosteronism

Clinical presentation
This syndrome was first described by Conn in 1955. When fully developed the affected individuals suffer from moderate hypertension, periodic muscular weakness, intermittent tetany, hypokalaemia, hypernatraemia, impaired glucose tolerance, polyuria and polydipsia. It is almost three times commoner in females than in males and the peak incidence is between 30 and 50 years of age.

The frequency of these findings is as follows:

(a) More than 75 per cent suffer from hypertension.
(b) Between 50 and 75 per cent suffer from weakness, polyuria, headache and retinopathy.
(c) Between 25 and 50 per cent suffer from polydipsia and cardiomegaly.
(d) Approximately 25 per cent suffer from paraesthesia, disturbances of vision, intermittent muscular weakness, tetany, fatigue, cramps and impaired glucose tolerance.

Pathology
Primary aldosteronism is most commonly associated with a solitary adenoma of the cortex. Only rarely is it associated with hyperplasia or a cortical carcinoma. In 75 per cent the adenoma is less than 3 cm in diameter and less than 6 g in weight.

The adenoma forms a bright yellow lesion within which are areas of dark brown discoloration due to lipid and lipofuscin. The yellow areas consist of lipid-filled cells similar to the clear cells of the zona fasciculata, the brown areas consist of compact cells similar to those of the zona reticularis.

Diagnosis
The important diagnostic features of primary aldosteronism are:

(a) Biochemical tests:
 (i) routine electrolyte estimations establish that the serum (Na^+) and (HCO_3^-) are raised and the (K^+) concentration lowered. Typical results in a patient treated by the author were (Na^+) 142, (HCO_3^-) 33 and (K^+) 2.2;
 (ii) the plasma aldosterone level is higher than normal as also is the amount of water-soluble glucuronide in the urine;
 (iii) plasma renin activity is lower than normal, the normal value does not exceed 32 iu/l;
 (iv) the urinary excretion of 17-oxogenic steroids should be within normal limits;
 (v) selective adrenal venography can be performed thus permitting the specific measurement of the adrenal output of aldosterone.

Primary aldosteronism must be distinguished from secondary hyperaldosteronism. This condition can complicate a variety of conditions including advanced pregnancy, congestive heart failure, cirrhosis of the liver and renal artery stenosis. A common feature of all these conditions is that they are accompanied by ascites and a reduction in the plasma renin concentration.

(b) Localization of the adenoma:
- (i) the introduction of CT scanning has made the localization of aldosterone secreting tumours much easier;
- (ii) if this technique is not available but satisfactory radiological facilities are available together with a capacity to perform satisfactory steroid analysis selective caval venography can be used, anticipating that higher concentrations of aldosterone will be found in the venous blood draining the affected adrenal gland;
- (iii) operative exploration—in some patients failure may be encountered either because the condition is due to hyperplasia or the adenoma is too small to be detected without dislocation and devascularization of the gland.

Operative results in primary aldosteronism
In approximately 75 per cent of patients both the hypertension and electrolyte imbalance associated with the condition resolve, in 25 per cent the patients remain hypertensive but the symptoms associated with electrolyte imbalance disappear and in 5 per cent both the symptoms and hypertension persist.

4 Overproduction of glucocorticoids

The excessive secretion of glucocorticoids produces Cushing's syndrome, first described by Harvey Cushing in 1932 in a patient suffering from a pituitary tumour. Any patient suffering from the stigmata of this disease due to adrenal cortical activity is deemed to be suffering from Cushing's syndrome. Adrenocorticotrophic-like polypeptides simulating adrenal overactivity can be produced ectopically by a variety of tumours including oat cell cancers of the bronchus, thymic tumours, pancreatic islet cell tumours and also ovarian tumours.

Clinical picture
Although affecting both sexes this condition is commoner in women than in men and is most frequent between the third and fifth decades. When developing in childhood it is almost always due to a malignant tumour of the adrenal cortex.

The following features suggest the diagnosis:

(a) obesity. This is of proximal distribution and occurs particularly over the supraclavicular fossae, arms, thighs, and over the upper dorsal spine producing the so-called buffalo hump. Associated but not proportional to the obesity are purple striae.
(b) hirsutism. This is due to the associated excessive secretion of androgens.

(c) insulin-resistant hyperglycaemia. This occurs in approximately 20 per cent of patients.
(d) muscular weakness. This particularly involves the proximal muscle masses and when extreme may lead to the patient being unable to rise from the knee–elbow position without assistance.
(e) hypertension.
(f) mental disturbance. In approximately one-quarter of affected individuals a frank psychosis occurs.
(g) investigation reveals osteoporosis which, in turn, leads to the onset of backache, loss of height and kyphosis.
(h) failure to respond to infection.

In addition to the above symptoms menstrual disturbances are common in women and males usually become impotent.

The underlying cause of the phenomena described is the overproduction of cortisol by the adrenal cortex and as a primary cause of this a tumour of the cortex is responsible in approximately 20 per cent. In the remainder, i.e. the majority, a pituitary tumour is present although both ectopic ACTH production by tumours elsewhere in the body or the overadministration of cortisone may both produce Cushingoid phenomena.

Pathology

In the 20 per cent of patients suffering from Cushing's syndrome of primary adrenal origin either a benign or malignant cortical tumour is present. In childhood the tumours are predominantly malignant and since steroid synthesis is relatively ineffective in the malignant cell they tend to be considerably larger than the benign adenoma.

Adenomas usually weigh between 5 and 30 g and because of the autonomous secretion of cortisol, pituitary ACTH production is suppressed. This results in atrophy of the normal adrenal cortex on the affected, as well as on the opposite, side. Benign tumours are normally bright yellow in colour with dark brown areas.

Adrenal carcinomas resemble adenoma and it may be difficult for the histopathologist to distinguish a benign from a malignant tumour. Areas of necrosis and haemorrhage and nuclear pleomorphism are more likely to be seen in adrenal carcinoma but despite the malignant nature of the tumour mitotic figures may be difficult to find.

In some patients Cushing's syndrome is due to cortical hyperplasia. This may be uniform or nodular in character, the latter term being applied when the nodularity is evident to the naked eye.

Diagnosis

The important diagnostic features of Cushing's syndrome are:

(a) Biochemical tests:
  (i) plasma ACTH assay. The concentration of the circulating ACTH varies with the circadian rhythm. The level is determined by either biological or radioimmunoassay techniques. Whereas in Cushing's disease caused by primary pituitary disease the plasma ACTH level

exceeds the normal range in Cushing's syndrome due to primary adrenal disease the ACTH level will be reduced and the normal circadian rhythm lost.

(ii) plasma cortisol concentration. Two specimens are required daily, the first taken between 8.00 and 10.00 hours and the second between 20.00 and 22.00 hours so that the presence or absence of the normal diurnal variation can be established. The normal value lies between 110 and 525 nmol/l, 10 and 25 µg/dl and the most marked difference from the normal value is observed in the late evening specimen when the reduced production of cortisol observed in a healthy individual does not occur.

(iii) dexamethasone suppression test. The administration of dexamethasone, 0.5 mg every 6 hours, in a patient suffering from cortical hyperplasia, an adenoma or carcinoma fails to reduce the cortisol output and hence no alteration in the urinary excretion of 17-oxogenic steroids occurs. In Cushing's disease, primarily due to pituitary disease, the administration of this drug produces some indirect suppression of adrenal function by suppressing ACTH production.

(iv) measurement of the urinary 17-oxosteroids, formerly known as the 17-ketosteroids. These compounds are the excretory end products of the androgens and are, therefore, derived from the adrenal cortex and testes of the male and from the adrenal cortex and possibly an abnormal ovary in women. A marked rise above the normal value of 20–60 µmol/24 hours occurs in females who show marked masculinization in addition to Cushingoid features, in whom the primary pathology is nearly always a carcinoma of the adrenal cortex.

(b) Radiological identification of the adrenal tumour:

(i) intravenous pyelography combined with tomography. In the presence of an adrenal mass downward displacement of the kidney, usually more obvious on the right than the left may be observed. This investigation is of little use in the presence of adrenal hyperplasia or an adenoma since little anatomical distortion is produced by these conditions. This technique can also be combined with retroperitoneal air insufflation but different authors have reported very different results.

(ii) suprarenal angiography. This technique is of little use since the rich arterial supply of the adrenal makes the differentiation of an abnormal from a normal gland difficult to detect. Similarly, suprarenal venography is a difficult technique to interpret due to the ease with which the extravasation of dye can be produced by the too vigorous injection of too great a volume of dye.

(c) Computerized axial tomography: this technique is available only in those centres in which a whole body scanner is available. Although extremely sensitive, an adenoma 1 cm in diameter can be identified; it is important that the surgeon should inspect both glands at the time of operation. It should be noted that adrenal cortical carcinomata are so inefficient at producing cortisol that they are usually more than 6 cm in diameter by the time the clinical picture of Cushing's syndrome is finally established and in some cases the tumour may even be palpable in the loin.

Treatment

All patients in whom a firm diagnosis of Cushing's syndrome due to primary adrenal disease has been made should be explored. This can be achieved by bilateral flank incisions but the technique which is now most commonly used is an upper transverse abdominal incision passing from the tip of the 10th rib on the left to a similar point on the right side of the abdomen.

In all cases because a bilateral adrenalectomy may be required if no obvious tumour has been located or is found after exposing the adrenal glands, see *Tutorials 3*, p. 145, the patient should be prepared for surgery with cortisone and at the time of operation hydrocortisone should be intravenously administered. It should also be noted that if an adrenal adenoma or carcinoma is present the remaining cortical tissue will have undergone atrophy and cortisone will be required for some time in the postoperative period. After some months the plasma cortisol level following suspension of the drug should be measured.

When bilateral adrenalectomy has been performed the administration of glucocorticoids and sometimes mineralocorticoids is required throughout life.

Prognosis

Benign hyperplasia or adenoma. The surgical removal of a benign adenoma or if necessary bilateral adrenalectomy is gradually followed by a complete remission of the symptoms and signs of the disease. Whilst complete cure is the rule it may take several weeks before an objective response is seen. A major long term problem is the possible recurrence of the disease due to the retention of abnormal adrenal tissue.

Apart from the possibility of adrenal insufficiency following surgery, patients suffering from Cushing's syndrome commonly suffer from the following postoperative complications: wound infection, peptic ulceration and pulmonary problems.

A less well known long term problem if adrenalectomy is required is the development of Nelson's syndrome which is due to pituitary hypersecretion. It includes hyperpigmentation, headaches, exophthalmos and heightened sex hormone effects.

Malignant cortical tumours. Only approximately 25 per cent of patients suffering from an adrenal cortical carcinoma are cured. Recurrence as long as 12 years after apparent clinical and biochemical cure has been recorded. If the tumour is clearly incompletely resected death is inevitable, the tumour eventually invading the inferior vena cava and metastasizing to the liver, causing hepatomegaly and/or to the lungs, causing respiratory difficulties. Some symptomatic relief may be gained in such patients by the administration of aminoglutethimide 0.75–1.0 mg daily. This compound blocks the production of steroids of all classes. It may produce drowsiness and in some patients a morbilliform rash which disappears if treatment is continued.

5 Phaeochromocytoma

The term 'phaeochromocytoma' to describe tumours of the adrenal medulla was coined by Pick in 1912. The association of hypertension with tumours of chromaffin tissue was described by Labbé in 1922 and in 1927 Mayo reported the first successful resection of a tumour in a patient suffering from paroxysmal hypertension.

Clinical presentation

The outstanding symptoms in patients suffering from a phaeochromocytoma are as follows: headache, sweating, palpitation, pallor, nausea, vomiting, tremor, weakness and fatigue. Also encountered in about one-quarter of all cases are anxiety, abdominal pain, chest pain, dyspnoea, flushing attacks, visual disturbance, polyuria and polydipsia.

The characteristic signs are hypertension which may be periodic at first but is usually constant by the time a clinical diagnosis has been achieved. Tachycardia, reflex bradycardia, arrhythmias, hyperhidrosis, tremor, glycosuria and an abnormal glucose tolerance test all can be found.

So far as hypertension in general is concerned the frequency with which a phaeochromocytoma is responsible varies between 0.4 and 2 per cent of all patients found to be suffering from this condition depending upon the series examined.

Pathology

In 90 per cent of patients the primary tumour is in the adrenal medulla but in 10 per cent of patients the excessive catecholamines are formed in the chromaffin paraganglia.

The majority of phaeochromocytomata are benign, the frequency of malignancy varying between 2.5 and 13 per cent according to the series examined. In 10 per cent of patients the tumours are bilateral and in childhood bilateral tumours are almost as common as unilateral.

Phaeochromocytoma form well circumscribed masses within the cortex. The cut surface of a typical benign tumour is grey or brown and both cystic and haemorrhagic areas are common. Microscopically the tumour consists of irregularly shaped cells enclosed in a fine network of reticulin and collagen fibres. If a fresh specimen is fixed in a bichromate solution the cytoplasm is coloured brown. Occasional immature ganglion cells are sometimes found among the chromaffin cells.

All the symptoms described above are due to the excessive production of catecholamines. These act on either the α- or β-receptors and according to the dominant secretion the symptoms associated with this type of tumour can vary considerably. If the tumour is large enough to be felt by bimanual examination palpation may cause hypertension.

Occasionally phaeochromocytomata are associated with neurofibromatosis, medullary carcinoma of the thyroid and rarely there is a family history.

Diagnosis

Biochemical

(a) In 90 per cent of all phaeochromocytomata raised levels of VMA in a series of 24-hour specimens of urine can be detected. Normally less than 35 μmol/24 hours (7 mg/24 hours) of VMA is excreted but in an active tumour the rate of excretion may rise several fold. Prior to collecting urine specimens the administration of monoamine oxidase inhibitors should cease otherwise an abnormally low result may be obtained. In addition because several screening tests for VMA also detect other phenolic acids the patient should omit foods such as coffee, vanilla, citrus fruits and chocolate from the diet.

(b) As an alternative to the estimation of VMA the total catecholamines in 24-hour specimens of urine can be measured. These normally are between 1.5 and 4.5 μmol and this value may also rise several fold. If indicated this investigation can be still further refined by the measurement of urinary metanephrine and nor-metanephrine.

(c) If the above investigations are negative but the history is highly suspicious a 'provocation test' may be used. In general this type of test should only be used when the blood pressure is found to be normal or only slightly raised and an α-adrenergic blocking agent should be available in case an unexpectedly large rise in the blood pressure occurs. Typical of this type of test is the histamine test. Urine should be collected for 2 hours prior to the test and for 2 hours immediately following the injection, the dose of histamine being never greater than 25 μg. Almost immediately following its injection if the test is positive both the systolic and diastolic pressures will rise and headache, flushing and possibly nausea will develop. The urine is collected and assayed for the catecholamine level which will be found to be elevated.

(d) Plasma catecholamine levels. It is now possible to assay dopamine, adrenaline and noradrenaline levels and in the presence of a phaeochromocytoma the values of all three will be found to be raised. Commonly the noradrenaline level is much more markedly raised than that of dopamine or adrenaline.

Localization of the tumour. Four methods can be used but not all may be available:

(a) intravenous pyelography. In the presence of a large tumour a soft tissue mass may be seen on tomographs taken using a low kilovolt peak. Some caudal displacement of the kidney with distortion of the renal calyces may also develop in some patients.

(b) arteriography. This investigation was very commonly used prior to the introduction of computerized axial tomography. The investigation is extremely sensitive but tumours less than 1 cm in diameter are not readily identified by this method. The use of a 'scout' aortogram, injecting some 60 ml of 70 per cent contrast medium into the aorta at the level of the renal vessels allows ectopic tissue to be located. This investigation should not be performed unless phentolamine is available to control a possible hypertensive crisis. Certain radiological problems do, however, remain:

(i) the presence of a relatively avascular tumour may make radiological interpretation difficult;
(ii) the presence of multiple tumours may escape notice;
(iii) associated stenosis of the renal artery which may be occasionally encountered.

(c) ^{131}Iodocholesterol scan. This test is now being increasingly used to localize the site of the tumour.

(d) CATscan. If available this method should identify the presence of a suprarenal or ectopic abdominal mass in the para region.

Treatment

The treatment of all phaeochromocytomas is surgical excision but prior to surgery an attempt must be made to bring the blood pressure under control and it is also essential to control the blood pressure during and after the completion of the operation since the two great dangers are:

(a) dangerous levels of hypertension during the operation due to handling of the tumour;
(b) a precipitous fall in the blood pressure after the removal of the tumour.

Preoperative preparation

The incidence of severe hypertension during surgery can be reduced by the administration of phenoxybenzamine 10–20 mg daily increasing to a maximum of 240 mg a day according to need. Alternatively, this drug can be administered intravenously in a dose of 0.5 mg/kg in 250 ml of 5 per cent dextrose over 2 hours each day. At the same time 40 mg of propranalol should be given orally at 8-hourly intervals.

Operation

Although the tumour can be approached through a tenth rib incision it is now generally considered that a transverse supraumbilical incision is more acceptable since by this approach both adrenal glands can be explored at the same time.

During the operation the blood pressure may rise, particularly when the tumour is handled. This should be controlled by the intravenous infusion of sodium nitroprusside, at first 0.5–1.5 μg/kg per minute and then after controlling the crisis a dose according to necessity, normally between 0.5 and 8 μg/kg per minute. The tumour should be dissected free and removed as gently as possible. If both adrenals appear to be normal it must be assumed in the presence of adequate biochemical evidence, that the tumour lies elsewhere and the common extra-adrenal sites, particularly those around the origin of the inferior mesenteric artery, must be explored.

Postoperative course

In many patients recovery is uneventful but some patients may become hypotensive and this should be controlled by the intravenous infusion of noradrenaline in a dose of 4 mg/l in isotonic saline and in addition plasma expanders may be necessary.

If the hypotension is refractory to both noradrenaline and plasma a dose of hydrocortisone, 100 ml intravenously, will frequently produce a beneficial effect.

Several days after surgery, even in the absence of symptoms, the urinary VMA and plasma catecholamine levels should be assayed. Abnormal results indicate that a reassessment of the patient is required.

Prognosis
In the absence of secondary vascular changes the prognosis is excellent. Occasionally the tumour is irremovable because it is malignant or is removable but malignant metastases may be present. In this situation all that can be attempted is a control of the hypertensive symptoms by means of α- and β-blockers or alternatively, by alphamethyltyrosine, between 2 and 3 g a day being required. This drug blocks catecholamine synthesis but is associated with a variety of side effects which may require reduction of the dose.

6 Advanced breast cancer

The topic of adrenal surgery cannot be dismissed without reference to bilateral adrenalectomy for advanced breast cancer. This was in the past the commonest indication for adrenal surgery.

This treatment was proposed and subsequently performed by Huggins, in 1951 as a result of his studies on tumour growth and hormonal secretion; first, in carcinoma of the prostate in males and, later, carcinoma of the breast in women. However, Huggins' work was preceded by an earlier observation, made in 1895 by Beatson, who noted that oophorectomy brought some relief to certain patients suffering from inoperable breast cancer.

A remission, usually defined as an objective improvement lasting for at least 6 months, occurs in only about one-third of women following adrenalectomy and oophorectomy, although a further group have some subjective improvement. In general terms benefit is most frequent in women who:

(*a*) are premenopausal;
(*b*) have a long disease-free interval between primary treatment and the development of metastases;
(*c*) have had a positive response to oophorectomy;
(*d*) have local or skeletal metastases rather than soft tissue secondaries.

These statements are broad generalizations and many exceptions occur.

However, in an attempt to establish which particular patient would respond to adrenalectomy, always accompanied by bilateral oophorectomy, a variety of tests were devised. These included the so-called Bulbrook discriminant, a low 24-hour output of urinary 11-deoxy-17-oxosteroid associated with a relatively high output of 17-OHCS indicating that a nil response to operation would occur whereas the converse indicated a favourable response could be expected.

A second discriminant test was the use by Bonser and her co-workers of combined biochemical and histological methods. This group came to the conclusion that the minimum oestrogen levels required to sustain a hormone-dependent breast tumour resulted in a 24-hour urinary oestrogen output of 3 μg/24 hours. They also concluded that pituitary dependence, as opposed to ovarian and adrenal, could be estimated by the degree of lobular development in a biopsy of uninvoluted breast tissue. Thus patients who had a high oestrogen output in the absence of lobular development were chosen for adrenalectomy.

Neither of these sophisticated methods has stood the test of time and neither came into general clinical use but perhaps of greater importance is the recent development of the drug, aminoglutethimide, by CIBA which inhibits the synthesis of adrenal steroids. Clinical trials to date have demonstrated the value of this drug in postmenopausal and oophorectomized premenopausal women suffering from widespread metastases. In addition some remissions have been reported in premenopausal non-oophorectomized women.

Treatment should commence with 250 mg twice daily for 2 weeks after which if no side effects are observed the dose may be increased to 250 mg four times daily. Since the drug suppresses the production of glucocorticoids 20 mg of hydrocortisone should be given twice daily. A careful watch should be kept on the level of sodium and potassium since the suppression of aldosterone production may result in both hyponatraemia and hyperkalaemia.

The principal clinical side effects of aminoglutethimide are transient drowsiness and lethargy which may proceed to dizziness. This syndrome occurs in about 40 per cent of patients and usually abates spontaneously or can be abolished by reducing the dose.

Thus disseminated breast cancer is now no longer regarded as an indication for bilateral adrenalectomy.

2.5 Endocrine-secreting tumours of the gastrointestinal tract

CARCINOID TUMOURS

The argentaffin cell was first distinguished from other cells in the depths of the intestinal crypts by Kulchitsky in 1897. It is now recognized to be but one of a family of specialized endocrine cells that have the dual secretory function of producing polypeptide hormones and biogenic amines. These cells are collectively known as APUD cells, the letters indicating their chief properties, i.e. amine content, amine precursor uptake, and decarboxylation. In an ordinary histological preparation all members of this family are similar, the cells are low columnar or roughly triangular with the broadest part of the cell in contact with the basement membrane, the nucleus is centrally placed with small eosinophilic granules lying between the nucleus and the base of the cell. Various cell types forming the APUD family can be distinguished on immunological and ultrastructural grounds but not by conventional histological methods and included within this family are the cells of the islets of the pancreas, certain cells in the tracheobronchial mucosa and the calcitonin secreting (C) cells of the thyroid. Collectively this whole series of cells are now referred to as the 'endocrine cells'.

Whilst the argentaffin cell was first recognized in 1897 and tumours were known to arise from them they remained clinical and pathological curiosities until the early 1950s when a series of papers from different parts of Europe drew attention to the so-called carcinoid syndrome which accompanies about 10 per cent of these tumours.

Clinical presentation of tumours producing the carcinoid syndrome

The diagnosis should be suspected if a patient with gastrointestinal symptoms such as colic, borborygmi and diarrhoea also suffers from atypical flushing attacks in which the face may, at first, be bright red and, later, pink with areas of blueness. These attacks may be associated with wheezing and may be precipitated by alcohol or, during investigation, by 1–5 µg of adrenaline or 5–15 µg of noradrenaline. A pellagra-like change in the skin may develop from a relative insufficiency of nicotinic acid in consequence of the excessive utilization of dietary tryptophan in the synthesis of 5-HT by the tumour cells.

Cardiac valvular lesions are not infrequent, in particular both the pulmonary and tricuspid valves may be involved, the former becoming stenotic and the latter incompetent.

When a carcinoid tumour is inactive it may be found as:

1 an incidental finding at laparotomy;
2 an occasional cause of acute obstructive appendicitis;
3 a rare cause of intestinal obstruction.

Physiopathology
At least 50 per cent of carcinoid tumours are hormonally inert, but the remainder secrete 5-hydroxytryptamine and a variety of other kinins including serotonin.

To produce the symptom complex described above, the active tumours must either be ectopic or have metastasized to the liver because 5-hydroxytryptamine is broken down in this viscus.

It is now believed that bradykinin is the major factor that produces flushing and that 5-hydroxytryptamine produces the marked cyanosis and hyperventilation. The diarrhoea is believed to be due to the direct action on the bowel of serotonin, which stimulates small bowel motility and causes the colonic muscle to relax so that there is an increased intestinal flow rate due to a decrease in the intraluminal resistance in the colon.

Pathology
The common sites of origin of carcinoid tumours in descending order of frequency are the appendix, in which they are commonly found in patients between 20 and 30 years of age. Tumours at this site are usually solitary and

rarely metastasize. The small intestine, usually the lower ileum when their highest incidence is in the seventh decade and they commonly metastasize; the colon, stomach, a Meckel's diverticulum and ovarian teratoma.

The term argentaffinoma was applied to this cell when it was observed that fresh tissue fixed in aldehyde such as formalin resulted in a reaction forming a β-carbolic complex which can reduce silver salts without the addition of any other reducing agent. (Note: other members of the APUD family do not give this reaction but may be argyrophile, i.e. metallic silver is deposited in their granules from a solution of silver salt in the presence of an extraneous reducing agent.)

The gross appearance of these tumours varies from white to a distinctive yellow colour. In the appendix they form small circumscribed growths invading the submucosa but rarely giving rise to metastases whereas in the ileum they are commonly multiple and commonly produce gross enlargement of the mesenteric lymph nodes as they metastasize.

Investigation

1 Measurement of 5-hydroxytryptamine concentration in the blood, normal value less than 0.280 mg/l.
2 Measurement of urinary excretion of 5-hydroxyindole acetic acid, normal value less than 12 mg/24 h (60 μmol/24 h), 70 mg/24 h (350 μmol/h) is pathognomonic of this condition. This test is invalidated if the patient has eaten foods containing large quantities of 5-HT e.g. bananas, pineapples or tomatoes. A false negative reaction is possible if the patient is taking phenothiazine derivatives.
3 A small bowel meal may demonstrate a non-obstructing tumour in the small bowel.
4 Liver scan may demonstrate secondary deposits.
5 Coeliac axis angiography may be used to assess the possibility of resecting hepatic metastases.

Treatment

Surgical

Resection of primary lesion, if possible. When hepatic secondaries are present, hepatectomy is advised in order to reduce the bulk of active tumour tissue because removal of the tumour mass reduces the kinin levels, thereby reducing the symptoms. Intestinal resection may, of course, be followed by a cholerhoeic enteropathy.

The prognosis after resection is fair, 70 per cent of patients surviving for 5 years. If hepatic metastases are present at the time of resection 20 per cent of patients still survive for 5 years.

Medical

When the tumour cannot be resected, some relief may be obtained by medical treatment.

1 Methyldopa may prevent flushing by preventing kinin release.
2 Wheezing may be reduced by administration of isoprenaline by an aerosol.

3 Methysergide or parachlorophenylalanine, which are both serotonin antagonists, may control the diarrhoea and colic.

INSULIN-SECRETING ISLET CELL TUMOURS OF THE PANCREAS

Insulin-secreting tumours are mainly composed of β-cells although it is rare for there to be only one cell type present. Ten per cent of these tumours are multiple, consisting of two or more tumours, and 10 per cent frankly malignant. The islet cell tumour may merely represent one facet of the pluriglandular syndrome. The tumours are usually vascular and yellowish or brownish in colour.

Physiopathology
The cause of symptoms in this syndrome is inappropriate rather than excessive secretion of insulin. Long-continued output of insulin causes inhibition of hepatic glucose release by:

1 direct action of the insulin on the liver;
2 depression of glucagon release from the α_2 cells of the pancreas worsens the hypoglycaemia until it produces characteristic neuroglycopenic symptoms.

The greater part of the insulin produced by β-cell tumours is often proinsulin, the plasma concentration varying from about 8 to 78 per cent of the whole, whereas in healthy normal subjects the proinsulin content forms only 20 per cent or less of the total insulin content of the plasma.

Ectopic sources of insulin-like substances capable of producing hypoglycaemia are tumours in the thorax and retroperitoneal tissues. These are nearly always fibrosarcoma, and although hypoglycaemia may exist the immunoreactive insulin level remains normal.

Causes of hypoglycaemia

All other causes of hypoglycaemia must be considered before reaching the diagnosis of a β-cell tumour.
The commoner causes are:

1 iatrogenic, e.g. excess insulin;
2 factitious;
3 toxic, e.g. monoamine oxidase inhibitors;
4 spontaneous;
5 excessive loss or utilization of glucose due to relative failure of the compensatory mechanisms; e.g. starvation or prolonged exercise, though this is rare.

Islet cell tumours belong to the fourth group, which can again be subdivided into:

(*a*) fasting group, which includes islet cell tumours, liver diseases, endocrine conditions and glycogen storage diseases;
(*b*) reactive group, which includes such conditions as postgastrectomy hypoglycaemia, the prediabetic state, and the reaction to substances such as leucine, galactose, and alcohol.

Clinical presentation of insulinoma

A wide range of symptoms are met with and a high level of clinical suspicion is required, especially when a patient suffers from seemingly inexplicable bizarre psychiatric symptoms associated with neurological signs.

As the disease progresses the patient recognizes that the symptoms of which he or she complains are brought about by starvation or fasting, the onset of symptoms usually taking place when the blood sugar falls to around 40 mg/dl (2.2 mmol/l).

Hence the triad described by Whipple in 1935, which consists of:

1 symptoms induced by fasting;
2 symptoms associated with hypoglycaemia;
3 symptoms relieved by glucose.

Hypoglycaemia from any cause may result in the following symptoms:

1 anxiety, panic or restlessness;
2 hunger;
3 palpitations;
4 abnormal behaviour;
5 coma.

In chronic hypoglycaemia an insidious change in behaviour and personality may take place so that the patient exhibits psychotic or paranoid features with mental deterioration leading to dementia.

Pathology
β-cell tumours are most commonly recognized between 40 and 50 years of age, the sex incidence is equal. They occur with equal frequency in all parts of the pancreas and although usually solitary 10 per cent are multiple, two or more tumours being present. The majority of tumours are from 1 to 2 cm in diameter. Usually the growth is not visible on the surface of the gland but may be palpable once the pancreas has been mobilized. The cut surface of the tumour may have a pinker surface than the surrounding glandular tissue. The tumour may or may not be encapsulated. About 10 per cent of β-cell tumours are malignant but this diagnosis may be difficult for the histopathologist to make and the only certain evidence of malignancy is the presence of metastatic disease.

Microscopically the tumour is composed of cords of islet cells separated by vascular connective tissue. As the tumour ages the stroma undergoes extensive hyalinization. β-granules can be demonstrated within the cells if the tissue is first fixed in Zenker–formal solution and then stained by the Gomori–aldehyde–fuchsin technique.

Assuming that other causes of spontaneous hypoglycaemia have been considered and eliminated, the following investigations are required to confirm the diagnosis.

Biochemical tests

1 *Overnight starvation*, in patients suffering from tumours. Ninety per cent will become sufficiently hypoglycaemic after a night of starvation to produce symptoms.
2 *Intravenous tolbutamide test* together with simultaneous insulin assays.

The patient fasts overnight after which 1 g of tolbutamide dissolved in 20 ml of distilled water is administered intravenously.

Results

1 In a healthy individual there is a moderate fall in the blood glucose, the lowest point being reached within 20–30 minutes. The blood sugar returns to normal, or near normal, fasting levels within 3 hours.
   At the same time the immunoreactive insulin level rises from a mean value of $10.8 \pm 1.2\,\mu U/ml$ to $42.9 \pm 4.8\,\mu U/ml$.
2 In patients with insulinoma the IRI level may start at $40.8 \pm 8.1\,\mu U/ml$ and rise to $160 \pm 30\,\mu U/ml$ within 5–20 minutes; if the tumour is malignant, the IRI levels may rise as high as $1260\,\mu U/ml$. The test can be made even more selective by assaying the different levels of proinsulin and insulin. Benign tumours tend to secrete insulin in response to tolbutamide, whereas in malignant tumours there is a greater proportion of proinsulin.

Disadvantages of tolbutamide test

(a) In approximately 20 per cent of patients suffering from insulinoma the tolbutamide test is negative; in addition, a positive response may be obtained in cirrhosis, Cushing's disease, acromegaly, and lipodystrophy.
(b) It is dangerous, due to the extreme hypoglycaemia that may take place. For this reason intravenous glucose should always be available and the test should *not* be carried out in patients who are extremely hypoglycaemic after overnight fasting.

3 *Glucagon test.* This is a much safer test than the tolbutamide test. One mg of glucagon administered intramuscularly into a normal individual results in a rise in the blood sugar of not less than 40 mg/dl (2.2 mmol/l), after which there is a gradual return to normal. In the presence of a tumour the blood sugar rises but is followed by an abnormal fall within 90–120 minutes.

Of patients suffering from insulinoma, 70 per cent show an exaggerated rise in the plasma insulin within 5–10 minutes of the injection, with a delayed return to normal levels.

4   L-*leucine test*. This test is less sensitive than the tolbutamide test but it is more specific. In 50 per cent of patients oral L-leucine produces a fall in blood sugar and a rise in the radioimmunoactive insulin levels.

Localization of the tumour
Coeliac axis angiography. Selective angiography, examining the arterial, parenchymatous and venous phases is extremely useful in localizing tumours. A negative result, obtained in 25–50 per cent of patients is, however, of no diagnostic importance.

Treatment

1   Surgical

When the tumour has been accurately localized, the problem of removal is equal in difficulty to the surgical removal of a parathyroid tumour. If accurate localization has not been accomplished it may be necessary to mobilize the entire pancreas because tumours occur with equal frequency in all parts. Occasionally, the tumour is extrapancreatic and may be situated in the duodenal wall, the splenic hilum or, very rarely, it may be found in a Meckel's diverticulum.

When no tumour can be found, even after extensive mobilization of the pancreas, modern surgical opinion is against subtotal pancreatectomy or the even more radical 95 per cent resection. Instead, opinion suggests that the abdomen should be closed, the symptoms controlled medically, and the situation reviewed after a prolonged interval.

2   Medical

The symptoms may be controlled by diazoxide, 300–800 mg a day, orally. The major adverse effects of the drug are nausea, dizziness, hypotension, and sodium retention.

GASTRIN-SECRETING TUMOURS OF THE PANCREAS (ZÖLLINGER–ELLISON SYNDROME)

This syndrome was first described by Zöllinger and Ellison in 1955 but not until the work of Gregory and his co-workers in 1967 was it finally established that the condition was due to the production of gastrin by an islet cell tumour.

Since the original description, two types of syndrome with similar clinical features have been recognized:

1   Type I syndrome, in which there is a short history, high serum gastrin levels, and profound hyperplasia of the antral G cells;

2 type II syndrome, in which there is a long history, relatively lower serum gastrin levels, normal antral G cells, and pancreatic D cell hyperplasia or tumour.

Clinical syndromes associated with excess gastrin production

1 *Ulceration.* One of the most common syndromes is peptic ulceration, which is found in all parts of the duodenum and sometimes in the jejunum. Multiple ulcers are not uncommon. The ulcer or ulcers are uncontrolled by both medical and surgical treatment. Partial gastrectomy may even be followed by recurrent ulceration while the patient is still in hospital.
2 *Diarrhoea.* This usually fails to respond to the ordinary antidiarrhoeal drugs such as Lomotil. Typically, the motion is watery due to the impairment of absorption of water and electrolytes, and as a result there may be fluid losses in excess of 5 l/day. Death has been reported from potassium deficiency. The diarrhoea is produced by an acid enteritis because the volume of extremely acidic gastric juice is too large to be neutralized by the normally alkaline duodenal and pancreatic juices. In many patients a true steatorrhoea develops due to the acid inactivation of the pancreatic lipase and the precipitation of bile salts.
3 *Protein-losing enteropathy.* This may take place in the presence of the hypertrophied gastric mucosa, because of the abnormal loss of protein from the mucosal surface and the absorption defect in the small bowel. This syndrome is associated with a reduced plasma albumin level and may lead to gross oedema of the feet and legs. Hypoproteinaemia can only exist when protein catabolism exceeds synthesis and an enteropathy should be suspected in a patient with a reduced serum albumin in the absence of proteinuria.

Pathology
Approximately two-thirds of these tumours are microscopically malignant and one-third in visible metastases, usually in the liver, are present when first seen. The rate of growth may, however, be extremely slow so that the patient may survive for several years after the initial diagnosis has been made.

The condition may be only one facet of the syndrome of multiple endocrine adenomata which is inherited as an autosomal dominant. In one of the author's patients, recurrent ulceration was thought to be due to hyperparathyroidism because the serum calcium levels were high and four hyperplastic parathyroid glands were removed. Approximately one year later the patient developed a mass in the abdomen due to a malignant islet cell tumour. Other organs in which adenoma are to be found are in the anterior pituitary and the adrenals.

Diagnosis
Any patient who develops recurrent ulceration soon after apparently adequate surgery should be treated with suspicion. The investigations of value include:
1 *radiology.* The barium meal may show the classical changes of hyper-rugosity together with massive or multiple ulceration of the upper gastrointestinal tract.

2 *gastric secretory tests*. Aspiration of the intact stomach may well reveal an acid secretion in excess of 15 mmol/h (mEq/h) or if a previous gastrectomy has been performed 9 mmol/h (mEq/h) and above.

The abnormal rates of acid secretion are unaffected by administration of histamine or pentagastrin because the gastric mucosa is already under maximal stimulation.

3 *immunoassay of circulating gastrin levels*. The normal value lies between 80 and 170 pg/ml, the value in the ZES may rise as high as 10 000 pg/ml.

4 *localization*. Localization of a tumour may be possible with abdominal angiography.

Treatment

If an islet cell tumour is found by biopsy to be malignant the rational treatment of the condition is removal of the target organ by total gastrectomy. The progression of hepatic secondaries and indeed of the primary tumour may be so slow that the patient may live for several years.

VERNER–MORRISON SYNDROME

Since the recognition of the Zollinger–Ellison syndrome a second syndrome has been described known as the Verner–Morrison syndrome. This syndrome is associated with profuse watery diarrhoea accompanied by hypokalaemia unaccompanied by peptic ulceration and associated with a normal or even reduced gastric secretion. In addition approximately half the patients suffering from this syndrome have associated hypercalcaemia and about one-third hyperglycaemia.

Histologically the responsible tumour is indistinguishable from those causing gastric hypersecretion but there is evidence that they secrete secretin or a gastric inhibitory polypeptide related to enterogastrone. In addition a vasoactive intestinal peptide similar to glucagon has also been identified.

3 Surgical Oncology

3.1 Classification, pathology, clinical presentation and treatment of bone tumours
3.2 Investigation, pathology and treatment of the thyroid nodule
3.3 Common benign swellings of the breast
3.4 Different methods of staging breast cancer and factors affecting the prognosis
3.5 Tumours of the lymphoreticular tissues with special reference to Hodgkin's disease
3.6 Diagnosis and treatment of bladder tumours
3.7 Pathology, clinical presentation and treatment of pigmented lesions of the skin

3.1 Classification, pathology, clinical presentation and treatment of bone tumours

Bone tumours may be divided into:

1 primary tumours of the bone forming cells themselves:
   (a) benign—osteoma, osteoid osteoma;
   (b) malignant—osteogenic sarcoma, giant cell tumour of the bone;
2 primary tumours of the cartilage cells found in bone:
   (a) benign—osteocartilagenous exostosis (ecchondroma), enchondroma, chondromyxoid fibroma;
   (b) malignant—chondrosarcoma;
3 miscellaneous primary tumours of bone which include: fibrosarcoma, Ewing's tumour, chondroma;
4 tumours arising from the bone marrow: myeloma;
5 metastatic bone tumours.

TUMOURS ARISING FROM CARTILAGE

Tumours and tumour-like lesions arising from cartilage cells are found in bone formed in cartilage. They include chondroma which, if situated in the medulla, are known as enchondroma or, if projecting from the surface, ecchondroma, benign chondroblastoma, chondromyxoid fibroma, and chondrosarcoma.

Many pathologists would argue that only the chondrosarcoma can be accepted as a true neoplasm.

Chondroma

These tumours are usually centrally situated, although in thin flat bones, e.g. ribs or scapula, the exact origin may be indeterminate. Multiple chondromata form the clinical entity known as endochondromatosis, dyschondroplasia, or Ollier's disease. Multiple enchondromata usually appear in childhood and lead to swellings or bosses on the affected bones, retardation of bone growth, and their progressive thickening or bending.

Solitary chondromata are relatively rare but they are the most common tumour of the small bones of the hand, particularly of the phalanges. These tumours develop from the metaphyses, near to, but not involving, the epiphyseal plate. As the tumour grows in size the cortex is destroyed, leading to the development of spontaneous pathological fractures.

Pathology
These tumours are composed of lobulated masses of hyaline cartilage. The microscopic appearance is one of mature hyaline cartilage and the degree of cellularity is variable, making a histological differentiation from chondrosarcoma difficult.

Radiological appearance
Chondromata normally appear as well-circumscribed central areas of rarefaction. When the tumour forms in a long bone there is prominent stippling, or calcification. They may cause the cortex to expand, often eccentrically.

Treatment
This consists of curettage and, when necessary, the defect should be filled with bone chips. Alternatively, when the tumour is in a bone that can be sacrificed, e.g. a rib, it may be removed *en bloc*.

Chondromyxoid fibroma

These are rare. The tumour was formerly known as Codman's tumour but the terminology now used was introduced in 1942 by Jaffe and Lichtenstein to describe a rare, benign bone tumour that appears in the second decade, usually at the lower end of the femur or the upper end of the tibia in the metaphyseal region which tends to be transformed into hyaline tissue with the passage of time. The resulting defect is usually an eccentrically placed area of rarefaction; microscopically the tumour may resemble hyaline cartilage or even fibrous tissue.

Chondrosarcoma

This tumour occurs in adult life. The patient usually presents with swelling and pain: in the presence of a pre-existing lesion the history may be of long duration but in the absence of such a lesion the clinical history may be very short. The antecedent lesion may be an enchondroma or exostosis. Common sites are the trunk and the upper ends of the long bones, e.g. the femur and humerus. Peripheral chondrosarcoma are exceptionally rare.

Pathology
These tumours are composed of proliferating cartilage tissue. They may be divided into central and peripheral varieties. Macroscopically the coalescing lobules of the tumour may be necrotic or even cystic. In the long bones the cortex is thickened and will usually show macroscopic evidence of invasion or may even be completely disrupted.

Microscopically the histological diagnosis of malignancy may be difficult because mitoses may be infrequent.

Radiological appearance
The common finding is one of bone destruction in the area of the lesion combined with mottled densities due to calcification and/or ossification. A central chondrosarcoma involving a long bone may produce a fusiform expansion of the shaft of the involved bone together with thickening of the cortex.

Treatment
These tumours are not radiosensitive and, therefore, the only beneficial treatment is adequate removal. Radical removal of tumours of the scapula, thoracic cage, clavicle, and some tumours of the pelvis may be possible without gross deformity or loss of function, but tumours of the upper end of the femur or humerus may require either hindquarter or forequarter amputation. The prognosis, if adequate surgery is possible, is relatively good because these tumours are slow to metastasize by the blood stream. There may, however, be local recurrence even after a period of 10 years.

TUMOURS ARISING FROM BONE

Osteosarcoma (osteogenic sarcoma)

This is the most important primary malignant tumour of bone. According to the dominant cellular component these tumours have been divided into osteoblastic, chondroblastic or fibroblastic. Although they occur in relatively early childhood and early middle age the maximum incidence of these tumours is between 10 and 20 years of age and over 50 per cent present before the epiphyses close. Osteosarcoma also occur in old age when they are normally a complication of Paget's disease. The most common sites are in the metaphyseal area of the lower end of the femur, approximately 50 per cent, and at the upper end of the tibia, approximately 25 per cent, the remainder being scattered throughout the various bones of the body.

Aetiology
In the older literature reference was commonly made to injury but this has now been dismissed. However, one causative agent is radiation; this may be by thorium, but more important are the fission products of a nuclear explosion, in particular ^{90}Sr which has a half-life of 7 years. External irradiation given for causes other than osteogenic sarcoma may precipitate sarcomatous change in bone and, lastly, Paget's disease may be complicated by this condition.

Symptomatology
Pain, intermittent at first, later becoming continuous together with swelling. The development of a spontaneous pathological fracture is rare despite the gross destruction of bone that ensues.

Physical findings
In the affected area a painful tender mass may be felt. Because of its propensity to metastasize at an early stage to the lungs, physical signs in this area may also be present, e.g. signs of an obvious pleural effusion.

Pathology
Usually, by the time a clinical diagnosis can be made the tumour has breached the cortex and may even encircle the bone. It may be soft, friable and excessively vascular, or show areas of irregular ossification. Sclerosis when present tends to involve the central part of the tumour, the peripheral zones being softer. Metastatic lesions come about by haematogenous spread and produce pulmonary metastases. Microscopically there is a great variation in structure, depending on the dominant cellular pattern. Neoplastic osteoblasts may be large with hyperchromatic nuclei and are commonly spindle-shaped, hence the term 'sarcoma'. Bone formation varies from small spicules of osteoid to calcified osseous tissue. Characteristically, the blood vessels are thin walled, or merely channels lined by tumour cells.

Radiological appearance
A wide variety of radiological appearances can be seen because the tumour may produce a lytic, sclerotic, or a mixed reaction. The majority of osteogenic sarcoma begin in the endosteal region and, later, spread within the interior of the bone. Finally, they destroy the cortex, so separating the periosteum from the bone, and then break out into the soft tissue. The precise borders of the lesion may appear indistinct, and non-neoplastic bone may be deposited by the elevated periosteum. A characteristic radiological feature is the appearance of radiating spicules of bone at right angles to the shaft.

Treatment
The treatment of this particular tumour has radically altered over the last

decade. Initially it was the practice to amputate the affected limb. It was then appreciated that the overall results were exceedingly poor, the majority of patients dying of pulmonary metastases. However, it was also observed that metastatic disease usually appeared within 18 months and that only in approximately 5 per cent of surviving patients did metastases occur after this period. The assumption was, therefore, made that in the great majority of patients the osteosarcoma had already disseminated at the time of recognition of the primary tumour even though no clinical or radiological evidence of metastases could be found. With the recognition that early amputation, however radical, was inadequate, the next phase in the treatment of this tumour was to administer high energy irradiation and then wait for several months before advising amputation.

The third phase now under intensive examination is a combination of early amputation combined with perioperative and postoperative chemotherapy. Early chemotherapy is administered:

1 to control microscopic neoplastic emboli which might be shed at the time of operation. In some series chemotherapy is combined with heparinization since thrombus formation is known to protect the neoplastic cell, either by shielding them from the body's natural defences or from administered cytotoxic agents;
2 on the basic premise that it is likely to be more successful when the tumour mass is small;
3 because in human osteosarcoma pulmonary metastases have been seen to grow rapidly after treatment of the primary lesion by operation or radiotherapy.

Among the many regimens which have been suggested the following drugs have been included: methotrexate dose $10 \,mg/m^2$ together with heparin beginning 12 hours before operation and continuing at 6-hourly intervals for 8 doses. After radical surgery courses of vincristine $1 \,mg/m^2$ and Adrimycin $15 \,mg/m^2$ are given over five days at 14- or 21-day intervals with methotrexate being given every 3 weeks. Because the bone marrow is particularly sensitive to the toxic effects of methotrexate, folic acid is administered and the intervals stated are interposed between each treatment schedule.

Using such chemotherapeutic regimens some increase in survival time has been reported with delay in the appearance of pulmonary metastases. However, once metastases appear they develop with great rapidity unaffected by further chemotherapy.

Giant cell tumour (osteoclastoma)

The exact cell of origin of the giant cell tumour is unknown. The term osteoclastoma was used to describe this tumour in the mistaken belief that the cell of origin is the osteoclast. This view is now no longer generally accepted although the ubiquitous giant cell is the most characteristic cell of this tumour.

Many bone tumours contain similar cells, e.g. osteogenic sarcoma, aneurysmal bone cysts.

The peak incidence of these tumours is in the third and fourth decades, usually in the epiphyses of the long bones, particularly around the knee, although any bone may be affected.

Symptomatology
The usual clinical presentation is with pain, sometimes swelling and, occasionally, with a pathological fracture. A hard mass may underlie the painful swelling and, because of the proximity of the 'tumour' to the joint surface, it is not uncommon to find a joint effusion.

Pathology
The gross appearance of an osteoclastoma is of a soft friable mass, often blood red in colour. The osseous tissue in the neighbourhood of the tumour is expanded and destroyed although the periosteum is usually intact. The thinning of the cortex may rarely give rise to physical signs of 'egg shell' crackling.

Histological examination shows that the basic cell of the osteoclastoma has an oval or spindle-shaped nucleus. Mitotic figures are usually frequent. Little intercellular substance is produced, and scattered among the small cells are the giant cells that resemble the osteoclasts.

Radiological appearance
An expanding zone of radiotranslucency is seen, usually at the end of a long bone. The margin between the tumour and the surrounding normal bone may be indefinite and there may be no evidence of reactive sclerosis. A characteristic soap bubble appearance may be seen.

Treatment
Surgical treatment of osteoclastoma consists of curettage of the tumour. The defect is then filled with bone chips. Unfortunately, this treatment is followed by recurrence in a fairly large percentage of patients. If the tumour involves an unimportant bone, e.g. the fibula or radius, complete excision is the treatment of choice.

Occasionally, the cause of recurrence is the frankly malignant nature of the original tumour but this is fortunately very rare.

Ewing's sarcoma

In 1921 Ewing described a tumour of bone which he thought originated from the endothelial cells of the bone marrow but there still remains no general consensus of opinion as to the cell of origin.

Symptomatology
This tumour accounts for between 10 and 15 per cent of all primary bone tumours, the majority occurring below the age of 30 and although any bone

may be involved the majority occur in the midshafts of the long bones of the extremities. Clinically these tumours present as rapidly increasing, painful swellings attached to bone and in some patients general symptoms such as fever and general malaise are present associated with a leucocytosis.

Pathology
The tumour may be greyish white and translucent with zones of necrosis, haemorrhage, and even cyst formation. Metastases may be found in the lung and other bones, the latter leading to the suggestion that Ewing's tumour may have a multicentric origin. Willis regarded these tumours as either metastatic neuroblastoma—and indeed some of these tumours cannot be histologically differentiated from the bony metastases that may arise from proven neuroblastoma—or as reticulum cell sarcoma. These tumours produce neither a chondroid nor osteoid matrix and they are essentially composed of solidly packed small round cells containing a high glycogen content with an occasional tendency to rosette formation. It is the latter appearance that suggests the origin is from a neuroblastoma.

Radiological appearance
These tumours tend to be extensive. Lytic destruction is commonplace and when the tumour has burst through the cortex multiple layers of subperiosteal new bone are found, giving rise to the characteristic 'onion skin' appearance.

Treatment
Surgery plays little part in the treatment of Ewing's sarcoma apart from obtaining tissue for histological confirmation of the tumour type. Thereafter the primary treatment was radiotherapy, high energy irradiation being delivered to the whole bone. However, the prognosis was poor, death occurring in nearly all patients within 5 years usually due to pulmonary metastases.

Intensive cytotoxic therapy has greatly improved the prognosis since this particular tumour is sensitive to a wide variety of agents including cyclophosphamide, vincristine and actinomycin. These drugs are normally given in combination and the 5-year survival has increased considerably, approximately 50 per cent of affected individuals surviving for at least 5 years.

Myeloma

This tumour arises from the haemopoietic cells of the bone marrow and is the most common single neoplasm of bone. It arises in areas of haemopoietic marrow, especially the lumbar spine, ribs, and pelvis.

Symptomatology
Common presentation is after the age of 50. Usually, the patient complains of pain, often backache situated over the lumbar or thoracic spine. In the course of the disease weakness and loss of weight occur. Neurological symptoms

either due to pathological fractures of the spine or extraosseous extension of the neoplasm may develop.

Pathology
Myelomatous deposits are grey and friable, resembling the type of tissue observed in a malignant lymphoma of the lymph nodes. Histologically the tumour cells vary in appearance from mature plasma cells to cells indistinguishable from reticulum cell sarcoma.

Radiological appearance
These tumours produce multiple lytic areas in the affected bones, especially in the skull. The lesions are distinctive in that there is no surrounding zone of sclerosis and they therefore appear to have been punched out.

Diagnosis
This can nearly always be confirmed by the accompanying biochemical changes. These include a raised ESR, hypercalcaemia accompanied by hypercalciuria and the demonstration of abnormal proteins including IgG and the Bence Jones protein in the urine.

The latter occurs in approximately 50 per cent of patients and may eventually produce the condition of myeloma kidney due to its precipitation in the tubules. The presence of hypercalcaemia may lead to nephrocalcinosis which may ultimately damage renal function.

Treatment
If the lesion is solitary, irradiation is the treatment of choice. If neurological complications have come about due to spinal cord compression a laminectomy may be necessary prior to treatment. When the disease is diffuse, chemotherapy is often effective in controlling the symptoms of the disease. The alkylating agent, L-phenylalanine mustard, or chlorambucil may be effective, together with prednisone which may control the hypercalcaemia. However, the prognosis is poor, few patients surviving for longer than 2 years.

Metastatic tumours of bone

These are much more common than primary tumours. They generally involve the red marrow and, therefore, there is a predilection for the bones of the vertebral column, ribs, sternum, pelvis and the proximal ends of the femora.

Symptomatology
The osseous lesions of secondary metastases commonly produce pain and/or a pathological fracture. The classic primary sites from which osseous metastases arise are breast, prostate, thyroid, kidney, and adrenal.

Radiological appearance
Metastatic tumours of bone produce irregular destructive lesions in bone.

Most are osteolytic, but occasionally carcinoma of the prostate produces osteoblastic secondaries.

Treatment
Secondary bone tumours are now treated by a variety of methods. Radiotherapy may alleviate bone pain or the development of a pathological fracture. If the latter occurs internal fixation should first be used followed later by radiotherapy. Widespread bony metastases may be relieved by the administration of ^{32}P given intravenously for several days.

The widespread metastases of breast cancer may be controlled in about one-third of all patients by hormonal manipulation using drugs such as tamoxifen which is an antioestrogen or aminoglutethimide. The latter produces a 'medical' adrenalectomy and since it destroys all adrenal cortical activity must be administered together with cortisone.

Prostatic secondaries may respond to either irradiation or oestrogen therapy although it is not uncommon to find that one area appears to respond whereas in another area actual growth continues to occur.

Thyroid metastases can sometimes be controlled by the administration of L-thyroxine or radioactive iodine.

Occasionally when a solitary metastasis develops following the excision of a hypernephroma its excision may be followed by long term survival.

3.2 Investigation, pathology and treatment of the thyroid nodule

THYROID NODULE

Definition. A solitary thyroid nodule is any localized enlargement within the gland that is not associated with increase in size or nodularity of the remaining thyroid tissue.

Presentation

Solitary nodules are between seven and ten times commoner in the female than the male in keeping with the usual female predominance of thyroid disorders.

The majority are found by the patients themselves when some incidental movement of the neck throws the developing deformity into relief or they may be found on incidental palpation of the neck. It is unlikely that any nodule less than 1 cm in diameter will be detected in this manner. Less commonly a solitary nodule developing in a retrosternal position may give rise to such a degree of tracheal deformity that classically on turning over in bed at night onto the affected side the patient develops breathing difficulties. Less commonly haemorrhage into a solitary nodule may produce sudden dyspnoea, probably due to a combination of tracheal compression and laryngeal oedema or a solitary nodule may occasionally cause the clinical symptoms and signs associated with thyrotoxicosis. Lastly, if the solitary nodule is malignant the patient may present not with a swelling in the neck but with overt metastases.

However, clinical examination and assessment of thyroid nodules, both of their nature and number, is notoriously inaccurate and if all apparently solitary thyroid nodules are explored between 10 and 50 per cent, according to the series examined, will be found to be part of a multinodular goitre.

Of greatest concern to the surgeon, however, is the incidence of malignancy in apparently solitary nodules. This is variously reported in different series as between 1 and 33 per cent, suggesting that thyroid histology is difficult to interpret.

Investigation

Plain X-ray of the neck and superior mediastinum
This may reveal displacement and/or compression of the trachea. A nodule which enlarges, particularly from the lower pole downwards, passes into the superior mediastinum and forms a soft tissue shadow with sharply defined convex lateral margins. In addition to forming a soft tissue mass, calcification is commonplace in thyroid masses, particularly when such enlargement is due to a multinodular goitre. Such calcification may be dense, nodular, spherical or curvilinear and very rarely psammoma bodies typical of papillary carcinoma of the thyroid may be seen.

Scintiscanning
This can be performed using either ^{131}I- or ^{99}Tc^{m}-pertechnate, although either method is limited in the resolving power and nodules less than 1 cm in diameter cannot be detected by this technique. This places the nodule into one of three categories.

1 *The hot nodule.* This type of nodule takes up more of the isotope than the surrounding normal thyroid tissue. The majority of hot nodules synthesize thyroid hormones independently of pituitary TSH, and pituitary TSH secretion is at first inhibited and, later, ceases. When this happens there is no iodine uptake in the remaining normal thyroid tissue. Such patients may remain euthyroid or show evidence of toxicity.

Further investigations of value are:

(*a*) TSH stimulation. This shows that the remaining, apparently non-functioning, thyroid tissue is normal.
(*b*) T_3 suppression test. This demonstrates that a hot nodule has not fully suppressed TSH and that the surrounding thyroid tissue is still functional. A nodule showing the latter characteristics is sometimes classified as warm.

2 *The 'normal' nodule.* In this group are those nodules which present clinically as discrete masses but in whom the scan appears normal because the isotope is evenly distributed throughout the gland.

3 *The 'cold' nodule.* This group comprises the largest number in any series, accounting for between 70 and 85 per cent of the whole. In this variety neither isotope is taken up by the nodule.

Clinical implication of the isotope study

The clinical importance of isotope study lies in the knowledge that, although hot nodules may occasionally be responsible for thyrotoxicosis, they are never malignant, whereas the incidence of malignancy in a cold nodule is reported to be as high as 12.8 per cent. The true incidence is probably considerably lower, however, because of the high proportion of cold nodules which are found at the time of operation to be a part of a multinodular goitre. It is in this group of patients that a third investigation has proved useful, i.e. ultrasound scanning.

Ultrasonography

By means of ultrasonography 'cold' nodules can be divided into two categories, the cystic and the solid.

Treatment

1 Should the nodule appear cystic and unilocular it is possible in a large proportion of cases to treat the condition by aspiration, a method first introduced by Crile in 1966.

Aspiration can be performed using local anaesthesia only attaching a 20 gauge needle to a 10 ml syringe. The method is particularly successful if when withdrawing the plunger greenish or brown fluid is aspirated but in some patients, i.e. those with a colloid nodule in a multinodular goitre, the material in the cyst is too viscid to be aspirated. Following aspiration of a unilocular cyst the cavity can be obliterated by the injection of a small quantity, 1–2 ml of sodium tetradecylsulphate (STD).

To be considered successful the palpable swelling should disappear completely and cytology of the aspirated fluid should be negative, i.e. acellular, or show no evidence of containing exfoliated malignant cells. If any palpable swelling remains following aspiration this is an indication for immediate exploration of the neck.

2 When ultrasonography indicates that a solitary nodule is solid the possibility of malignancy arises, this then forms the major indication for exploration of the neck, some 10 per cent of solitary solid nodules being finally classified as malignant.

Pathology of the cold nodule

Excluding degenerative cysts in multinodular goitres the following conditions may cause a solitary nodule in the thyroid gland.

Neoplastic	
Benign	(a) follicular adenoma
	(b) papillary adenoma
Malignant	(a) follicular carcinoma
	(b) papillary carcinoma
	(c) medullary carcinoma
	(d) undifferentiated carcinoma
Autoimmune	Hashimoto's disease
Inflammatory	Solitary metastatic abscess

In this section only the neoplastic conditions will be described.

NEOPLASTIC TUMOURS

1 Benign

(a) Follicular adenoma

Pathology
This tumour has many synonyms, including terms such as colloid adenoma, Hürthle cell adenoma, fetal adenoma, and microfollicular adenoma. By definition, it is a benign epithelial neoplasm with a tendency to form follicles. A typical follicular adenoma is solitary, has a well-defined capsule, and is rubbery hard.

The appearance of the cut surface varies with the amount of colloid; it is often brown and may show degenerative changes including softening, cyst formation, haemorrhage, infarction, and calcification due to interference with the blood supply.

Histologically there is a variety of growth patterns; the embryonal, fetal or microfollicular, the macrofollicular, the oxyphil and, lastly, the atypical adenoma in which there may be a good deal of cellular pleomorphism. The subgrouping is descriptive and has no bearing on the clinical course except that atypical adenomas should be very carefully examined for evidence of invasiveness.

Clinical presentation
Follicular adenoma form solitary slow-growing tumours in the thyroid. Rarely, they may produce sufficient thyroid hormone to cause thyrotoxicosis.

Treatment
If the nodule is producing thyrotoxicosis it should be excised. In the absence of hormonal changes a hemithyroidectomy should be performed.

(b) Papillary adenoma

Pathology
This benign neoplasm may form cysts, several centimetres in diameter,

containing a brownish fluid, a tendency that is an aid in distinguishing this type of tumour from the follicular type.

Microscopically the individual cells, which resemble resting thyroid epithelium, are arranged in single layers on thin vascular connective tissue stalks.

Clinical presentation and treatment
The papillary adenoma is exceptionally rare, even though papillary carcinoma is the most common malignant tumour of the thyroid. It should be treated by hemithyroidectomy and a careful histological search made for evidence of malignancy, of which it is often a precursor. A finding of especial significance is that of calcospherites (psammoma bodies) which are particularly common in papillary carcinoma.

2 Malignant

Malignancy of the thyroid is uncommon, the annual deaths in the United Kingdom due to cancer of the thyroid being $4/10^6$ for males and $10/10^6$ for females. It may occur at any age but the prognosis deteriorates with advancing age because well differentiated tumours are more common in the young.

Aetiological factors
1 *Origin in benign adenomata.* This is probably extremely rare because although papillary carcinoma is the commonest malignant tumour, papillary adenomata are rare.

2 *Adenomatous goitre.* In the experimental animal both adenomatous goitres and thyroid tumours may be induced by a low iodine diet. Wegelin of Berne also reported that there is a high incidence of thyroid cancer in areas of endemic goitre. This observation has not, however, been confirmed, and in the United States a careful comparison was made between the incidence of thyroid cancer in Chicago and Detroit, both of which are endemic goitre areas, and 10 other large non-goitre cities. This survey revealed no difference in the incidence of thyroid cancer.

3 *Previous local irradiation.* It was first pointed out by Duffy and Fitzgerald, in 1950, that of 28 cases of childhood cancer of the thyroid, 10 had previously received therapeutic irradiation to the thymus. A larger review of 562 children suffering from thyroid cancer showed that 38 per cent had been previously irradiated. The dose received had varied from 200 to 600 rads and the period between irradiation and the diagnosis of thyroid cancer was 36–64 years. In the experimental animal a similar effect is produced if, following irradiation, the thyroid is stimulated by continuous administration of thiouracil.

Papillary cancer

Clinical aspects
This tumour accounts for approximately 70 per cent of all thyroid malignancies and is the most common thyroid cancer of childhood.

The clinical course is often very long, and 20 years may elapse between the initial diagnosis and death which may result from local recurrence in the neck, pulmonary metastases or, finally, widespread blood-borne metastases. The 10-year survival, assuming there has not been extrathyroidal spread, may be as high as 80 per cent.

Pathology
(a) *Macroscopic appearance.* Although small tumours may be encapsulated the majority of papillary carcinomata are unencapsulated. There is a strong tendency for cyst formation, the cysts being filled with a brownish fluid and papillary projections may be seen projecting from the lining membrane.
(b) *Microscopic appearance.* The tumour epithelium is arranged on fibrovascular stalks which project into cystic spaces. In 40 per cent of papillary tumours, laminated, calcific spherocytes, called psammoma bodies, are found. These are pathognomonic of this type of cancer.

Whilst occasionally the whole tumour has a papillary pattern most are a mixture with papillary fronds in some areas and colloid filled follicles in others. In some tumours a follicular pattern predominates but if any papillary structure is present the tumour should be classified as a papillary carcinoma.

Treatment
1 *Surgical.* The treatment of this tumour remains somewhat ambiguous. Some surgeons would recommend a total thyroidectomy with the removal of all thyroid tissue. The rationale for this operation is the frequency with which intraglandular metastases occur. If this operation is performed one or more parathyroids should be identified and those removed from the neck can be reimplanted in the muscles of the forearm. The author has performed this operation on three occasions only but in all no substitution therapy other than L-thyroxine was required which suggests that the grafts were successful. Other surgeons recommend a near total thyroidectomy, removing the whole of the lobe on the side of the tumour but preserving a fraction of the superior pole on the opposite side in order to retain an intact blood supply to the superior parathyroid gland on this side of the neck.

Whilst prophylactic block dissection of the deep cervical lymph nodes is not recommended the removal of the juxtathyroidal nodes on the affected side together with any pretracheal lymph nodes which can be identified is advised.

If, however, one of the nodes removed appears suspicious a frozen section should be performed and a radical block dissection performed at the same time as the thyroidectomy.

L-Thyroxine should be administered not only because it is necessary following total thyroidectomy but because it will suppress the production of TSH and thus the stimulation of any remaining thyroid tissue if a near total thyroidectomy has been performed.

2 *Radioactive iodine.* Although papillary carcinoma and its metastases do not readily take up radioactive iodine, Pochin has shown that some tumours can be stimulated to do so by administering TSH. This, therefore, becomes a possible method of treating metastases.

3 *External irradiation.* External irradiation is useful if the tumour cannot be excised.

Follicular carcinoma

Clinical aspects
The incidence of follicular carcinoma increases with age and because of its slow development a swelling may have been present in the neck for as long as 10 years. Even so, the possibility of transition from a benign adenoma to malignancy is regarded as rare.

Pathology
(*a*) *Macroscopic appearance.* The macroscopic resemblance between a follicular adenoma and carcinoma is so close that it may be impossible to distinguish them by the naked eye. Unlike papillary carcinoma, however, follicular carcinoma appear to be encapsulated although in some patients the presence of intrathyroidal or extrathyroidal invasion is clearly apparent.
(*b*) *Microscopic appearance.* The histological structure is similar to that of follicular adenomata. Some tumours are nearly solid, only microfollicles being present, whereas others are so well differentiated that they form follicles resembling normal thyroid tissue.

In some tumours the only evidence of malignancy lies in the infiltration of the capsule or surrounding veins which can only be detected after very careful histological examination.

Metastases
The degree of invasiveness of follicular carcinoma is variable but when it happens it is nearly always evident in the blood vessels. Osseous or pulmonary metastases may cause the presenting symptoms and signs even in the absence of any apparent goitre. Radiologically the bony metastases produce osteolytic lesions and the lung secondaries rounded 'cannon ball' type defects in the lung fields.

Treatment
Since this tumour and its metastases take up radioactive iodine with much greater avidity than does a papillary tumour the administration of the isotope becomes an important aspect of the treatment of this condition.

However, the first measure must be a total thyroidectomy followed by adequate replacement therapy in order to make such treatment effective. Following surgery a whole body scan should be performed in order to detect any metastases which are capable of taking up radioiodine which have not been seen on plain radiographs.

If the tumour is inoperable external HER should be used since this will nearly always reduce the swelling and relieve, for a time at least, dyspnoea and dysphagia.

Undifferentiated carcinoma

An undifferentiated thyroid carcinoma may be defined as one in which neither papillary nor follicular structures are seen and amyloid is not deposited. They comprise between 5 and 15 per cent of all thyroid malignancies.

Clinical aspects
This type of tumour is usually seen in older patients and there is often a long history of goitre. The mass in the neck is nearly always poorly defined because of spread to adjacent structures, and invasion of the trachea with the development of dyspnoea and stridor is not uncommon.

Treatment
Exploration nearly always reveals a locally inoperable tumour. In such patients a tracheostomy may be necessary prior to HER. The prognosis is poor, only about 50 per cent of patients surviving for 6 months following diagnosis.

Medullary carcinoma

The incidence of this tumour is variously reported as being between 5 and 15 per cent of all thyroid neoplasms.

Pathology
Macroscopically the tumour is often composed of one single, apparently unencapsulated, grey-white mass in which degenerative changes are rare.

Microscopically the tumour consists of sheets or rounded masses of round or fusiform cells in a stroma of amyloid.

Clinical aspects
This is the only tumour of the thyroid more common in men than women. It may be familial and it is occasionally associated with phaeochromocytoma (always bilateral), cutaneous tumours of the neurofibromatous type, parathyroid tumours, and structural abnormalities such as a high, arched palate and pes cavus.

This tumour may secrete a variety of polypeptides which produce a variety of symptoms. Thus, prostaglandin secretion may cause diarrhoea; 5-hydroxytryptamine, flushing; an ACTH-like material, Cushing's syndrome; and calcitonin, hypoglycaemia, and tetany.

Slow growing, they metastasize via both lymphatics and blood vessels, and at the time of diagnosis approximately a half have lymphatic metastases.

Treatment
Although the tumour may appear to be a solitary nodule in one lobe, pericapsular lymphatic spread or a multicentre origin may lead to involvement of the opposite lobe. For this reason hemithyroidectomy on the affected side and subtotal lobectomy on the contralateral side is necessary.

Both external irradiation and ^{131}I may be useless for the treatment of this tumour because of its insensitivity.

3.3 Common benign swellings of the breast

ANATOMY OF THE BREAST

1 Gross anatomy

The breast is divisible into three zones:

(a) the nipple and areola;
(b) the breast disc, which is a thick white fibrous structure containing all the ducts and lobules;
(c) the skin and subcutaneous fatty tissue that surrounds the disc.

2 Microscopic anatomy

Ductal system
The ducts of the breast fan out into the breast disc from the lactiferous sinuses on the undersurface of the nipple. Each duct is lined by pseudostratified columnar epithelium outside which is a thin layer of myoepithelial cells together with a network of loose connective and elastic tissue in which there is a subepithelial lymphatic plexus. External to these is a final layer of rather denser connective tissue. The main ducts are connected by the terminal ducts to the lobules, in which lie the acini embedded in loose intralobular connective tissue. As the terminal duct reaches the acinus it loses the various connective tissue layers and is eventually surrounded only by a thin basement membrane. Throughout active 'hormonal' life the epithelium of the ducts and lobules secretes and absorbs its secretions.

Structure of lobule
Each lobule contains a variable number of acini, from less than 10 to more than 100. Each acinus is lined by a double layer of cells; the cells resting on the basement membrane have a relatively clear cytoplasm whereas the inner layer of cells are more deeply staining. In the active lactating breast, distension of the acini reduces the lining membrane to a one-cell structure.

Involution
Involution is a process caused by lack of hormonal stimulus during which the breast passes into the postmenopausal state. In normal circumstances the growth of the breast disc is controlled by somatotrophic hormone and oestrogen and acinar development by prolactin and progesterone. All four hormones are

required to maintain the normal architecture of the breast following development.

During involution, the breast may enlarge because of the deposition of fat, but the glandular tissue, as represented by the number of acini per lobule, decreases and the fibrous tissue becomes increasingly dense and hyalinized.

In about one-third of women between 30 and 40 years of age the lobules shrink and collapse, only an occasional acinar-like structure persisting, often with cyst-like dilatation. The latter change is possibly brought about by the involuting acini coalescing to form small intralobular cysts which then enlarge.

As involution progresses, the lobular elements continue to disappear and the surrounding stroma increases in density.

The proliferation and deposition of fibrous tissue within the lobules and its fusion with the basement membrane has been named 'lobular sclerosis' by some pathologists. Excessive fibrosis or sclerosis often appears to halt the development of involution so that even in old age small clumps of cells may be seen within a dense stroma. By the middle 50s sclerosis and obliteration of the small ducts has usually taken place even in a perfectly normal breast.

BENIGN SWELLINGS

The nomenclature and nature of benign swellings of the breast have been bedevilled by the multiplicity of terms and eponyms that have been used to describe similar conditions. Further, the term 'chronic mastitis' applied to certain benign conditions of the breast wrongly suggests that many of these conditions are inflammatory in origin.

Based on physical findings at the bedside benign breast swellings may be classified as follows:

1 *discrete with well-circumscribed margins*
   (*a*) Solid—fibroadenoma
   (*b*) Cystic— (i) tension cysts
             (ii) lymphatic cysts
             (iii) galactocele
2 *diffuse, ill defined swellings*
   (*a*) irregularities of breast without histological change
   (*b*) uneven involution across the breast disc
   (*c*) cystic disease leading to—
      (i) excessive fibrous (lobular sclerosis)
      (ii) cystic lobular sclerosis
      (iii) cystic lobular degeneration
   (*d*) duct ectasia
   (*e*) fat necrosis
   (*f*) breast abscess

Further consideration will now be given to the aetiology of these various conditions.

1 Discrete breast swellings

Fibroadenoma
These develop in the breast prior to the menopause, pericanalicular tumours usually being found below the age of 30 and intracanalicular thereafter. Either tumour may be multiple, and successive tumours may develop in the same or contralateral breast. The pericanalicular tumour forms a firm discrete mass which is freely mobile in the breast tissue, hence the term 'breast mouse'.

The intracanalicular tumour tends to be softer and may grow to such a size that there is necrosis of the overlying skin. To such a condition the terms serocystic disease of Brodie or cystosarcoma phylloides have been given. However, despite the implications of malignancy in the latter term the tumour is benign.

Pathology. This swelling has been variously regarded as a simple hyperplasia of the epithelial and/or connective tissue elements, or as a composite neoplasm of the breast tissue in which the epithelial and mesenchymal components grow simultaneously.

Treatment. Treatment consists of excision.

Tension cysts
These are relatively common and may be both bilateral and multiple. They form smooth obviously cystic swellings, usually in the central or middle zones of the breast tissue.

Pathology. Cysts of this type probably arise from obstruction to the ducts of a breast which is already in a state of cystic lobular degeneration. Such cysts are usually surrounded by a dense connective tissue stroma which may obliterate the lymphatic drainage with the result that, although secretions may form, they cannot be absorbed. Large cysts may be formed from coalescing microcysts rather than by the dilatation of a single acinus.

The lining membrane of a tension cyst is often apocrine in type and many cells show intense eosinophilic staining due to pink cell metaplasia.

Treatment. Cysts should be treated by simple aspiration. The aspirate is commonly light yellow, green or brown in colour, and is normally acellular.

All should be sent for exfoliative cytology. If suspicious cells are found or a palpable mass remains after aspiration the affected area of the breast should be excised. This is extremely rare.

Lymphatic cysts
These are clinically indistinguishable from the common tension cysts but the diagnosis may be suspected if the aspirating needle meets no resistance as it penetrates the cyst wall.

Galactocele
These are probably formed by obstruction to a duct in the puerperium. The milk retained proximal to the obstruction eventually becomes cheese-like. This condition has become less frequent in the UK and USA as better ante-and postnatal care has become available to the general population. The common complication of this type of swelling is infection.

2 Diffuse and ill defined swellings

Routine examination of the breasts, particularly in women who have borne children, often reveals painless irregularities in the breast tissue. In approximately 25 per cent, these irregularities, particularly those situated in the upper and outer quadrant of the breast, are painful and tender, especially in the week preceding menstruation.

The term mastodynia was applied to such a breast by Geschiekter in 1945 but the term is virtually meaningless since nodular breasts are not necessarily painful, and in young women the breast may be painful in the absence of any palpable abnormality. These common irregularities in the breast are often without a radiological or histological basis, but in older women uneven involution may lead to a nodularity that has a true structural basis.

When the breast is painful some relief may be achieved by the administration of bromocriptine (Parlodel) which inhibits the secretion of prolactin by the pituitary. Controlled trials in some centres have shown that it is better than a placebo in relieving breast pain but it is only useful in cyclical pain, i.e. pain immediately prior to the onset of menstruation. Constant breast pain remains unaffected. It is recommended that 1.25 mg are administered at bedtime, increasing the dose after 2–3 days to 2.5 mg at bedtime and then after an interval to 2.5 mg twice daily. Various series suggest that between 70 and 80 per cent of women will achieve symptomatic improvement on this medication.

Variants of involution
The variants of involution, regarded by some pathologists as distinct entities, include lobular sclerosis and cystic lobular degeneration. Both conditions present clinically as irregular ill defined swellings in the breast which are *not* associated with any of the classic signs of malignancy.

Lobular sclerosis is a condition in which excessive fibrosis is followed by hyalinization within the lobules, in which some acini persist. Once cystic changes take place in the persistent acini the condition may be regarded as cystic lobular degeneration.

In the past, such changes have been variously known as chronic mastitis, adenosis, and cystic hyperplasia.

Treatment. A mammogram is sometimes necessary in this type of breast to eliminate cancer. If the mammogram is negative the decision to excise the affected area depends upon the degree of localization of the pain, tenderness, and swelling. When diffuse, relief can often be obtained by the use of diuretics during the week prior to the period. If the swelling is well localized and extremely tender it can be excised.

Duct ectasia
Clinically, this condition presents as solitary or multiple tender swellings in the sub- or periareolar region of the breast. Palpation reveals a number of cord-like swellings which radiate from the areola, a physical finding which led Bloodgood to apply the term 'varicocele tumour of the breast' to this condition.

The ducts are dilated and contain an inspissated yellow cheesy material that can be expressed like tooth paste from the cut end of a duct. The periductal elastic tissue is destroyed and the surrounding tissues are infiltrated with lymphocytes and plasma cells.

Occasionally, the inflammatory response may be so acute that skin changes occur and the condition may be mistaken for a breast abscess.

Fat necrosis
This is traumatic in origin and is met with only in women with large fatty breasts. Clinically, the patient develops severe bruising after a moderately severe injury. When the bruise settles the woman notices a swelling which it is clinically impossible to distinguish from carcinoma of the breast because the irregular mass is often attached to the skin.

The excised lesion is an infiltrative yellowish white mass. Microscopically a central area of necrotic fat cells are surrounded by a granulomatous reaction consisting of macrophages and mononuclear cells.

Breast abscess
This condition is usually found during lactation. As a rule the infecting organism is *Staphylococcus aureus*, less commonly *Streptococcus pyogenes*. The usual mode of infection is by the nipple, the infection being carried by the suckling infant in the nasopharynx. In maternity wards the condition may occasionally reach epidemic proportions. The infection is at first limited to the segment drained by the lactiferous duct but it may subsequently spread to involve other areas of the breast.

The majority of breast abscesses present clinically as ill localized areas of painful cellulitis, often associated with redness of the overlying skin and general malaise.

In the early stages the inflammation may respond to antibiotic therapy, but as oedema of the overlying skin develops drainage is required. All loculi must be broken down, and under antibiotic 'cover' the dead space can be closed and the wound sutured without drainage. Alternatively, the abscess can be treated on traditional lines by 'saucerizing' the cavity and allowing it to heal by secondary intention.

3.4 Different methods of staging breast cancer and factors affecting the prognosis

STAGING METHODS

In order to compare methods of treatment and prognosis various methods of staging breast cancer have been designed. These methods rely upon accurate clinical assessment, and one that gained almost universal acceptance until recently was the Manchester system, in which the following stages were recognized:

Stage I   Tumour is 5 cm or less in diameter. Skin involvement, if present, is limited to that overlying the tumour.
Stage II Tumour is 5 cm or less in diameter with skin involvement still limited to the tumour area. The ipsilateral axillary lymph nodes are involved but mobile.
Stage III Tumour is larger than 5 cm in diameter. It is fixed to the underlying pectoralis major, and the ipsilateral lymph nodes are also fixed to the chest wall.
Stage IV Regardless of the local signs in the breast there is evidence of generalized dissemination.

Recently, a more sophisticated staging procedure, which is known as the TNM classification, has been introduced. This staging procedure can also be applied to tumours of the larynx, stomach, cervix, and body of the uterus. In this method four references are made to the breast tumour and four to the lymph nodes.

The breast lesion is staged as follows:

1 T1 tumour 2 cm or less in diameter.
2 T2 tumour larger than 2 cm but less than 5 cm.
3 T3 tumour larger than 5 cm in its greatest diameter.
4 T4 tumour a tumour of any size with direct extension to the chest wall or skin.

A tumour of less than 2 cm in diameter that is fixed to the underlying pectoral fascia and/or muscle is classified as T1b. Similarly, a T2 tumour with the same attachment is classified as T2b. If there is widespread oedema and infiltration or ulceration of the breast in a T4 tumour it is classified as T4b.

The nodes are staged as follows:

N0 no palpable homolateral axillary nodes.
N1 mobile homolateral axillary nodes.
N2 homolateral nodes fixed to one another or to other structures.
N3 homolateral supraclavicular or infraclavicular nodes or oedema of the arm.

Distant metastases are nominated as M:

M0 no evidence of distant metastases.
M1 distant metastases present including skin involvement beyond the breast area.

If the TNM classification is to be adopted it is essential that a 'box' chart is used, otherwise the great variety of options will lead to inaccurate recording of the clinical data.

Survival at different stages

There is little doubt that even the comparatively simple Manchester classification gives a reasonable idea of the outlook. The accepted 5-year survival for the four stages is 85, 45, 20 and 10 per cent respectively, at 10 years the overall survival of Stage I tumours has fallen to 65 per cent and of Stage II tumours to 26 per cent.

These simple statistics prove that Stage I tumours, usually regarded as curable, are incurable in about a half of the cases. They also suggest that staging procedures may be fallacious, and of the many fallacies associated with classification the following are the most important.

Fallacies associated with staging

1 *Observer variation*
Observation variation particularly affects two factors: the size of the tumour and the presence or absence of enlarged axillary glands. Whether the latter are felt or not is dependent upon the skill and care of the examiner and the physical make up of the patient. An error of about 40 per cent can be expected from this one aspect alone.

2 *Internal mammary lymph nodes*
Internal mammary lymph nodes are particularly liable to involvement when the tumour is present in the medial quadrants of the breast, but unless an open biopsy is performed this mode of dissemination will go unrecognized. Investigation of this particular problem indicates that as many as 50 per cent of patients may have internal mammary involvement when the tumour lies in the medial quadrants, falling to only 20 per cent when the primary is in the lateral quadrants.

3 *General dissemination*
The finding that approximately 20 per cent of Stage I patients are dead within 5 years, rising to 35 per cent after 10 years, suggests that many patients presenting with a swelling in the breast are already suffering from disseminated disease. Unfortunately, the various techniques available to discern the presence or absence of dissemination are as yet fairly crude and most have been directed to the detection of skeletal secondaries.

The following investigations are possible:

(a) *skeletal survey*. Conventional radiographic techniques are notoriously unreliable, for over a half of the calcium content of the bone must have disappeared before radiological evidence of bone involvement appears on a plain skeletal X-ray.
(b) *bone scans*. This method of detecting bony metastases is more sensitive than plain radiographs. However, the available reports suggest that both false positives and false negatives occur.

(c) *biochemical tests*. Recently, interest has centred on the measurement of the urinary hydroxyproline. This amino acid in the body is almost entirely in collagen, about one-third of which is in bone. The urinary hydroxyproline level is a measure of collagen metabolism. Any condition in which increased bone destruction is taking place, e.g. osseous metastases, is associated with an increase in urinary hydroxyproline above the normal level of 35 mg/day.

(d) *protein markers*. Recent investigations have shown that malignant disease of the breast is associated with the appearance of abnormal protein markers in the plasma. Complete elimination of the tumour tends to remove the marker, while persistent or recurrent tumour produces either no decline in concentration or a marked upswing.

4 *Palpable but uninvolved lymph nodes*

Recent experience in the King's trial, in which enlarged lymph nodes were left untreated, suggests that not all these nodes are involved, since many disappeared within 3 months of treating the primary tumour. It is also well established that the routine section of lymph nodes by the histopathologist is very inaccurate, numerous false negatives being reported. Harnell found as many as a third.

FACTORS INFLUENCING PROGNOSIS OTHER THAN STAGING

1 The characteristics of the tumour

(a) *Histological grading*

An attempt to grade breast tumours by an examination of histological features was first made by Greenhough in 1925, followed by Patey and Scarff in 1928.

These workers assessed three histological characteristics separately and then combined the results to give a composite histological picture.

The three aspects were as follows:

(i) degree of structural differentiation as shown by the presence of tubular arrangement of the cells;
(ii) variation in size, shape and staining of the nuclei;
(iii) frequency of hyperchromatic and mitotic figures.

This method of grading was further refined by Bloom and Richardson (1957) who used a points system based on each of the above criteria to arrive at an overall estimation of the degree of malignancy.

Tumours were graded from I to III and Bloom found that when no nodal involvement is present 94 per cent of patients suffering from Grade I tumours were alive and well after 5 years, whereas only 16 per cent of patients with Grade III tumours survived for this period.

In general, Bloom found that the presence of tubule formation produced a favourable prognosis, that great cellular pleomorphism led to a worse prognosis, and that the more hyperchromatic the nuclei the more gloomy the outlook.

Bloom and Richardson also investigated the possibility that metastatic tumour developed a different histological grade from the primary growth. Their findings showed that the pattern was identical in 82 per cent, higher than the primary in 12 per cent, and lower in the remainder. Thus, the distant metastases may show remarkably little change even though there may have been an interval of many years between the removal of the primary tumour and the appearance of the metastases.

(b) Elastosis

The amount of elastic tissue, as estimated from sections stained by the Van Gieson method, has been shown to influence prognosis, increasing amounts of elastic tissue being associated with an overall better prognosis.

(c) Rate of tumour growth

Gershon-Cohen considers that the rate of tumour growth is all important in determining prognosis. He considers that survival may not be due to cure or total elimination of the tumour by treatment but, rather, an expression of the extremely slow tumour growth rates. He considers that the growth rate of tumours is exponential and constant. From an analysis of available data he estimated that the doubling time for breast tumours may vary from 23 to 209 days. Assuming that the parent cell is 10 µm in diameter and the doubling time is 200 days, a tumour of 1 cm in size would develop only after 17 years. However, if the doubling time is as little as 23 days, the tumour could reach a size of 1 cm after 2 years, after 30 doublings. Three more doublings taking 2 months would then result in a 2 cm tumour. Gershon-Cohen considers that an important factor governing the development of metastases is the doubling time. This is probably so because the percentage of axillary metastases is low if the primary tumour is small, whereas tumours of 2.5 cm in diameter are associated with axillary nodal involvement in 60 per cent of cases. It is, however, highly probable that as tumours increase in size the exponential growth pattern is lost because the decreased oxygen tension in the interior of the tumour leads to necrosis.

(d) Oestrogen receptor status

A breast tumour is defined as oestrogen receptor positive (RE^+) by the Tenovus Institute in Cardiff when it contains more than 5 fmol specific oestradiol binding per mg cytosol protein. The amount of receptor is measured by a dextran-coated charcoal technique.

There is some conflict of opinion between various observers as to whether in potentially curable cancer of the breast i.e. (T1–3, N0–1, M0) the presence of oestrogen receptors in the primary tumour significantly delays the time of appearance or the total incidence of metastases. Evidence has been produced both in favour of and against this hypothesis with perhaps the majority favouring the view that the presence of oestrogen receptors favourably influence the disease-free interval by prolonging it. However, when the axillary nodes are already involved at the time of the initial operation there appears to be little difference in the disease-free interval and only a slight overall prolongation of survival.

However, it does appear to be generally acknowledged that RE⁺ tumours tend to metastasize to bone whereas RE⁻ tumours appear to have a specific affinity for viscera. Patients suffering from osseous metastases appear to have a somewhat higher response rate to endocrine therapy and therefore, a better chance of palliation than those with visceral metastases.

The presence of oestrogen receptors appears to be related to their histological structure, poorly differentiated tumours and tumours which have a more rapid rate of cellular replication tending to be RE⁻.

(e) Tumour type
One of the common histological types of breast cancer recognized by the WHO tumour division is that of colloid cancer, in which islands of tumour cells lie in a mass of mucinous material. When this tumour is graded according to the histological criteria already described it is found that three-quarters are of the Grade I variety. However, both Grade I and the less common Grade II tumours have almost the same prognosis, indicating that the specialized behaviour of these tumours specifically alters their behaviour.

2 Cell-mediated immunity

In 1922, MacCarty concluded that the prognosis in breast cancer was determined not only by the degree of cellular anaplasia of the tumour but also by certain stromal features such as fibrosis, hyalinization, and lymphocytic infiltration. Although this work aroused considerable criticism, Black and his co-workers found that a well-marked lymphocytic infiltration of the primary tumour together with sinus histiocytosis was associated with high survival regardless of the presence or absence of axillary metastases.

This work has continued to receive attention from many workers, and one of the latest papers on the subject, by Paola and others in 1974, showed that it was possible to grade the 'cellular host resistance' into three divisions.

To achieve this, the degree of lymphocytic infiltration in and around the tumour and the degree of follicular hyperplasia and sinus histiocytosis in the regional lymph nodes was scored from 0 to 3. The sum of the scores then became the HDF (Host Defence Factor).

Paola found a good correlation between punitive host resistance and long term survival. If those patients with an extremely good host reaction are discounted because of the smallness of their numbers, there still remained two large groups in which either host reaction was poor or moderately good. In the former, the overall 5-year survival was approximately 40 per cent as compared to nearly 70 per cent in the latter.

3 Treatment

Many surgical operations have been designed to treat the early stages of cancer of the breast. Simple mastectomy, radical mastectomy, modified simple mastectomy, and supraradical mastectomy are all in common use. In addition to surgery, both pre- and postoperative radiotherapy as an adjuvant have been widely canvassed.

Supraradical mastectomy has had few protagonists in the United Kingdom but has been extensively practised in the United States and, in general, argument has mainly revolved around the merits of simple and radical mastectomy. Between the years 1948 and 1955, McWhirter of Edinburgh questioned the necessity for radical mastectomy which, until then, had been the standard treatment of breast cancer since its introduction by Halstead in 1894. McWhirter's argument was based on the contention that, if the surgeon was prepared to trust radiotherapy to 'sterilize' the lymph nodes of the supraclavicular fossa and the internal mammary chain, it seemed only reasonable that it might also be expected to produce the same effect on the axillary nodes. McWhirter's arguments have now been accepted by many surgeons, particularly in Europe, and simple mastectomy is probably the most commonly practised operation for carcinoma of the breast today.

In the majority of centres in which only a simple mastectomy is performed a sample is taken of the axillary nodes by opening the axillary fascia. Individual surgeons differ in how radical this sampling procedure should be, some removing only the lowermost pectoral lymph nodes and others removing the whole of the axillary contents. The importance of this manoeuvre lies in the fact that the majority of surgeons and radiotherapists would not administer high energy irradiation if the lymph node sample contained no tumour tissue. Furthermore, prognosis can be predicted on the basis of the number of nodes involved, the critical figure appearing to be four or more nodes.

The reasons for a watch and wait policy are the general belief that irradiation in any case will only prevent the development of chest wall metastases and, secondly, that widespread irradiation involving the chest wall, axilla, supraclavicular region, and internal mammary chain does considerable harm to the immunological status of the patient by reducing the cell-mediated immune response.

It could be argued that the original surgical operation has little bearing on the ultimate survival of the patient although it does have some effect on the immediate outlook, for without any treatment whatsoever the mean survival time of women in all stages is only 31 months.

Typical of the published results comparing simple with radical mastectomy are those of Rissanen of Helsinki who treated two groups of 500 patients suffering from Stage I cancer. The first group was treated by radical mastectomy, and the second by simple mastectomy followed by postoperative radiotherapy.

The 5-year survival in each group was 79 and 82 per cent respectively and the 10-year survival was 71 per cent for both.

There is growing evidence that even simple mastectomy is too radical an operation and that the surgeon should resort only to removing the cancer together with a relatively small area of surrounding normal breast tissue. This is then followed by a radical course of HER, the patient receiving 4000–6000 rads in 4–6 weeks using daily fractions. However, this type of treatment is only valid in the treatment of T1 and T2 lesions and much depends upon the configuration of the breast as to how much or how little breast deformity is produced.

Adjuvant therapy

Since the recognition that undetectable systemic disease is present in at least 25 per cent of women suffering from cancer of the breast even when the regional lymph nodes are not involved the search has gone on for some form of general treatment which will either suppress the growth of the occult metastases or totally ablate them.

Two main lines of treatment have been adopted:

1 hormonal.
2 cytotoxic chemotherapy.

1 *Hormonal.* An early attempt at adjuvant hormonal therapy was to perform a bilateral oophorectomy at the time of the initial operation in premenopausal women. Although this produced some prolongation of the disease-free interval there was no increase in overall survival. A further disadvantage was the induction of a premature menopause accompanied by all the psychosexual problems this may produce.

Recently an antioestrogen drug known as tamoxifen (Nolvadex) has been introduced by Imperial Chemical Industries. It was first shown that this drug had few side effects and could produce remarkable remission in advanced breast cancer. This has stimulated a prospective trial of the drug in early breast cancer, commencing therapy at the time of the initial treatment. This trial commenced in 1977 and up to and including February 1981, 1285 patients were entered, one half receiving 10 mg of the drug twice daily and the other half no treatment. So far the preliminary results of this trial support the view that the administration of the drug produces a prolongation of the disease-free interval but with no significant decrease in mortality. Analysis of the study group shows somewhat surprisingly that menopausal status has little significance and furthermore, the initial results appear to indicate that the presence or absence of oestrogen receptors is of little importance although the amount may be significant.

2 *Cytotoxic chemotherapy.* The concept of using cytotoxic chemotherapy is simply that occult metastases present at the time of operation should be killed and the emboli occurring due to handling of the tumour during surgery should also be ablated. Three names dominate the field of perioperative chemotherapy; they are Fisher, Nissen Meyer and Bonnadonna. All unfortunately have used different drugs and different regimens. Fisher has used thiotepa 20 mg preoperatively and 10 mg in the first two postoperative days in one trial and 5-fluorouracil 75 mg daily for 4 days from the seventh to the tenth postoperative days in another trial. Nissen Meyer used 250 mg cyclophosphamide for 6 days postoperatively and Bonnadonna of Milan used a combination of cyclophosphamide orally on Day 1 and Day 14 and methotrexate and 5-fluorouracil intravenously on Day 1 and Day 8 of a 4-week cycle for 12 cycles covering 1 year.

All these modalities of treatment appear to increase the disease-free interval but ultimate survival does not so far appear to have been affected. Continuation of such trials using other drug combinations and cytotoxic agents together with hormone therapy continues.

4 Early detection

There is, as yet, no 'hard' evidence that early detection leads to an increasing survival. However, an extensive investigation of this has been mounted in New York in which some 31 000 females between the ages of 40 and 64, chosen at random, have been divided into two equal groups. These women are being screened either by 3-yearly clinical examinations or mammography. So far, the rate of cancer detection is approximately 2.04 per 1000. Interestingly, the palpating hand has proved a better guide to the necessity for biopsy in the small breast, and mammography superior in the large fat breast.

3.5 Tumours of the lymphoreticular tissues with special reference to Hodgkin's disease

Common causes of painless, localized lymph node enlargement include:

1 Infective: *Mycobacterium tuberculosis*; tuberculous enlargement. *Wuchereria bancrofti*: filariasis.
2 Non-infective: secondary metastatic involvement.
3 Lymphoproliferative disorders. Hodgkin's disease. Non-Hodgkin's lymphomas (NHL).
4 Reactive hyperplasia.

It is with this type of lymphadenopathy that the surgeon is commonly concerned, not necessarily from the viewpoint of curing the patient since none of the diseases noted above can be cured by surgical treatment but chiefly in order to establish the correct diagnosis and in the case of the lymphoproliferative disorders to 'stage' the disease.

Although the clinical history in a patient in whom a localized painless lymphadenopathy is present can be exceedingly helpful, physical examination may be of little value although the nodes involved in tuberculosis will commonly be matted together and adherent, sometimes fluctuant if central caseation has occurred and a collar stud abscess formed, whereas the nodes in the lymphoproliferative disorders are commonly rubbery hard and discrete, especially in the early stages, whilst later they may become harder and matted together but never fluctuant. However, it is impossible by palpation to distinguish between a lymph node involved in simple reactive hyperplasia, early tuberculosis or lymphoproliferative disease and indeed a carotid body tumour may well be mistaken for an enlarged solitary cervical lymph node.

Tuberculous lymphadenopathy

All forms of tuberculosis have become increasingly uncommon in the highly industrialized societies due to a combination of factors which include the rapid rise in the general living standards, the elimination of tuberculosis from the milk herds and the use of BCG inoculation in childhood.

Tuberculous lymphadenopathy is most frequently seen in childhood when the cervical nodes are affected by the bovine type of the disease. In the past, subclinical infection of the mesenteric lymph nodes was also commonplace and occasionally infection of the inguinal nodes occurred. In a child there may be no other evidence of tuberculosis but in the adult cervical lymph nodes are frequently associated with an active pulmonary lesion.

At an early stage the nodes may be discrete but as the disease advances so they coalesce and when central caseation occurs it is only a matter of time before the caseous material breaks through the deep cervical fascia to produce a so-called collar stud abscess. When resistance to the disease is poor, or inadequate therapy given, a chronic discharging sinus eventually develops.

Specific investigations required to establish the tuberculous nature of the involved nodes include:

1. a Heaf test performed with purified protein derivative (PPD). Since skin necrosis may occur in an extremely hypersensitive individual a dose of PPD not exceeding 0.0001 mg of PPD should be administered at first.
2. plain X-rays of site or the involved nodes and of the chest. In the older age groups the reactivation of old tuberculous nodes is not uncommon. Such nodes are often partially calcified and, therefore, visible on a plain X-ray. So far as the chest X-ray is concerned the radiological appearances depend upon the chronicity and severity of the disease.
3. aspiration. If the disease has advanced to the stage at which a fluctuating mass can be felt in the neck the diagnosis can sometimes be made quite easily by aspirating the pus and examining it for the presence of *M. tuberculosis* after staining the aspirate by the Ziehl–Neilson hot carbol fuchsin stain. If no bacilli are seen by direct examination a specimen of pus or aspirate must be cultured on a selective medium such as the Lowenstein–Jenner, a medium which contains malachite green to suppress the growth of all other organisms. On this type of plate the colonies of mycobacteria are dry, buff coloured and wart-like. When no growth occurs within 8 weeks the culture can be regarded as negative.
4. biopsy. This may be undertaken not only as a diagnostic manoeuvre but also as part of a therapeutic programme. In the neck, care must be taken not to damage the accessory nerve or the large veins with which the lymph nodes lie in contact. The histological hallmark of a tuberculous infection is the presence of the tuberculous follicle which consists of three elements, an inner central area of caseation, an intermediate zone of epithelioid cells and an outer peripheral layer of densely packed small round cells which are mostly lymphocytes. Between the intermediate and peripheral zones some macrophages fuse to become Langhans' giant cells, the nuclei of which are disposed around the periphery of the cell in the form of a horseshoe or ring.

Secondary metastatic involvement

A metastatic lymph node may develop in the absence of any detectable primary source. However, more commonly such a source can be identified, for example, the enlargement of the left supraclavicular nodes in patients suffering from cancer of the stomach, Troisier's sign, enlargement of the cervical nodes in patients suffering from carcinoma of the larynx, thyroid or lung, enlargement of the axillary nodes in breast cancer.

In the majority of patients the diagnosis may be accepted without a biopsy, assuming that the clinical history and demonstrable physical signs substantiate the diagnosis. In other patients a biopsy may be required or some form of abdominal investigation such as peritonoscopy or laparotomy. Lymph node biopsy, assuming secondary carcinomatosis is suspected, may be performed by either needle or open biopsy, the latter being preferable if the biopsy is to be followed by a 'block' dissection of the neck or groin.

A node involved in secondary neoplasia may be soft and fleshy but is more commonly hard in consistency with a whitish cut surface. The actual cytopathology may give a clue to the nature of the primary lesion but on occasions such is the degree of dedifferentiation no clue can be obtained as to the site of origin of the primary.

Lymphadenopathy due to lymphoproliferative disorders

The lymphoproliferative disorders are those malignant conditions arising from the lymphoid tissues. They may all be associated with nodal enlargement although in chronic lymphocytic leukaemia this is only a minor facet of the disease.

The lymphoid cells from which these disorders arise can be distinguished by certain markers as T (thymus derived), B (bursa/bone marrow derived) or null (neither T nor B).

Characteristically the B-cells have a surface immunoglobulin marker (SIg) whereas the T-cells attract sheep red cells *in vitro* with 'E rosette' formation and null cells lack these markers.

Excluding the various forms of lymphocytic leukaemia the lymphoproliferative diseases are subdivided into two main groups, Hodgkin's disease and the non-Hodgkin's lymphoma although the position becomes more complex when it is appreciated, first, that cells of non-lymphoid origin (e.g. histiocytes) may sometimes be the origin of a malignant clone and secondly, that the discovery of new immunological markers is resulting in an increasing subdivision of the major groups of diseases.

HODGKIN'S DISEASE

This disease was first described by Dr Thomas Hodgkin in 1832. It accounts for only about 1 per cent of all malignancies and is commoner in males than females. It has a bimodal age distribution, the first peak occurring between 15 and 35 years of age and the second over 50 years of age. The approximate incidence is 20 per million at 25 years and 60 per million at 60 years of age.

Aetiology

The aetiology of this condition is unknown but it has recently been suggested that a viral infection may play some part.

Clinical presentation

The commonest mode of presentation is by the asymptomatic enlargement of one or several nodes in a single group with or without splenic enlargement. Examination of large series of patients has shown that the order of frequency of the enlarged nodes is as follows:

1   cervical,   60–80 per cent;
2   axillary,   6–20 per cent;
3   inguinal,   6–12 per cent;
4   mediastinal, 10 per cent.

This last group tends to be particularly involved in the nodular sclerotic variety of the disease, and its development is usually first appreciated when pressure effects or general symptoms develop.

Involved superficial nodes are characteristically rubbery hard and discrete but with the passage of time they become much firmer and may be matted together, thus resembling old tuberculous nodes.

The systemic manifestations of the disease include weight loss, anaemia, fever and, very rarely, pain in a deposit following alcohol.

In advanced disease pruritis is common and in the later stages of the disease, particularly when there is visceral involvement, opportunistic infections develop due to reduced resistance caused by immunodeficiency.

Constitutional (B) symptoms occur usually in late and widespread disease. These include weight loss, fever and sweats, the fever commonly being of the Pel-Ebstein variety.

Splenomegaly of moderate proportions, possibly only discerned by a CAT scan occurs in the majority of patients at some time and hepatomegaly is even more frequent, sometimes giving rise to jaundice.

It is worth observing that Hodgkin's disease can involve many tissues other than the lymph nodes and thus can present in a number of bizarre ways. Thus involvement of the lungs may lead to a dyspnoea or a pleural effusion, involvement of bones, a pathological fracture and lastly, involvement of the central nervous system leading to a progressive leucoencephalopathy or compression of the cord with a resultant paraplegia.

Pathology

The original pathological classification of the disease into two types, paragranuloma and Hodgkin's sarcoma, has now been superseded by the Rye classification in which four cellular patterns are recognized:

1 lymphocytic predominant: in which the lymphocyte forms the main cellular element of the enlarged lymph node. In this group Sternberg–Reed cells are present but infrequent. However, a histiocyte component is present in about a half of the nodules belonging to this group.
2 nodular sclerotic: in which cellular foci composed of lymphocytes, eosinophils, plasma cells, Sternberg–Reed and reticulum cells are enclosed in interlacing collagenous bands. This is the commonest histological type and accounts for approximately 40 per cent of all cases.
3 mixed cellular: accounting for about 25 per cent of all cases. In this group all forms of cell are found and a variable, though not severe, degree of disorderly fibrosis runs through the affected nodes.
4 lymphocytic depleted: in which lymphocytes are few in number. This group is highly malignant and is really equivalent to Hodgkin's sarcoma. It is now considered that the changing histological pattern observed is an expression of the host's response to the tumour, the different histological types representing differences in the effectiveness of the host's attempts to prevent induction of malignant neoplasia.

Diagnosis

The diagnosis is normally established by removing an enlarged node when the pathological changes noted above will be seen. In addition the following haematological and biochemical tests should be performed:

1 Full blood count. This will often reveal a moderate to severe normochromic, normocytic anaemia, an eosinophilia and a lymphopenia. The platelets are commonly increased in number in active disease.
2 Biochemical tests may demonstrate the following:
   (*a*) a rise in the serum caeruloplasmin and acute-phase reactant proteins;
   (*b*) a rise in alkaline phosphatase if the liver is grossly involved;
   (*c*) hyperuricaemia which reflects the degree of cellular proliferation and catabolism.
3 Erythrocyte sedimentation rate, this is normally elevated in active or recurrent disease.

Once a positive diagnosis has been achieved it is necessary to stage the disease in order to determine the type and intensity of treatment.
   The following are the stages recognized at the Ann Arbor Conference (1971):

Stage I   Involvement of a single lymph node region (LNR) or single localized extralymphatic site (ELS).
Stage II Involvement of two LNR or one localized ELS plus one or more LNR on the same side of the diaphragm.
Stage III Involvement of LNR on both sides of the diaphragm—involvement of the spleen (IIIS).

Stage IV Diffuse/disseminated involvement of one or more ELS—liver, marrow, pleura, lung, bone, skin.

In addition each stage can be again subdivided into:

(a) absence of qualifying B symptoms
(b) presence of qualifying symptoms
  (i) unexplained weight loss, 10 per cent of total body weight in 6 months;
  (ii) unexplained fever with pyrexia of 38°C or over;
  (iii) night sweats.

In order to stage the disease, in addition to the investigations described, it is necessary to proceed with the following:

1. chest X-ray with tomography.
2. skeletal survey. An almost pathognomonic lesion of the vertebral column is an osteolytic lesion which spares the intervertebral discs but may involve the adjacent ribs.
3. bipedal lymphography. This is regarded as essential since in 25 per cent of patients with clinical Stages I and II with apparently supradiaphragmatic disease only, para-aortic node involvement is demonstrable. When a fat-soluble medium is used the normal lymph node appears homogeneous throughout. When the lymph node is involved it becomes enlarged, greater than 2.6 cm in diameter and appears foamy. In advanced involvement non-filling may occur.
4. CAT scan. This is of particular use in evaluating the size and, therefore, possible involvement of the spleen and also the size of the para-aortic nodes high in the abdomen and in the thorax. Lymphography is not of great value in assessing nodal status at a higher level than the lower para-aortic nodes.
5. 'staging laparotomy'. This was initially introduced when it was shown that in the presence of a positive lymphogram only 75 per cent of the lymph nodes were, in fact, involved in disease and that nearly 50 per cent of apparently normal nodes on lymphography were involved in the pathological process. Essentially at a staging laparotomy the spleen is removed, a liver biopsy is performed and the higher para-aortic nodes are removed for histological examination. Thus, in addition to the clinical stage, laparotomy together with marrow biopsy provides a pathological staging as well.

A recent communication, Gazet *et al.*, *British Journal of Surgery*, 1982, has shown that of 310 patients in whom a staging laparotomy was performed 51 per cent had positive findings and that in 30 per cent of patients the initial staging was altered.

Such an operation is not, however, without some morbidity; approximately one-third of the patients developed complications, chiefly chest and wound infections, and about 4 per cent developed serious complications requiring further surgical intervention.

Staging laparotomy should not be performed in the presence of medical contraindications or in the very young in whom splenectomy carries an increased risk of overwhelming pneumococcal infection.

Treatment

This involves surgery, radiotherapy and chemotherapy.

Surgery
At the present time, surgical interference is confined to the initial biopsy and the 'staging' laparotomy. In the past, however, radical dissection of the affected lymph nodes was extensively practised.

Radiotherapy
It is now clear that Stages I and II disease can certainly be cured in a high proportion of cases by radiotherapy, delivering 4000 rads to the affected tissues over a period of 3–4 weeks. Various published series indicate that the survival curve for these patients flattens and parallels the natural death rate for the general population between the tenth and fifteenth year, at which point some 70–80 per cent of the patients are still alive.

Chemotherapy
This is indicated at any stage with B symptoms. When B symptoms are absent it is used for Stages III and IV and it is, of course, the remaining hope in patients who relapse after adequate radiotherapy.

At the present time, sequential chemotherapy employing a number of different agents, each with an independent action on the tumour cell, is the method of choice. This has been shown by De Vita and Carbone to be far superior to single drug regimens. Illustrative of the type of drug schedule used are the following:

Drug	*Dose*
Nitrogen mustard	6 mg/m^2 i.v. on days 1 and 8
Vincristine	1.4 mg/m^2 i.v. on days 1 and 8
Procarbazine	100 mg/m^2 orally on days 1–4 inclusive
Prednisone	40 mg/m^2 orally on days 1–4 inclusive

Six courses are given, with 2 weeks' rest between the end of one course and the beginning of the next.

As an alternative, vinblastine may be substituted for vincristine. The former is less neurotoxic than the latter but has a more serious effect on the bone marrow. Such chemotherapeutic regimens have completely altered the prognosis of the more advanced and malignant forms of Hodgkin's disease, and at the present time survival rates of 40 per cent over 5 years are being reported in patients whose prognosis would once have been considered hopeless.

NON-HODGKIN'S LYMPHOMA (NHL)

The following are brief notes on the non-Hodgkin's lymphoma (NHL). Like Hodgkin's disease this group of lymphoproliferative diseases has undergone radical changes of classification in recent years particularly as the cell of origin of the tumour has been identified and its particular characteristics defined. Thus the newer classifications take into account the nature of the cell, i.e. whether it is a B-cell, T-cell or null cell tumour, the majority being of B-cell origin, and the stage of maturation and transformation of the cell.

This group of diseases is much more heterogeneous than Hodgkin's disease itself, occurring not uncommonly in childhood but predominantly in middle and later life. Nodal presentation is much less frequent than Hodgkin's disease and extranodal sites are common, including such sites as the orbit, nasopharynx, tonsil, gastrointestinal tract, skin and bone.

Although relatively benign forms of disease do occur, treatment is usually indicated, except for asymptomatic well differentiated follicular lymphoma, otherwise known as Brill–Symmer's disease, in which observation is only necessary unless malignant transformation occurs.

For the malignant varieties of NHL radiotherapy may be effective in localized disease otherwise chemotherapy is used. Two combinations in common use at the present time are cyclophosphamide, vincristine and prednisolone (COP) and another used for non-localized types of disease with a poor prognosis is the addition of hydroxydaunorubicin to this combination.

BURKITT'S LYMPHOMA

This malignant lymphoproliferative disease is of particular interest in that it was only recognized in 1957 by Burkitt and was at first thought to be restricted to African children in particular localities. Epstein–Barr virus antigens have been detected on, and virus-like particles within, Burkitt's lymphoma cells.

Clinically the disease is rapidly progressive with a predisposition to extranodal involvement, including especially the facial bones and the central nervous system.

Histologically the tumour consists of malignant B-lymphocytes with cytoplasmic basophilia arranged in such a manner that they produce a 'starry sky' effect. Normally the initial response to chemotherapy is good with an 80 per cent rate of remission but if the condition involves the central nervous system the prognosis is generally poor.

3.6 Diagnosis and treatment of bladder tumours

The incidence of carcinoma of the bladder is 30 per 100 000 and overall, bladder tumours are three times commoner in males than females. Three per cent of all deaths from cancer are due to malignant bladder tumours. The following predisposing factors have been identified:

1. ectopia vesicae. This is a rare congenital abnormality resulting from a developmental failure of the anterior abdominal wall which also involves the anterior wall of the bladder with the result that the trigone opens directly onto the anterior abdominal wall below the umbilicus. In the male this condition is accompanied by epispadias and in the female by a split clitoris and in both sexes the pubic bones fail to develop. Exposure of the trigone leads, if the affected individual lives long enough, to metaplasia occurring in the transitional cell epithelium to both a squamous and a columnar mucus-secreting epithelium. This is generally followed by the development of a squamous carcinoma.
2. infection with *Schistosoma haematobium*. The adult female deposits her eggs which are ovoid in shape and about $100 \times 50\,\mu m$ in the small venules of the bladder in which site the embryo develops. Some of the eggs erode through the bladder wall to be discharged in the urine whilst others which escape from the venules provoke a granulomatous reaction which terminates in ulceration, hyperplasia and finally malignant changes in the mucosa. The diagnosis of schistosomiasis is usually made on finding ova or embryos in the urine, by complement fixation tests or by intradermal tests using an antigen prepared from the adult worm.
3. exposure to urinary tract carcinogens:
   (a) smoking; tobacco smoke contains the carcinogen 2-naphthylamine;
   (b) aromatic amines
      (i) l-naphthylamine;
      (ii) benzidine.

Clinical presentation

The commonest presenting symptom is intermittent painless haematuria which is a feature in 50 per cent of patients. However, in some patients in whom invasive, ulcerating malignancy develops frequency of micturition and dysuria occur due to the associated infection. Should a malignant tumour invade one or both ureteric orifices pain in the loin or loins may occur due to developing hydronephrosis.

Pathology

Macroscopic appearance
The growth pattern of vesical tumours can take a variety of forms:

1. they may be non-papillary and non-infiltrating. In such cases the changes are confined to the mucosal layer. Such tumours are very rare.
2. the most common type of bladder tumour is the papillary exophytic variety.
3. a less common variety is the infiltrating endophytic tumour.
4. mixed endophytic and exophytic types.
5. diffuse papillomatosis. This is a very rare variety.

Well differentiated tumours are papillary in type with long fronds but with decreasing degrees of differentiation the fronds become shorter and thicker and finally an undifferentiated tumour forms a solid, frequently ulcerating plaque. The tumours may be single or multiple, show different degrees of differentiation in various parts and progress with the passage of time from being well differentiated to dedifferentiated.

Of all the epithelial tumours of the bladder approximately 90 per cent are basically transitional cell carcinomata, 7 per cent are squamous and the remainder are adenocarcinomata, the last arising from urachal remnants at the fundus of the bladder.

Whether truly benign papillomata of the bladder really occur is questionable. This diagnosis is always suspect since a high proportion of patients in whom such a diagnosis is made later develop invasive cancer.

Diagnosis

Clinical examination reveals nothing until the tumour has advanced to Stage T2 (invading mucosa) and, therefore, a precise clinical and pathological diagnosis is normally made only after the performance of one or more of the following investigations.

1 *Exfoliative cytology*

An early morning specimen of urine is collected and, because tissue cells rapidly degenerate, it is immediately fixed by adding an equal volume of 50 per cent ethyl alcohol. Smears, a paraffin block of the sediment, or a filtered preparation are stained by Papanicolaou's stain. The histopathologist must distinguish between tumour cells and other cellular elements that may be found in urine such as collecting tubule cells, transitional cells, and squamous cells from the prepuce or vulva.

In experienced hands, an accurate diagnosis of bladder tumour can be made in 90 per cent of all suspected cases.

2 *Cystourethroscopy*

Both the wall of the urethra and the bladder should be examined. The following features of the tumour should be recorded:

(a) site, size and whether solitary or multiple;
(b) appearance: solid, papillary, ulcerated;
(c) the condition of the apparently uninvolved mucosa.

This investigation ends with two further manoeuvres:

(a) biopsy, by resection of some or all of the tumour whichever is appropriate. Some thickness of the wall of the bladder should be taken to ascertain the degree of infiltration.
(b) after completely emptying the bladder and withdrawing the instrument a bimanual examination of the bladder should be performed. If the tumour is palpable it can be assumed that it is of the infiltrating malignant endophytic type.

3 *Radiological investigation*
(a) Intravenous pyelography. This may demonstrate:
   (i) renal function;
   (ii) the presence or absence of unilateral or bilateral hydronephrosis;
   (iii) coexisting urothelial tumours of the upper urinary tract;
   (iv) the presence or absence of a filling defect or calcification of the tumour. The latter is an indication of malignancy.
(b) Cystography. This technique may be used to estimate the degree of infiltration of the bladder wall. Less commonly used radiological methods are:
   (i) antegrade ureteropyelography using a needle nephrostomy;
   (ii) angiography, a possible aid for the estimation of extravesical spread;
   (iii) lymphangiography, by which method lymph node involvement may be observed.
(c) Chest X-ray.

Once these investigations have been completed it should be possible to classify the tumour according to the TNM classification of the UICC.

T refers to the primary tumour. The suffix (m) may be added to the appropriate T category to indicate multiple tumours e.g. T2(m).

T1. On bimanual examination a freely mobile mass *may* be felt. Nothing should be palpable after complete transurethral resection of the lesion and microscopic examination of the resected tumour should show that it has not extended beyond the lamina propria.

T2. On bimanual examination there is induration of the bladder wall which is mobile but no residual mass is present following resection. However, histological examination shows that the tumour is invading the superficial muscle.

T3. On bimanual examination induration persists after transurethral resection of the exophytic portion of the tumour and histological examination shows that there is invasion of the deep muscularis.

T4. The tumour is fixed to or invading adjacent structures.

In a similar manner the regional and juxtaregional lymph nodes can be categorized according to their degree of involvement and the presence or absence of distant metastases recorded.

The performance of multiple biopsies is essential to the proper assessment of any bladder tumour since it gives the surgeon an indication of the degree of invasion and also the presence of anaplasia, the degree of which is recognized from the following features: increased cellularity, nuclear crowding, disturbance of cellular polarity, failure of differentiation from base to surface, pleomorphism, irregular cell size, variation in nuclear shape and abnormal mitotic figures.

It is important to recognize that there are no lymphatics in the mucosa, submucosa and superficial muscularis. Therefore, it is only when the deeper layers of the bladder muscle have been invaded that lymphatic metastases begin to make their appearance.

If the bladder is not inflamed, such changes in the mucosa justify a diagnosis of carcinoma. Anaplastic changes are found in approximately 40 per cent of bladder tumours, but many biologically malignant tumours show little evidence of anaplasia in the early stages.

Treatment of bladder tumours

The spectrum of treatment of bladder tumours includes the following:

1 *Endoscopic fulguration or resection*

The former should not be practised until adequate knowledge of the degree of infiltration of the bladder wall and histological grading have been obtained. At the present time its use, if used at all, is limited to the treatment of small satellite tumours a few millimetres in diameter. In general terms for all practical purposes fulguration has been abandoned and replaced by endoscopic resection. Nevertheless, even those tumours which do not invade the bladder tend to recur after resection, figures as high as 60 per cent being reported. Furthermore, some of these recurrent tumours become difficult to treat either because of multiple recurrences or because of invasion.

2 *Intracavitary chemotherapeutic agents*

This treatment is probably best reserved for those patients who develop multiple recurrences or whose tumours are difficult to control by endoscopic resection. One drug which appears to have been used with considerable success is Adriamycin (doxorubicin). One regimen described is the instillation of 50 mg of Adriamycin in 50 ml of saline for 30 minutes. This drug appears to be differentially concentrated in bladder tumours and involved lymph nodes without being systemically absorbed, thus systemic toxicity is minimal. Reports suggest that 60 per cent of T1 tumours undergo partial or complete remission following this type of treatment and that the appearance of T1 tumours which rapidly occur following transurethral resection can be delayed by means of this treatment if it is performed after resection.

3 *Radiotherapy*

The exact place of high energy irradiation (HER) in the treatment of bladder cancers has yet to be determined. This type of treatment is reserved for T3 tumours in the hope that cure may be achieved and for T4 tumours in which irradiation may be associated with palliation, relieving the patient of such distressing symptoms as haematuria, dysuria and frequency. However, in T3 tumours this form of treatment competes with total cystourethrectomy with the formation of an ileal loop for urinary diversion as the treatment of choice.

In addition either of these treatments, i.e. radical irradiation and radical surgery, may be combined with systemic adjuvant chemotherapy. In such adjuvant studies cytotoxic agents are usually begun 3 or 4 weeks after the patient has recovered from the primary treatment.

In practice there appears, as yet, to be little difference in the survival rates in patients treated by HER alone, HER plus adjuvant chemotherapy using Adriamycin and 5-fluorouracil and cystectomy, only 50 per cent of patients surviving for 2 years and between 20 and 30 per cent at 5 years.

External irradiation is not without its complications, the most important of which include:

(*a*) sigmoid or small bowel damage producing later cicatrization and/or perforation;

(b) vesical telangiectasia. This may sometimes lead to such severe bleeding that a cystectomy will be required;
(c) rectal telangiectasia.

However, if HER has been used as the primary treatment, recurrence or severe bleeding following the development of vesical telangiectasia are an indication for cystectomy although this is always a more difficult technical exercise following irradiation than when performed as a primary procedure.

4 Cystectomy

Simple cystectomy has now been replaced by radical cystectomy in which the plane of dissection follows the muscular and bony walls of the pelvis. The operation involves removal of the bladder, together with the peritoneum overlying it, and the perivesical fat. In the male, the prostate and seminal vesicles and, if necessary, the entire urethra are removed, and in the female, the urethra and anterior vaginal wall, anterior fornix, uterus, and adnexa.

The regional lymph nodes are removed from the bifurcation of the common iliac artery downwards. An ileal conduit is fashioned. If the tumour is confined to the bladder mucosa and superficial muscle the results are good, but in patients in whom deep infiltration of the vesical muscle or perivesical tissues has taken place the 5-year survival rate is between 18 and 38 per cent.

The reasons for tumour recurrence after cystectomy are:

(a) failure to remove the tumour;
(b) dissemination of the tumour at the time of operation, which produces lymph or blood stream metastases;
(c) direct implantation of tumour cells at the time of surgery.

The complications of cystectomy include:

(a) cardiopulmonary complications;
(b) prolonged ileus;
(c) wound infection, particularly if cystectomy follows external irradiation;
(d) wound disruption;
(e) anastomotic leaks at the ureterointestinal junctions;
(f) difficulties associated with the ileal conduit.

Methods which have been described but which have been abandoned include:

(a) the introduction of a balloon into the bladder and applying pressure onto the bladder mucosa for several hours, a method described by Helmstein of Sweden in 1966. He reported very satisfactory results even in deeply invasive anaplastic tumours claiming that the distended balloon reduced the blood supply to the tumour and hence caused necrosis and that in some inexplicable fashion this method might also stimulate the immunological system. Case reports in the UK indicated that moderately satisfactory results could be obtained by this method in multiple long fronded T1 tumours but that the method was useless for the treatment of T2 and T3 tumours.

(b) intracavitary radiation using a radioactive cobalt source in a Foley catheter.
(c) local implantation of a radioactive source using ^{198}Au.
(d) partial cystectomy.

3.7 Pathology, clinical presentation and treatment of pigmented lesions of the skin

PIGMENTED NAEVI, OTHERWISE KNOWN AS MOLES, NAEVUS CELL MOLES OR MELANOCYTIC NAEVI

These are benign tumours composed of melanocytes, pigment containing cells which, although most numerous in the basal layer of the epidermis also occur in the dermis. These tumours, which are all benign, are commonly classified according to their site of origin into junctional, compound or intradermal. This classification is purely descriptive and has no pathological significance.

In the junctional naevus the melanocytes appear to proliferate at the epidermodermal junction. All pigmented lesions on the palms, soles and genitalia are of this type. The lesion, clinically, is usually flat and deeply pigmented and should be removed if it develops in an area liable to irritation.

When the cells appear to 'drop' into the dermis a compound naevus is produced; 98 per cent of moles in children and 12 per cent in adults are of this type. In this position the cells may disappear, producing a zone of depigmentation, the Sutton's naevus.

Naevi arising from the dermal melanocytes are rare and produce the clinical lesion known as the Mongolian spot, usually found in Mongolian and Negro infants and only occasionally in Caucasians. Such naevi commonly occur in the sacral area and commonly disappear at about 4 years of age. Arising in other sites such as the face and forearms they may persist throughout life.

When pigmented lesions develop from melanocytes in the epidermis they produce lesions such as the common freckle, lentigo senilis and the café au lait spots found in association with neurofibromatosis.

Macroscopically moles vary from flat to warty and may even be pedunculated; some are associated with excessive hair, producing the 'hairy naevus'. Microscopically there is a considerable variation in the amount of melanin in pigmented naevi and occasionally special stains such as the Masson–Fontana may be necessary to demonstrate its presence.

MALIGNANT MELANOMA

This is a rare form of malignancy accounting for approximately 3 per cent of all skin tumours. They arise from the melanocytes previously described in connection with naevus cell moles either *de novo* or within a pre-existing lesion. The chances of malignancy developing in a pre-existing benign lesion are unknown but modern opinion suggests that it is very small, whereas it was once thought that as many as 40 per cent of malignant lesions arose in this manner.

As well as occurring in the skin malignant melanoma may occur in the uveal tract of the eye which comprises the choroid, ciliary body and iris. In addition they are also found in the mouth, vagina and upper respiratory tract.

There are two types of malignant melanoma *in situ* in which the melanoma cells remain confined to the epidermis.

1. lentigo maligna also known as Hutchinson's freckle. This lesion forms an unevenly pigmented macule extending over several centimetres in diameter from which an invasive lesion may take between 10 and 20 years to develop. Indicative of this change is an increasingly rapid rate of spread and the development of superficial nodularity. This type of tumour occurs most commonly in the elderly and rarely metastasizes.
2. pagetoid malignant melanoma *in situ*. This is a macular lesion developing usually on unexposed skin areas. It is smaller than lentigo maligna and becomes overtly malignant at an earlier stage.

When either of the above lesions become malignant they are known respectively as lentigo maligna melanoma and pagetoid malignant melanoma.

Invasive malignant melanoma

The clinical signs of malignant change in a pre-existing lesion are:

1. increasing pigmentation in a pre-existing lesion;
2. ulceration accompanied by bleeding and crusting;
3. the development of satellite tumours in the surrounding skin;
4. overt evidence of metastases.

The clinical signs of malignancy arising *de novo* are the appearance of a dark area in previously normal skin which ulcerates and bleeds shortly after its appearance.

Predisposing factors and especially vulnerable situations include:

1. exposure to ultraviolet light. Malignant melanoma are more common in Australia and the southern states of the United States of America. The death rate from this condition trebles between Hobart and Brisbane;
2. ectopic pigmentation on the soles or palms of Negroes;
3. commonest sites include the face, genitalia and feet.

Pathology
The growth of all malignant melanomata starts at the epidermodermal junction with the exception of the rare melanomata arising from the dermal melanocytes. Histologically, junctional changes are seen, i.e. proliferation of nests of melanocytes in the basal layer of the epidermis. These cells tend to be more

pleomorphic than the naevus cells of the benign moles and mitotic figures are normally present. In some melanomata the tumour cells are spindle-shaped and may resemble the cells of a sarcoma but normally they are round and polygonal. Malignant melanomata are more cellular than simple moles and the cells show no signs of becoming effete as collagen develops in the underlying dermis, as occurs with a benign mole.

The quantity of pigment produced varies from case to case and between the primary and secondary tumour. Some tumours produce no melanin or so little that special staining is required to demonstrate it. These tumours are the amelanotic melanomata. There is absolutely no relationship between pigment formation and the degree of malignancy. So much melanin may be produced that in the presence of liver metastases the whole of the patient's skin becomes secondarily pigmented. The pigment may be excreted unchanged in the kidneys or alternatively a colourless melanogen is excreted in the urine which darkens on exposure of the urine to air or an oxidizing agent.

Malignant melanomata rapidly spread by the lymphatics to regional lymph nodes and by the blood stream to the lungs and liver.

One peculiar characteristic of malignant melanoma is the occasional tendency for highly invasive metastases to appear many years after the apparently adequate excision of the primary and further spontaneous regression of this tumour has been well documented, particularly in association with pregnancy in women.

Prognostic indicators

Bodeham divided melanomata into two large groups, the 'good' and the 'bad'.

The 'good' tumours, that is to say those which remain localized and rarely metastasize, are tumours arising in an area of lentigo, slow growing tumours producing little mass in relation to their surface area and the very rare, ring melanoma. Included perhaps in this group should also be tumours arising on the extremities which in general always have a better prognosis than tumours arising on the trunk.

The 'bad' tumours metastasize early. In this group Bodeham included tumours which ulcerate rapidly, those whose bulk is out of proportion to their surface area and lastly, diffuse tumours with satellite formation. Also included in this group should be tumours of the trunk.

Recently Bodeham's somewhat empirical classification has been refined by two different pathologists in two entirely different ways. First, Clark and his colleagues related the prognosis of malignant melanomata to the level of invasion, so-called Clark's microstaging and secondly, Breslow related prognosis to the actual thickness of the lesion, Breslow's microstaging. By most UK pathologists who have made a special study of malignant melanoma tumour thickness as a method of microstaging appears to be preferred to the depth of invasion.

In the Breslow classification three thicknesses are considered to be of importance:

1. a tumour thickness of less than 0.76 mm, the thin melanoma;
2. intermediate thickness tumours between 0.76 and 4 mm;

3   thick melanomata greater than 4 mm in thickness.

Reports from large series of cases suggest that the chances of metastases being present or developing following the excision of a thin melanoma, so long as this is adequately excised in the first place, are virtually nil. In keeping with this suggestion 98 out of every 100 patients treated will be alive and well after 5 years. With tumours of intermediate thickness there is an increasing risk, up to 80 per cent, of regional and/or distant metastases being present even though these may be micrometastases when the patient is first seen. In this group only 65 patients out of every 100 will be alive and well after 5 years. When the tumour exceeds 4 mm in thickness the risk factor of micrometastases being present at the time of initial consultation is 80 per cent or above, and in keeping with this the vast proportion of these patients are dead within 2 years of the diagnosis being made and the remainder die within the next 3 years.

Further factors which influence survival after treatment include:

1   pathological staging, i.e. whether involved lymph nodes are present at the time the patient is first treated.
2   the presence of ulceration; only 42 per cent of patients presenting with an ulcerating lesion are alive and well after 5 years compared to 77 per cent at the same interval when no ulceration is present. In general, however, the ulcerating lesions are also the thicker lesions.
3   position of tumour. Survival in patients presenting with trunk lesions is worse than that for patients presenting with lesions of the extremities.
4   pigmentation. Amelanotic melanoma appear to have a much worse prognosis than pigmented lesions.

Treatment
At various times the following modes of treatment have been applied to malignant melanoma.

1   Removal of the primary tumour and the surrounding skin, the actual area to be incised being a matter of considerable debate. This treatment must be followed by frequent observation of the regional lymph nodes; enlargement indicates that they should be removed.
2   Removal of the primary tumour and after some weeks the regional lymph nodes.
3   Removal of the tumour, the skin and underlying deep fascia and the nodes in one piece at the same operation, an operation pioneered by Sampson Handley.
4   Amputation.
5   Isolated limb perfusion with drugs such as melphalan.

It would now appear from the pathological data presented above that the treatment of malignant melanoma, particularly when occurring in the limbs can be placed on a more rational level.

With 'thin' lesions the risk of lymph node metastases is so rare that nothing is required other than radical local excision, i.e. a 5 cm margin of normal healthy skin should be removed around a tumour on a limb, possibly 15 cm on the trunk but on the face only 1 cm because of the cosmetic disability if more is removed.

When the lesion is of intermediate thickness there is a definite place of removing the regional lymph nodes particularly when the tumour is between 1.50 and 3.99 mm in thickness because in this group in particular the actuarial incidence of subsequent lymph node involvement within 3 years is almost 60 per cent.

When the lesion is greater than 4 mm in thickness the benefits of regional node excision are much less apparent because of the high risk of distant blood-borne metastases at the time of the initial diagnosis.

Wide excision implies the use of grafts to close the defect. Regional lymph node dissection, particularly when concerned with the inguinal nodes, is associated with considerable morbidity. Necrosis of the skin flaps is common however they are constructed, a lymph fistula may develop and lymphoedema is commonplace. In the upper limb the same morbidity is not encountered and so far as the trunk is concerned lymph node dissection is impossible because the site of potential involvement is difficult to predict.

4 Orthopaedic Problems

4.1 Causes of an 'irritable' hip in childhood
4.2 Pathology, diagnosis and treatment of lumbar disc lesions
4.3 Pathology of osteoarthrosis with particular reference to the hip joint
4.4 Fractures and the general principles of treatment
4.5 Common complications of fractures
4.6 Fractures of the cervical spine, their complications and treatment

4.1 Causes of an 'irritable' hip in childhood

Definition. The term 'irritable' hip implies that an infant is exhibiting signs of restricted movement of the hip joint and evidence of pain on movement of the affected joint. The older child may spontaneously complain of pain and a limp may become obvious, examination revealing spasm of the periarticular muscles.

Because the obturator nerve supplies sensory branches to both the hip and the knee joint primary disease of the hip may result in referred pain in the knee.

Aetiology
An 'irritable' hip may be the result of the following causes:

1. transient synovitis of the hip, commonest about 5 years of age;
2. Perthes' disease, commonest about 5 years of age;
3. septic arthritis, can occur in the neonate and also throughout infancy and childhood;
4. tuberculosis, commonest in childhood;
5. rheumatoid arthritis, commonest in the juvenile;
6. slipped femoral epiphysis, commonest in adolescence;
7. brucellosis, rare;
8. salmonella, rare.

All these many causes, with the exception of transient synovitis, are now rare in Western society but each will be discussed in greater detail.

Transient synovitis of the hip

This is met with most frequently in children under 10 years of age. It affects boys more commonly than girls and is the commonest cause of a painful hip in childhood, accounting for as many as four cases out of five in most reported series describing this syndrome.

Aetiology
Despite numerous investigations the aetiology is unknown and for this reason a variety of names have been applied to the condition, including 'observation hip', irritable hip, coxitis fugax, coxitis serosa seu simplex, and acute transient epiphysitis. Some authorities believe that it is a form frusté of Perthes' disease but this is by no means a commonly held belief.

In 1970, Harding reported the results of a thorough investigation into a large number of children admitted to hospital complaining of painful hips, in which muscle spasm not only restricted movement in all directions but also held the hip in abduction and flexion. On all the children in the series the following investigations were performed: plain X-rays of the hip joint and chest, full blood count, erythrocyte sedimentation rate, throat swab, measurement of the antistreptolysin and antistaphylococcal titres, Mantoux skin test, latex fixation. A search was also carried out for viral antibodies to a wide range of viruses and, because allergy had often been suggested as a possible cause, the children were also examined for their response to a wide variety of allergens. None of these investigations threw any light on the aetiology of the disease.

The solitary pathological finding, regularly reported, is an occasional turbid, though sterile, aspirate from the hip joint.

Diagnosis
Because of the unhelpful nature of all investigations the diagnosis of traumatic synovitis is reached by exclusion, and usually becomes evident during the first 3 weeks.

The child complaining of hip pain is put to bed, rapid relief from the symptoms follows, and within 14 days the majority are weight-bearing in total comfort. Prolonged follow-up of such patients has revealed that in a few cases varying degrees of coxa magna, osteoarthritis, and broadening of the femoral neck occur.

Perthes' disease

This condition is also commoner in boys; it may occur as early as 2 years of age or as late as 18 years but the usual age pattern is between 4 and 9 years.

Aetiology
The cause is unknown although the basic pathology is an ischaemic necrosis of the upper femoral epiphysis. Harrison has recently shown that the skeletons of affected children are immature, ossification centres making a delayed appearance.

Symptomatology
The child complains either of pain which may have been present for days, weeks or months, or there is a disturbance of gait, a tendency, for example, to walk with the leg turned inwards.

The physical signs are variable. There is usually limitation of all axes of movement of the hip together with muscular spasm which particularly affects the adductors and psoas, producing a flexion deformity.

The differential white count and ESR are normal and there is no constitutional disturbance.

Natural history of Perthes'
This has been examined in great detail by Caterall, who tried to relate the initial radiological appearances of the hip joint with the final function. He divided the children into four groups according to the severity of the epiphyseal changes, which are themselves determined by the degree of vascular involvement.

Group I. This group contained children in whom only the anterior part of the epiphysis was involved, and if metaphyseal changes had taken place at all they were limited to the area immediately beneath the involved epiphyseal cartilage. Radiologically the course of the disease was one of absorption of the damaged segment of the head followed by regeneration from the periphery.

Group II. In this group, more than the anterior part of the epiphysis was involved. Anteroposterior and lateral radiographs show that the involved part of the epiphysis is a dense ovoid mass with viable fragments lying on the medial and lateral sides. Long term follow-up of this group showed that the involved portion of the epiphysis was slowly resorbed, after which there was regeneration.

Group III. In this group, only a small portion of the epiphysis escapes destruction and when the affected segment collapses the osteoporotic portion is displaced in an anterolateral direction producing gross broadening of the femoral neck.

Group IV. The entire epiphysis is involved and so the head flattens, which is revealed as an early loss of height between the growth plate and the roof of the acetabulum. Once the whole head is necrotic it is displaced *not* only anteriorly but also posteriorly, to produce the mushroom-like appearance. In this group extensive metaphyseal changes are met with.

Caterall found that whatever the extent of the disease, it apparently passes through four consecutive phases: first, a stage of ischaemia during which variable portions of the growth nucleus become dense, irregular in shape, and shrink; second, a stage of fragmentation and absorption during which the affected portion is eroded and removed; third, a stage of reossification; and lastly, a stage during which the head is remodelled.

Caterall found that the proportion of good results—defined as a hip with no symptoms, a rounded head, and full movement—decreased in orderly sequence from Groups I to IV and that, in general, the proportion of good results obtained in each group diminished once the child was over 5 years of age. Furthermore, for some inexplicable reason, the prognosis was worse in girls than in boys even though more girls fell into Groups III and IV.

The total length of time between the clinical onset of the disease and recovery was found to be most variable. In Group I it could be as short as 6 months, but as the amount of reconstruction necessary became greater, so the whole process lengthened and could take as much as 2 or more years.

Differential diagnosis
The differential diagnosis of Perthes' disease includes any other condition that can result in ischaemic necrosis of the femoral head, e.g. injury, infection, sickle cell anaemia, or manipulations of the hip. Most of these conditions can be distinguished by history-taking alone.

Treatment
The aim of treatment in Perthes' disease is to minimize the secondary changes in the femoral epiphysis which follow from collapse of the head. Since the magnitude of collapse varies with the mass of the involved epiphysis and the strains to which it is subjected, it is obvious that the fewer the initial changes the better the result. Caterall considers that regardless of the method of treatment the ultimate result is good in Group I.

In severer degrees of the disease it is now considered that the whole femoral head should be relieved of weight-bearing and contained within the acetabulum until the condition has progressed through its natural course. This containment can be achieved in a number of different ways, by the Synder sling, by containment in abduction using the abduction broomstick plaster described by Harrison, by the varus derotation osteotomy of Axer, or the pelvic osteotomy of Salter. Each method has its protagonists and each method appears to produce approximately the same proportion of good, moderate, or indifferent results.

Most observers consider that treatment is better than no treatment and that the aim of treatment must be to keep the hip abducted and medially rotated so that the head remains in the acetabulum during the recovery phase. The advantage of operative means to achieve this end is the shortened period of immobilization, although with newer forms of splintage, immobilization is avoided and the affected child can lead a relatively normal life.

Rheumatoid arthritis

This is comparatively rare in childhood, and the severest form of the disease, Still's disease, is even rarer. In this syndrome, multiple joints are involved with an associated hepatomegaly, splenomegaly, and lymphadenopathy together with fever and weight loss. The polyarticular nature of the disease in the majority of children allows the diagnosis to be made with comparative ease but in one-third of the children the condition is monarticular, in which case the diagnosis is more difficult.

In the monarticular patient, if the hip is affected, the child presents with a painful limp, and the most important differentiation is from tuberculosis. This requires a Mantoux or Heaf test and even a synovial biopsy. The latter, in a typical case, shows a thickened oedematous synovial membrane heavily infiltrated with lymphocytes and plasma cells. The presence of the latter distinguishes it from rheumatoid arthritis associated with hypogammaglobulinaemia. In the later stages the synovium is infiltrated with fibroblasts.

Laboratory investigations
The serum of most patients with rheumatoid arthritis contains rheumatoid factor, an IgM which behaves like an antibody and reacts with IgG, including the patient's own IgG. The factor is best demonstrated by using as 'antigen' IgG which has been altered by heating or by combination with inert particles, e.g. erythrocytes or latex. In the Waaler–Rose test, dilutions of the patient's heat inactivated serum are tested with sheep erythrocytes sensitized with rabbit IgG. However, in childhood some authorities would say that if the Waaler–Rose test was positive the disease could not be rheumatoid arthritis.
ESR. The erythrocyte sedimentation rate is essentially moderately or markedly raised and provides some evidence of the severity of the disease.

Radiology
Plain X-rays show no diagnostic features in the acute stage but as the disease progresses the bones on either side of the affected joint become osteoporotic and, as the articular cartilage is destroyed, the joint space narrows.

Treatment
When the child is suffering acute pain in the involved hip it should be treated on a frame or in a split plaster spica in 20 degrees of flexion and some abduction. In the majority, enteric-coated aspirin produces satisfactory pain relief. In the course of time the disease may become quiescent and may remain so. Severe disease is associated with a flexion adduction deformity due to contraction of the capsule, when a subtrochanteric abduction extension osteotomy may be indicated, fixation being achieved by a nail plate.

Acute septic arthritis

This disease occurs throughout childhood. Both the midwife and the surgeon must be aware that this condition can occur in the neonate usually associated with umbilical sepsis. In such cases there may be little systemic reaction but resistance to movement of the affected hip may be observed when changing a nappy. The older child presents with a painful limp which becomes rapidly worse, usually within a few hours. Examination reveals an ill child with an associated fever who has extremely limited hip movements.

Bacteriology
Most cases are due to metastatic infection by *Staphylococcus pyogenes*, less commonly by the streptococcus and, rarely, by the organisms of typhoid, brucellosis, pneumococcal pneumonia, and meningococcal meningitis. In the majority of the rare causes the arthritis is merely one facet of the total illness, but in staphylococcal and streptococcal infections the arthritis is usually the outstanding infective lesion.

Investigation
Radiology. In the early stages plain X-rays of the joint are of little use.
Blood count. The total white count is raised and the differential count reveals a relative polymorphonuclear leucocytosis.
Joint aspiration. When the diagnosis is suspected a specimen of synovial fluid should be obtained by aspiration and sent for immediate bacteriological examination.
Blood culture. This should be performed in all suspected cases.

Treatment
The most important aspect in the treatment of septic arthritis is to save the femoral head from destruction. The joint should be aspirated; if the surgeon is dissatisfied with aspiration or feels that it was unsatisfactory, the joint should be explored without hesitation.

The capsule is incised, left open to drain, and the skin and subcutaneous tissues closed. Because the majority of cases are due to infection with a Gram-positive organism, either staphylococcal or streptococcal, a suitable antibiotic should be easily found. Those appropriate for the treatment of this condition include cloxacillin, gentamicin or sodium fusidate.

Various published series indicate that when treatment is started within 48 hours the joint will be saved from destruction, whereas a greater delay than this nearly always ends in avascular necrosis of the head with subsequent absorption. If the joint is destroyed the ultimate disorganization may be such that arthrodesis is eventually required.

Tuberculosis

This once common disease has been almost completely eliminated in the highly industrialized societies by a combination of factors: elimination of *Mycobacterium bovis* from the dairy herds, the introduction of pasteurization, the development of Bacille-Calmette-Guérin inoculation in childhood and, lastly, bettering of living standards. The discovery of streptomycin and the many other antitubercular drugs has also had an effect by cutting down the massive reservoirs of infection. Nevertheless, the disease is still encountered, especially in immigrant communities.

Pathology of tuberculous arthritis
The joint is affected by haematogenous spread from a primary focus elsewhere in the body. Simultaneously, or separately, the synovial tissues and subchondral bone may be infected. There is a typical tuberculous reaction in the synovial membrane and multiple small grey tuberculous follicles develop on its surface, and as the tuberculous granulation tissue reaches the articular surface it spreads like pannus and erodes the cartilage. At the same time, the infection spreads in the subchondral bone, which rapidly becomes decalcified. Finally, the articular cartilage is sequestrated into the joint. Simultaneously, the infection spreads beyond the synovial tissues to involve the joint capsule and ligaments, and when the capsule is finally penetrated the disease extends into

the periarticular soft tissues, with eventual production of sinuses and the development of secondary infection. Before the advent of chemotherapy the end result of tuberculous arthritis was either a fibrous or bony ankylosis of the affected joint.

Clinical presentation

The symptoms of a tuberculous hip are usually of gradual onset. A child, usually less than 10 years of age, develops a limp which is frequently worse after exercise. In addition to the local symptoms the child may have had a prodrome consisting of a general decline in health accompanied by night sweats. In the early stages, when the child lies in the supine position the knee tends to lie in adduction, lateral rotation, and flexion; later, it becomes flexed, adducted and internally rotated, and in advanced disease there is both apparent and real shortening. If a periarticular abscess develops it usually points anteriorly or laterally.

Diagnosis

Radiological examination. The earliest evidence of a tuberculous infection on a plain X-ray of the hip is a generalized osteoporosis of the head and adjacent metaphysis. This usually takes place within months of the onset of symptoms. Later, the typical radiological features of a tuberculous hip are a blurring of the articular surfaces and localized destruction of bone. This leaves the subarticular bone ragged at the edges, the opposing surfaces often showing identical lesions.

Synovial biopsy. It is now accepted procedure to perform a synovial biopsy to establish the diagnosis well before the appearance of radiological changes.

Treatment

Treatment of a tuberculous hip now consists of antituberculous therapy together with local treatment to relieve pain and spasm. The measures designed to relieve pain are bed rest with skin traction, usually 2–4 lb in the line of deformity. Once spasm has disappeared splintage may be continued on a Jones abduction frame. When, despite chemotherapy, increasing destruction of the joint or the formation of localized abscesses in the bone develops the joint should be explored through an anterior incision.

The joint is opened, the pannus of thickened synovium is removed, and any local abscess curetted. Antitubercular therapy is then continued and the future management of the patient is determined by the presence of residual symptoms and the radiological appearances of the joint.

If the disease is only brought under control after considerable destruction, the joint must, if possible, be held in the optimum position for ankylosis, i.e. 20 degrees of abduction, 10–15 degrees of flexion, and 5–15 degrees of external rotation. In some patients an osteotomy is required to produce a satisfactory femoral position and to correct the deformity.

Before antimicrobial drugs were developed the hip was rested by performing an extra-articular arthrodesis. This can be performed in various ways. Two commonly used methods were either to turn down a bone graft from the ileum or, alternatively, to perform a subtrochanteric osteotomy and insert a bone graft through the line of the osteotomy into the ischium, the ischiofemoral arthrodesis of Brittain.

Slipped femoral epiphysis or adolescent coxa vara

This condition is a cause of limp in the somewhat older child, being commonest in boys between the ages of 12 and 14 years and girls between 11 and 13 years of age. The overall incidence is about equal to that of Perthes' disease. In about one-quarter of the patients the condition may become bilateral.

Aetiology
The cause of the condition is unknown but in about 25 per cent of affected male children there is some evidence of an endocrine abnormality. The children may resemble those suffering from dystrophia adiposa genitalis. Alternatively they may be excessively tall and slim.

Presentation
The boy or girl presents with a painful limp, the pain often being referred to the knee. In about three-quarters of patients the epiphyseal slip comes about gradually, and in the remainder suddenly. Examination reveals that the limb is held in external rotation and adduction with marked limitation of abduction. Internal rotation is limited. The shortening of the leg leads to a compensatory lumbar lordosis towards the affected side when the child stands, and sometimes the head can be felt as a hard mass.

Diagnosis
The diagnosis is confirmed by the radiological changes. In an early stage the epiphyseal line becomes slightly broadened and the sharp margin of the neck is lost. As the displacement continues the sharp upper margin of the neck and head is lost and in the affected hip the upper part of the natural curve of the femoral neck, which is normally concave, becomes flatter. Further deformity leads to the head moving backwards and downwards so that the lower half may project below the acetabulum.

Plain radiographs taken in external rotation appear to show the neck partly embedded in the head.

In the later stages, secondary effects, which include changes in the normal shape of the acetabulum, aseptic necrosis of the capital epiphysis, and early osteoarthritis, become evident.

Treatment
If the diagnosis is made when there is only a trivial degree of displacement, reduction need not be attempted. Instead, the epiphysis may be fixed in position by three or more pins.

If the displacement is acute, manipulative reduction may be successful. An arbitrary definition of 'acuteness' is a period of up to 3 weeks. To reduce the slip the pelvis is steadied by an assistant, the surgeon then exerts traction on the thigh, with the hip and knee flexed to 90 degrees. The thigh is then gradually and steadily rotated internally, then abducted, and finally extended. If the manipulation is successful the head is pinned. Fairbank has used this technique beyond the time interval mentioned. He claims that epiphyseal damage is not incurred if only gentle manipulation is used.

If, however, gross displacement remains unreduced by manipulative treatment the surgeon has a choice of three operative procedures: open reduction of the epiphysis which may damage the blood supply to the head, cervical wedge osteotomy which also suffers from the same disadvantage or a subtrochanteric osteotomy which does not suffer from this problem and avoids all danger of avascular necrosis of the head because the operative field is so far removed from the vessels supplying the head. However, with both the latter operations since the reduction is incomplete the joint surfaces remain incongruous.

The principle of both operations is to remove a wedge of bone from the lateral side of the neck or from the subtrochanteric position and at the same time correct the rotational deformity. The hip is then held in abduction by a plaster spica until the osteotomy unites. After the plaster is removed the hip adducts, bringing the epiphyseal line into a more horizontal plane, which reduces shearing strains on the epiphysis.

Brucellosis

Arthralgia or arthritis is a relatively rare complication of brucellosis which in Great Britain is usually acquired from cows, either by contact with an infected animal or by drinking raw milk contaminated with *B. abortus*. Arthritis is commoner when the infecting organism is *B. melitensis* which is transferred from sheep or goats.

The onset of arthritis is frequently preceded by general malaise, night sweats, rigors, the Pel–Ebstein type of fever and headaches which may last for weeks or months prior to the development of joint pain.

In approximately 50 per cent of patients the disease affects only one joint; others, apart from the hip, which may be affected are the knee, shoulder or sacroiliac joints.

When the hip is affected the arthralgia is usually transient lasting for only a few weeks. The diagnosis is frequently obvious in view of the preceding clinical history; it can be confirmed by the finding of a relative lymphocytosis, a raised ESR and a high or rising agglutination titre. In about one-fifth of patients the organism can be isolated from the blood stream or from the synovial effusion.

The treatment of this condition is rest and hip traction. The antibiotics which have been suggested include streptomycin and the tetracyclines. More recently Septrin 2 g daily for 4 weeks has been advocated.

Salmonella arthritis

Arthritis in the course of salmonella infections is rare and the hip is one of the least commonly affected major joints.

Severe pain in the hip is usually preceded by a period of diarrhoea although occasionally this may be absent. The condition should be suspected if patients involved in an epidemic of salmonella develop joint pain. The causative organism may be cultured from the blood and positive agglutination tests may be present with a rising titre of antibodies. Aspiration of the joint yields a purulent effusion with a high WBC and a positive culture.

Treatment consists of:

1 aspiration of the joint to reduce the effusion;
2 traction;
3 chloramphenicol.

4.2 Pathology, diagnosis, and treatment of lumbar disc lesions

Developmental anatomy

The intervertebral discs are formed from the axial notochord. By the time of birth the annulus fibrosus has differentiated from the primitive tissues and the nucleus pulposus has been formed, first by the rapid proliferation of notochordal cells, followed by the liquefaction of the surrounding fibrocartilage and the elaboration of a mucoid matrix. The nucleus pulposus of the infant is predominantly notochordal but cells of this nature disappear within the first decade of life, to be replaced by a sparse population of fibroblasts and cartilage cells within a soft matrix which is rich in randomly orientated collagen bundles. Persistence of the notochordal tract as a depression in the cartilaginous end-plate in association with midline weakness contributes to the frequent appearance of Schmorl's nodes in the adult.

Anatomy of the adult disc

The adult intervertebral disc is composed of several elements:

1 a thin layer of hyaline cartilage lying directly on the end-plate of the vertebral body;
2 the annulus fibrosus, which is divided into a peripheral laminated layer, an intermediate layer of collagenous fibres and, lastly, an inner layer of fibrocartilage;
3 the nucleus pulposus, which is contained within the annulus.

Age changes in the disc

In youth, the nucleus is composed of a three-dimensional collagen lattice in which is enmeshed a mucoprotein gel, and the efficient functioning of the discs is entirely dependent on the elasticity of the nucleus. This, in turn, is dependent on the water-binding properties of the mucopolysaccharide complex which is lost with advancing years, a change associated with a progressive decrease in the degree of hydration.

Cells derived from the annulus invade the nucleus, which slowly alters in colour and texture. There is still doubt as to whether the disc forms an osmotic system or whether it imbibes water. Degeneration of the nucleus leads to increasing stresses on the annulus which may split in a radial fashion allowing the escape of 'nuclear' material.

Types of lumbar disc protrusion

1 Projection, the fibres of the annulus bulge but are intact.
2 Intermittent, the protrusion cannot be detected at operation, which is usually performed with the lumbar spine in flexion.
3 Extrusion, the annulus is ruptured and nuclear material is found in the epidural space.
4 Scarred disc, the protrusion is no longer visible but there is a local arachnoiditis and the nerve roots are anchored to the disc.

When there is horizontal herniation or extrusion, it is commonly in the posterolateral position because the firm union of the posterior spinal ligament helps to prevent a direct posterior protrusion.

Sites affected

The most common discs in the lower back that are affected are the disc between L5 and S1, which is affected approximately twice as commonly as the L4, 5 disc; much less commonly affected is the L3, 4 disc. The annulus itself may form the protrusion because degeneration of the nucleus has led to a closer approximation of the vertebral bodies.

Symptomatology of disc protrusion

Symptoms of disc degeneration most commonly reveal themselves in the fourth decade, males being much more often affected than females. The most significant complaint is of pain, which may arise with extreme suddenness, or develop gradually over a period of days. In many patients a long history of intermittent backache (lumbago) precedes the development of sciatica.

The pain of a disc protrusion has three components:

1 aching in the back which is intensified by spinal movements;
2 a deep pain in the buttocks and thighs, aching in character, influenced by posture;
3 radiating pain extending a variable distance down the thigh, leg and foot which is increased by coughing, sneezing or evacuation of the bowels.

The main causes of pain are pressure on the dura mater, the cauda equina or spinal nerve roots. When the dura is under undue pressure, backache and local tenderness tend to develop. Pressure on the cauda equina may result in both motor and sensory disturbances. The motor effects produce weakness in the lower limbs and sphincters. Note, in the cervical region, because of the presence of the cord, similar pressure can produce a paraplegia or a tetraplegia. Pressure on the nerve roots gives rise to dural pain together with pain along the course of the nerve root under pressure.

In addition to pain, a patient may complain of weakness, paraesthesia or anaesthesia in the region supplied by the affected nerve. A protrusion may compress the spinal nerve running to the foramen one segment above or below the lesion, more often the one below. Thus, a lesion of the disc between L4, 5 affects the fifth lumbar nerve, whereas a protrusion of the disc between L5, S1 affects the first sacral nerve. In the former, therefore, the radiation of the pain is from the back of the thigh to the outer aspect of the leg and the inner aspect of the foot, whereas in the latter, pressure on the first sacral nerve leads to pain down the back of the thigh, leg and outer part of the foot.

Spontaneous remission is commonplace although it is often followed by an increased awareness of spinal movements leading to a patient being afraid to subject his back to undue strain.

Physical signs associated with protrusion

1 *Postural deformity*
During an acute attack, postural deformities and extremely limited spinal movements are experienced due to protective spasm in the erector spinae muscles. The lumbar lordosis is often flattened and the trunk may be tilted on the pelvis. The tilt may be either towards or away from the affected side and may sometimes be observed only on bending forwards. The direction of the tilt is in large measure determined by the relation of the nerve root to the protrusion. When the nerve is displaced laterally the tilt is usually to the side of the lesion but when the nerve is displaced medially the tilt is in the opposite direction.

2 *Sensation*
Sensory loss particularly to pin-prick is commonplace in the affected dermatomes but it is seldom complete.

3 *Muscle wasting*
This may develop in the glutei or muscles of the thigh and leg.

4 *Reflexes*
Compression of the first sacral nerve causes weakness of the calf muscles and a decreased or absent ankle jerk. Compression of the fifth lumbar root causes weakness of the peronei and, occasionally, a complete foot drop. The ankle jerk is preserved and the knee jerk may even be exaggerated due to relative

hypotonia of the hamstrings. Compression of the fourth lumbar nerve causes loss of the knee jerk.

Localization of the lesion

The localization of a disc lesion by clinical examination is notoriously inaccurate if there is no objective neurological defect, but various special clinical examinations have been described. One of these is Lasègue's sign, which consists of passive straight-knee leg raising. If 70 degrees of angulation or more can be achieved this is regarded as normal.

If angulation is limited by hamstring tightness it will not be reduced by either flexion of the neck or dorsiflexion of the foot, both these actions usually aggravating the pain associated with disc protrusions. This test permits horizontal localization of the disc in about 80 per cent of patients and, in addition, the examiner may be able to state whether the protrusion is central or lateral. In the former, straight-knee leg raising produces an exaggeration of back pain without radiation, presumably due to increased tension on the structures immediately overlying the disc.

Laseque's test is accurate in the vertical localization of a disc lesion in approximately 50 per cent of patients. Specific physical signs associated with various levels of root compression are described in Table 4.1.

Table 4.1 Chief findings according to the nerve root compressed

Nerve root	Referred pain	Weakness	Reflexes	Muscle wasting	Sensory loss
L2	Anterior upper thigh	Flexion and adduction of thigh	Not affected	Not present	Nil
L3	Anterior thigh and knee	Hip flexors and knee extensors	Weak knee jerk	Thigh	Nil
L4	Outside of thigh and inside of calf	Knee extensors; inversion of foot	Weak or absent knee jerk	Thigh	Medial aspect of calf and ankle
L5	Buttock, back and side of thigh; lateral aspect of lower leg	Knee flexors; dorsiflexion of ankle and hallux; eversion of foot	Ankle jerk weak	Calf	Lateral aspect of calf and medial half of dorsum of foot
S1	Buttock, back of thigh and calf	Knee flexors; eversion of foot; plantar flexion of ankle and toes	Ankle jerk weak or absent	Calf	Lateral aspect of ankle and foot; plantar aspect of foot

Screening investigations in patients suffering from low back pain

1 The most important is the erythrocyte sedimentation rate or plasma viscosity, a raised sedimentation rate suggesting an inflammatory or

neoplastic cause, whereas a normal result suggests a structural problem. Occasionally this investigation may be misleading, for example, in early ankylosing spondylitis and brucellosis the result may be within normal limits.
2 Serum calcium: hypercalcaemia suggests hyperparathyroidism or secondary carcinomatosis with osseous involvement.
3 Serum acid phosphatase: this is a valuable screening investigation in older men in whom back pain may be the first overt sign of carcinoma of the prostate.

Radiological investigation

1 *Plain films of the spine*
Standard anterior posterior views are taken with the patient supine, centring the film on L3, with lateral views centred on L3 and L5 with the patient lying on his side. These views are then supplemented by erect lateral films looking for alterations of posture and oblique views useful in looking for abnormalities of the vertebral arches as in spondylolisthesis.

It has, however, been shown that even in the presence of surgically proven disc prolapse the disc spaces may appear normal on plain radiography in approximately half the patients. Such films may, however, show a decrease in the vertical height of the disc space if a considerable loss of proteoglycans has taken place. This may take some time, and so an interval of 4–6 weeks commonly elapses between the onset of an attack and a visible reduction of the disc space on X-ray. Specifically, the lumbar disc spaces normally increase in a vertical diameter in a caudal direction. If, therefore, the disc space between L4 and 5 is only as wide as that between L3 and 4 it is probably a sign of pathology. However, 40 per cent of patients who have a lumbar spine X-ray for any symptoms show evidence of degenerative change in the form of marginal osteophyte formation since as the disc degenerates nuclear material migrates outwards and penetrates the fibres of the annulus fibrosus causing it to bulge. Periosteum is stripped from the vertical margin provoking the subperiosteal formation of new bone.

2 *Myelography*
This examination was first applied to the diagnosis of spinal tumours by Secard and Forestier in 1921. In the lumbar region, the medium passes down the sleeves of the arachnoid and dura which surround the nerve roots at each intervertebral foramen, forming little triangular peaks or tube-like extensions. The protruding disc gives rise to a clear-cut rounded defect, usually to one side of the midline. It is rare to find a complete block. In addition, the shadows of the root sheaths may be deformed or absent. Myelography is usually reserved for those patients in whom operation is contemplated or when one wishes to differentiate between a disc lesion and a tumour. Thus, in reported series, only approximately 15 per cent of patients are subjected to this examination. When a disc lesion only is suspected, water-soluble dyes are used. It is now generally accepted that this examination will correctly predict a surgically detectable disc

protrusion in nine out of ten cases. Furthermore, myelography may demonstrate multiple disc protrusions.

The use of water-soluble dyes rather than iodized oil allows a much better identification of lateral disc prolapse and also enables radiculography as well as myelography to be performed.

Treatment

The surgical treatment of 'prolapsed' intervertebral disc was introduced by Barr and Mixter in 1941. The original optimism that followed has been modified by two factors:

1. the realization that the majority of patients respond to conservative measures without operation;
2. reports of indifferent results following operation.

Acceptable indications for disc surgery are as follows:

1. the presence of a central prolapse associated with sphincter disturbance, widespread sensory loss and muscle weakness. This type of protrusion is found in 5–15 per cent of patients;
2. failure of conservative measures after a reasonable trial;
3. repeated attacks requiring time off work.

Conservative treatment of an acute disc lesion includes the following measures:

1. the provision of a Goldthwaite belt, which prevents forward flexion of the lumbar spine together with spinal exercises; alternatively, a full length plaster jacket may be applied from the nipples to just above the pubis;
2. bed rest with analgesics, tranquillizing drugs and the application of local heat;
3. bed rest with traction and analgesics.

Various opinions have been expressed as to how long such measures should be persisted with but, in the majority, pain is relieved following one or other of these measures.

Operative treatment
The original approach was via a formal laminectomy and through the dura. This has now been modified to an extradural approach. Many surgeons do not perform a laminectomy but, instead, approach the cord and its coverings by excising the ligamentum flavum from between adjacent laminae and then, if necessary, removing small portions of the laminae themselves. A further point of debate is the need or otherwise for spinal fusion following disc surgery. Recent series suggest that if the disc lesion is not associated with a congenital abnormality such as spondylolisthesis, fusion produces no overall benefit. In all reported series a certain proportion of patients are explored with negative findings.

Results

Overall, the majority of sufferers benefit from disc surgery, the greater proportion (60 per cent) having an excellent or good result defined as a total absence of residual symptoms or the presence of minimal residual symptoms with relief from backache or sciatica. Approximately 20 per cent achieve an intermediate result with residual paraesthesia, numbness and backache, and in approximately 5 per cent the results are poor, reoperation being required in approximately 10 per cent.

Complete failure may be due to one or more of the following causes:

1. too long a delay between the onset of symptoms and operative intervention;
2. neuroticism or accident neurosis;
3. degenerative changes in the spine;
4. removal of the wrong disc;
5. an incorrect diagnosis, e.g. a tumour of the spinal cord or spinal metastases are overlooked.

Complications of disc surgery

The common complications of disc surgery are pulmonary, i.e. atelectasis or pulmonary embolus. Muscular weakness may result if a motor root is damaged. Paralytic ileus is not uncommon and urinary retention may follow. Occasionally, either the aorta or inferior vena cava may be damaged, resulting either in immediate haemorrhage or the later development of an aneurysm. Injury to the dura may produce a dural leak and open the possibility of infection.

The late complications of disc surgery are recurrent backache, which may sometimes be severe enough to warrant spinal fusion.

Spinal stenosis

No essay on lumbar disc lesions and low back pain would be complete without reference to the condition of spinal stenosis. Although acquired types of this condition had been recognized and subjected to decompression laminectomy as early as 1911 it was the Dutch surgeon Verbiest in 1950 who established developmental spinal stenosis as a definite clinical entity. This condition, whether due to developmental causes or disease, produces a classic syndrome of low back pain and widespread pain in the legs especially on walking. The condition, therefore, resembles intermittent claudication but all the peripheral pulses are present even in the presence of pain. A further feature of the condition is that whilst the symptoms may be present on walking, the lumbar spine being in extension, activity in flexion, e.g. cycling, does not lead to the onset of pain.

Two varieties of spinal stenosis are now recognized:

1. primary narrowing of the canal which may be due to reduced sagittal diameter caused by short pedicles, reduced coronal diameter caused by

reduction of the interpedicular distance, the achondroplastic type caused by short pedicles and reduced interpedicular distance;
2 secondary narrowing of the canal which may be due to:
   (a) severe kyphosis with secondary lumbar lordosis;
   (b) severe degenerative spondylosis;
   (c) degenerative spondylolisthesis;
   (d) bone pathology;
   (e) trauma.

The diagnosis can be absolutely established by computerized axial tomography although some radiologists maintain that ultrasonography is equally valuable, a matter of dispute.

When the condition is disabling, operative relief may be achieved in some patients by laminectomy and possibly removal of the articular facets on the side of the lesion, the latter manoeuvre removing pressure on the lateral recess through which the spinal roots pass to the exterior.

4.3 Pathology of osteoarthrosis with particular reference to the hip joint

Definition. Osteoarthrosis is usually defined as a degenerative condition of the joint cartilage which develops particularly in joints that have been subjected to stress. However, there are other varieties of the condition:

1 A generalized polyarticular disease associated with Herberden's nodules in the fingers.
2 Primary osteoarthritis, in which a limited number of joints are attacked without apparent cause.
3 As a secondary arthritis due to one or more of the following causes:
   (a) Injury
      (i) A fracture may involve the joint surface or surfaces and produce an irregular articular surface.
      (ii) Chronic occupational trauma injures joints. Occupational osteoarthrosis is seen in the hands of pneumatic tool workers, the knees of coal miners, or following sporting injuries, e.g. the patellofemoral arthritis of footballers.
   (b) Joint disorders, e.g. a slipped femoral epiphysis or Perthes' disease.
   (c) Joint disease, e.g. rheumatoid arthritis, haemophilia.
   (d) Loss of joint sensation, e.g. diabetic neuropathy, syphilis, syringomyelia or peripheral nerve injury.
   (e) Metabolic disorders, e.g. alkaptonuria.
   (f) Developmental factors, e.g. multiple epiphyseal dysplasia.

In the majority of patients, however, osteoarthrosis develops in the absence of any demonstrable predisposing factor.

Prognosis

The progress of the disease, once symptomatic, is difficult to forecast. The results of one large survey showed that one-third of patients complaining of a painful osteoarthrosis of the hip had no measurable deterioration over a period of years, whereas another similar survey showed that the average time from the onset of hip pain to fixation was 8 years, with a range of between 18 months and 23 years.

Pathology

The initial changes of osteoarthrosis take place in the articular cartilage, which consists of chondrocytes embedded in a ground substance of mucopolysaccharides and collagenous fibres.

The earliest lesion of degeneration is softening of the matrix due to loss of chondroitin sulphate; whether because of breakdown or malformation is not yet clear. Once this process begins, regeneration is impossible because cartilage possesses no blood supply and under normal conditions gains its nutrition from the synovial fluid. As degeneration advances, in areas of greatest physical stress the superficial fibrils separate, break off from the surface, and are phagocytosed by the synovial cells.

Once the subchondral bone is exposed it grinds against the opposing articular surface, hardens, and becomes like polished ivory, a process known as eburnation.

Another characteristic feature of osteoarthrosis is the development of cysts which usually form away from the major lines of stress. Studies have shown that many of these communicate with the joint space via microfractures on the joint surface, possibly produced by changes in the intra-articular pressure that is exerted during movement.

At the periphery of the joint a typical proliferative change develops which results in the formation of bony nodular outgrowths, known as osteophytes. Studies with ^{32}P-labelled tetracycline show that there is considerable bone activity around both the cysts and the osteophytes, activity which it is thought represents an attempt at repair.

In primary osteoarthrosis there is no inflammatory reaction and no thickening of the synovium, findings that reflect the degenerative nature of the disease.

Symptomatology of osteoarthrosis of the hip

The condition is commoner in males than females and 20 per cent of sufferers eventually develop bilateral disease.

In the beginning, an insidious pain, aggravated by activity and relieved by rest, is felt in the affected joint. Pain from the hip and the knee share a common sensory nerve and the initial symptoms may be related to the latter joint. Eventually the pain may be felt even at rest and, indeed, it may be so severe at night that it may disturb sleep. As in all degenerative joint disease the joint stiffens with inactivity and slowly loosens with activity. Slowly, the hip joint becomes externally rotated, flexed and adducted, producing functional shortening and a shuffling gait, and as this comes about the glutei and quadriceps muscles waste, leading to a positive Trendelenburg sign.

Radiological diagnosis

The following evidence of osteoarthrosis may be present on plain X-rays of the hip joint:

1. narrowing or obliteration of the joint space due to disappearance of the articular cartilage;
2. sclerosis (denseness) of the articular surfaces;
3. subchondral cysts;
4. osteophytic formation at the joint margin;
5. irregularity of the joint surface.

Laboratory tests

The ESR is normal and the latex fixation test negative. The synovial fluid, if aspirated, contains less than 1×10^3 white cells/mm^3.

TREATMENT

Conservative

All patients suffering from osteoarthrosis of the hip should be treated conservatively until either the patient becomes intolerant of pain or is handicapped by lack of movement. The important aspects of conservative management of osteoarthrosis of the hip are:

(*a*) reduction in weight. This may itself produce a significant and prolonged relief of symptoms;
(*b*) the use of support, e.g. a walking stick;
(*c*) the use of analgesics. The anti-inflammatory drugs, e.g. phenylbutazolidine, are not usually so effective in this type of arthritis;
(*d*) local heat treatment, administered either as short-wave diathermy or radiant heat.

Surgical treatment

Surgical treatment was often a compromise between the relief of symptoms and the preservation of function.

Osteotomy
Subtrochanteric osteotomy, often called the McMurray osteotomy, did much to relieve the chief symptom of pain but if movement had already become restricted it did little to restore it. Relief of pain by osteotomy probably depends on a combination of factors. First, it results in a mechanical realignment of the joint. Second, it probably decompresses the affected bone, which has been shown by intramedullary phlebography to lack the venous channels that can be seen in the normal head of the femur. This anatomical defect is the probable cause of the high intraosseous femoral neck pressure, which may reach 40 mmHg when rest pain is present.

Either a valgus or varus osteotomy is indicated in patients under 50 years of age, who have been shown by plain X-rays of the hip in abduction and flexion, to have reasonable hip movements and good concentricity of the joint surfaces. A varus osteotomy should not be performed unless 20 degrees of active abduction is possible. It is now common practice to use internal fixation with compression so that the patient is able to walk on crutches after 4–5 days, and make a gradual change to sticks within 6–8 weeks.
Results. Approximately 75 per cent of patients gain symptomatic relief, and some authorities believe that an osteotomy actually delays the development of the disease. It is important to note that the prior performance of an osteotomy does not preclude the later performance of a total hip replacement.

Total hip replacement
Development of the concept. Direct surgery on the diseased hip joint began with reshaping of the femoral head and the acetabulum and the insertion of a cup between the two opposing surfaces, an operation that is still used in young patients. The main disadvantages of a cup arthroplasty are: the long wait of 4 months while a layer of fibrocartilage develops on the surfaces of the head and acetabulum, and a failure rate of some 25 per cent. This operation was succeeded by replacement of the femoral head by a prosthesis, first made of plastic and, later, of metal. The disadvantage of these manoeuvres was that unless the acetabulum was free from degenerative changes the area of load-bearing was small. The final development came in 1960, when Charnley described the use of the resin, methyl methacrylate, to produce adhesion between an artificial acetabulum and the pelvis and the head prosthesis and the femoral shaft.

Two main advantages are conferred by using resin:

1 It allows the artificial joint to be sited in a more or less normal anatomical position, thus allowing the muscles around the joint, particularly the abductors, to act in a normal way.
2 Depending on the prothesis used, it allows a much larger cup and head to be inserted, thus spreading the mechanical load over a larger surface area.

Many different prostheses have now been designed, the latest Charnley prosthesis consists of a thick plastic socket which is made of a high molecular weight polyethylene and a small diameter femoral head of stainless steel. To reduce the danger of prosthesis dislocation in the Charnley procedure the concavity of the socket is 2 mm deeper than its radius. The use of plastic produces a joint which, in the dry state, is self-lubricating. This reduces both wear and particle formation and permits a long wearing life because in a plastic bearing wear is more closely related to the total movement between the two components than the load. Thus a small head diminishes the amount of wear whereas a larger head would slide over a much greater area of plastic for the same distance walked.

The McKee–Farrar prosthesis, on the other hand, is made of chrome cobalt, which possesses the following advantages:

1 lower coefficient of friction;
2 no tendency to self-weld;
3 wears better than other metals.

The Charnley operation. This begins with an anterolateral approach to the hip joint which involves the detachment of the greater trochanter. Once exposed, the capsule is dissected from the joint and the head of the femur is then dislocated by a combination of traction, lateral rotation, and adduction.

The femoral head and neck are then removed with a Gigli's saw, after which any remaining acetabular cartilage is removed by a variety of special expanding reaming instruments. The surface is left in a rough state in order to produce better bonding with the resin. The artificial head and the acetabulum are now bonded into position, after which the hip is reduced and, if the greater trochanter has been detached, it is resutured into position. The wound is then closed. Active exercises may be started on the day after operation, and after one week the patient walks on crutches with partial weight-bearing. By the end of the first month the patient should be able to climb stairs unassisted.

Results of total hip replacement. Reported results confirm that 80 per cent of patients treated by total hip replacement are significantly improved in regard to stance, function, mobility, and pain relief. However, several factors have an important influence on the result including:

1 operative technique. Incorrect positioning of the head or the acetabulum may lead to a poor functional result.
2 loosening of the resin may result following undue trauma.
3 sepsis. As many as 10 per cent of operations may fail due to this factor alone. Infection may be introduced in the early postoperative phase or pursue a subclinical course with the onset delayed, in some 6 per cent, for as long as 3 months. In the latter the offending organism is usually *Staphylococcus albus*. The condition may not resolve until the prosthesis and all the resin have been removed. When this is done the end result approaches a Girdlestone type of arthroplasty.
4 the development of periarticular ossification. Although this may appear disastrous on plain X-ray it may not necessarily interfere with function.
5 metal sensitivity. Recent reports have shown that bone necrosis sometimes develops. In such patients high blood levels of chrome are found.

Further technical details concerning the Charnley operation are given in *Surgical Tutorials 3*, p. 182.

4.4 Fractures and the general principles of treatment

Classification

1 Type
Fractures may be classified as open or closed. The open type may be produced by a small spicule of bone puncturing the overlying skin or, alternatively, massive skin loss may have been sustained because of external or internal forces at the time of injury. Once the skin has been punctured, no matter what the size of the injury is, bacterial contamination of the wound may ensue, followed by overt bacterial infection of either the soft tissues, the bone, or both.
Stress fractures. This type of fracture is found in bones subjected to repeated minor trauma. An example is the March fracture of a metatarsal.
Pathological fractures. These are found in bones weakened by disease, in which case the force required is quite insufficient to break a normal bone. The common causes are senile osteoporosis, secondary metastases, and osteopenia.

2 Pattern of the fracture line
The specific pattern of the fracture line or lines is determined by:

(*a*) the forces that caused the bone to break;
(*b*) the internal structure of the involved bone.

Bone structure varies from the dense cortical type found in the shafts of long bones, to spongy or cancellous bone, found in the metaphyses of long bones, the bodies of short bones, and in flat bones.

Common terms applied to the fracture line are transverse, oblique or spiral, comminuted, compression, greenstick, epiphyseal fracture separation, avulsion and osteochondral.

3 Deformity
The subsequent deformity at the fracture site is described by a variety of terms such as angulation, shortening, distraction, and rotation.

Healing of fractures

1 Long bones
Immediately a bone is fractured the torn periosteum and the small blood vessels traversing the broken Haversian canals bleed and form a fracture haematoma. Repair cells derived from the endosteum and the periosteum invade the haematoma to produce both external and internal callus, which is at first radiotranslucent because it contains no calcium.

As time passes, this callus becomes firmer as it becomes more cellular. Some osteogenic cells differentiate into chondroblasts and so a variable quantity of cartilage is formed in the early callus. At the same time, new bone of the woven type is formed, first at a distance from the fracture line where there is least movement.

Later, this bone will be reabsorbed by osteoclasts and slowly replaced by lamellar bone. The healing process ends when gradual remodelling of the bone has restored the normal architecture, a process known as consolidation.

2 Cancellous bones
Cancellous bone, which consists of a sponge-like lattice of interconnected trabeculae, heals primarily through internal or endosteal callus formation which spreads across the fracture.

Healing is usually much faster than in the long bones because there is minimal bone destruction at the fracture site and, usually, a greater blood supply.

Factors influencing healing time

1 Age
Healing followed by final remodelling is always quicker in the young. Note, Perkin's formula, a spiral fracture in the upper limb unites in 3 weeks and consolidates in 6. Transverse fractures of the upper limb unite in 6 weeks and consolidate in 12; for lower limb fractures multiply by a factor of two, for children divide by a factor of two. A fracture of the femoral shaft at birth will unite in 3 weeks, at 8 years in 8 weeks, at 12 years in 12 weeks, and at 20 years in 20 weeks.

2 Blood supply
An adequate blood supply is essential for healing and, as a result, cancellous bones, which have a larger vascular network, heal sooner than cortical bones. If there is gross displacement in a fractured long bone the blood supply to one or several fragments may be jeopardized by damage to the nutrient artery. When this happens, the blood supply to the fragments is dependent on the periosteum which, in turn, derives part of its blood supply from the attached muscles. Because of these factors fractures of the lower third of the tibia are much slower in uniting than fractures of the upper third because the former has no muscles attached to the periosteum.

Fractures through the middle of the scaphoid often produce avascular necrosis of the proximal fragment because the greater part of the blood supply enters the distal half of the bone. Subcapital fractures of the femur interrupt all the blood supply to the head, with the exception of the vessels running in the ligamentum teres, which results in avascular necrosis of the head.

Avascular necrosis produces a 'relative' increase in the density of the bone on plain X-rays because, usually, there is osteoporosis in the immobilized surrounding bone. The first radiological signs of this complication may appear within 6 weeks.

3 *Configuration of the fracture*

In general, if there has not been soft tissue interposition, long oblique fractures heal more rapidly than do transverse ones. Associated with configuration is the initial displacement, and if the fragments are undisplaced they may have an intact periosteal sleeve, in which case healing from endosteal callus only is needed.

4 *Infection*

A fracture site may become infected because of the contamination of a compound fracture at the time of injury, or it may be a complication of the open reduction of a closed fracture. Commonly, acute infection is due to *Staphylococcus pyogenes*, but there can also be low-grade infections with Gram-negative organisms such as *Pseudomonas aeruginosa*, *Escherichia coli* and *Proteus mirabilis*. Infection delays or prevents healing, particularly if it is severe enough to give rise to acute or chronic osteomyelitis.

In addition to the types of infection already noted, the puncture wound overlying a compound fracture may form the point of entry for the two dangerous *Clostridia* infections, i.e. tetanus and gas gangrene, particularly if the wound is deep and heavily contaminated with soil or debris.

5 *Apposition*

If there is a gap between the bone ends, delayed healing or non-union is likely because callus can extend only over a few millimetres. One of the major aims of the surgeon is to produce reasonable bony apposition by reducing fractures in which apposition of the fragments has been lost.

In some fractures, successful reduction and apposition are frustrated by soft tissue interposition which cannot be overcome without open operation on the fracture site. Although apposition and reduction are usually associated with immobilization, the latter may not be necessary. Fractured ribs heal without immobilization, as also do fractures of the shaft of the humerus.

Treatment of closed fractures

The three major aims of treatment are:

1 to relieve pain;
2 to allow bony union;
3 to restore function.

In the majority of fractures bony union is facilitated by reduction, and if there is excessive angulation reduction may serve two other purposes. First, it may lead to better function in the future and thus prevent subsequent degenerative joint disease, and secondly, it may be cosmetically desirable.

Not all fractures need to be reduced; for example, reduction is unnecessary for compression fractures of the thoracolumbar spine, impacted fractures, crush fractures of the distal phalanx, or fractures of the ribs.

Some fractures, for example long bone fractures with good contact between the bony fragments and little associated rotation or angulation, do not require reduction but still require splintage in order to provide immobilization and union.

However, most fractures require both reduction and immobilization, and these may be achieved in the following ways.

1 *Closed reduction by manipulation followed by external immobilization*

Manipulation involves reversing the path of the original displacement, and method can be applied to all fractures in which accurate reduction can be achieved and maintained by external forces. This method, however, usually fails if the fracture line is spiral or comminuted. Further manipulation may also increase the damage already done to soft tissues. This could lead to progressive unrecognized swelling within a plaster and might end in a Volkmann's ischaemic contracture.

External immobilization of a fracture is usually achieved by the use of a plaster cast that must be accurately moulded to the limb. The use of plaster is not without hazard; the development of ischaemia has already been mentioned but, in addition, an ill-fitting plaster may fail to maintain reduction or immobilization, cause pressure sores, or lead to nerve palsies.

Fashions in external immobilization do not remain constant. For example, fractures of the lower third of the tibia which are notoriously difficult to unite due to their limited blood supply because of the absence of muscle attachments were commonly treated by a full length plaster. Recently Sarmiento has recommended the use of the so-called patella weight-bearing plaster leaving the knee joint free to move.

2 *Immobilization followed by early mobilization using cast bracing*

This method of treatment has been used for many years but recently has gained renewed popularity. It is a method which is particularly applicable to fractures of the lower third of the femur. The fracture is manipulated and maintained in position by traction for some weeks until the fracture line is 'sticky'. At this point the leg is released from traction and a series of plaster casts are applied. The first and upper segment is weight-bearing on the ischial tuberosity, this extends to just above the knee joint allowing sufficient space between it and the plaster surrounding the leg to contain a knee hinge which is fitted into the two plaster casts. At the lower end of the leg cast a further space is allowed so that a hinged foot piece can be fitted.

The advantages of cast bracing are:

(*a*) the duration of immobilization is much reduced;
(*b*) osteoporosis does not occur due to prolonged immobilization;
(*c*) muscle bulk and bone are retained;
(*d*) there is little, if any, stiffness of the joints following union of the fracture and full mobilization.

3 *Closed reduction followed by continuous traction to maintain position and immobilization*

There are many different ways of exerting traction. They include the use of adhesive plaster to the skin, or skeletal traction using a variety of pins passing through bone, e.g. the upper end of the tibia or the calcaneum.

Traction may be fixed or balanced. An example of the former is the treatment of a fracture of the shaft of the femur by tying the extension tapes over the end of a Thomas splint, the counterthrust being exerted by a padded ring encircling the thigh and pushing against the ischium.

Balanced traction implies the use of a system of splints, cords, weights, and pulleys. It is important to ensure that excessive traction is never exerted on the fracture, for this may produce distraction of the fragments, which is a cause of delayed union. If skin traction is used, the skin may be injured by excessive traction.

4 *Closed manipulative reduction followed by skeletal fixation*
An unstable fracture can usually be stabilized by internal skeletal fixation, using nails introduced via skin incisions. Examples of this are the use of pins and plates in the treatment of fractures of the upper end of the femur, or Küntscher intramedullary nails in the treatment of fractures of the shaft of the femur. Each method has its own specific complications in addition to the risks of infection of the fracture site.

5 *Open reduction followed by internal skeletal fixation with or without compression*
This method has strong protagonists and equally strong antagonists. The Swiss are particularly strong protagonists of precision reduction and compression internal fixation. Since the site is exposed surgically, and the fragments are reduced under direct vision, the fracture site becomes open to contamination and, possibly, infection. The metallic devices used to maintain rigid internal fixation include, pins, transfixion screws, plates held by screws, intramedullary nails, bands and wires. Usually, some form of external immobilization is also required. The method can be employed whenever closed reduction is impossible, e.g. in avulsion fractures, intra-articular fractures, fractures complicated by the interposition of soft tissues, and unstable fractures in which reduction cannot be maintained by any other method.

The complications of this method are infection, damage to the blood supply of bone fragments leading to delayed union, metal fractures, and postoperative adhesions leading to loss of function.

The chief advantage of internal fixation is early mobilization, which tends to prevent joint stiffness and muscle atrophy and thus permits a quicker return to normal function.

6 *Excision of fracture fragments*
This method is used when there is a high incidence of avascular necrosis associated with the particular fracture, e.g. in high fractures of the femoral neck, the head of the femur may be removed and replaced by a prosthesis.

Treatment of open fractures

Treatment of an open fracture depends in large measure upon the time interval between the injury and the beginning of treatment and the extent of the soft tissue injury. When the injury is seen within 8 hours, immediate primary closure of the skin, either by suture or by skin graft, can be attempted. When the wound is extensive, heavily contaminated, or seen late, débridement of the wound should be performed.

This is a most important aspect of the care of an open fracture. The skin should be sparingly excised but the underlying fascia must be extensively divided to prevent development of tension within muscular compartments, which may jeopardize the blood supply to the limb. In addition, all doubtfully viable or dead muscle must be excised in order to reduce the incidence of anaerobic infections.

After débridement, delayed primary suture is carried out, not later than 10 days from the time of injury. Internal fixation should, if possible, be avoided in this type of fracture.

At the time of admission, prophylactic measures should be taken to avoid both tetanus and gas gangrene (see Sections 5.5 and 5.6).

4.5 Common complications of fractures

The complications of fractures may be divided into early and late, local and general.

EARLY LOCAL COMPLICATIONS

1 Injury to the skin overlying the fracture

(a) Friction burns. Such burns should be thoroughly cleansed of the particles of dirt ground into the dermis, otherwise an ugly tattoo mark will develop.
(b) Compromised skin circulation. This is a result of gradual increase in internal tension. It can usually be avoided by padding the plaster adequately and taking care in applying it.
(c) Plaster sores. Badly applied and unpadded plasters may lead to plaster sores.

2 Vascular complications

Arterial
These are associated particularly with specific fracture sites, e.g. fractures or fracture dislocations of the head of the humerus may damage the axillary artery, supracondylar fractures the brachial artery, and fractures or fracture

dislocations around the knee joint the popliteal artery. Closed fractures may compromise the arterial supply in the following ways:

(a) by causing spasm of the appropriate artery;
(b) arterial tears;
(c) puncture wounds of the vessel by bone spicules;
(d) venous engorgement and/or oedema within a tight intact fascial compartment or a tight plaster.

Complete occlusion may be followed by gangrene of the limb, incomplete occlusion by Volkmann's ischaemic contracture.

An artery that is completely torn usually stops bleeding spontaneously. A partial tear may end in the formation of a false aneurysm (pulsating haematoma) or, alternatively, thrombosis may follow a partial tear and lead either to gangrene, Volkmann's contracture or, later, the development of intermittent claudication.

Venous
Any fracture requiring immobilization may be complicated by deep venous thrombosis which may be followed by a pulmonary embolus. Prophylactic measures such as the subcutaneous injection of small doses of heparin or intravenous dextran are used, particularly in elderly patients who are likely to be subjected to prolonged immobilization.

3 Neurological complications

Bony injuries involving the following sites may lead to nerve damage, particularly the following:

(a) cervical and thoracic spine—spinal cord;
(b) lumbar spine—cauda equina;
(c) posterior dislocation or fracture dislocation of the hip—sciatic nerve;
(d) fractures or fracture dislocations around the knee joint—the medial and/or lateral popliteal nerves;
(e) fractures of the shaft of the humerus—radial nerve;
(f) fractures of the medial epicondyle—ulnar nerve;
(g) supracondylar fractures of the humerus—medial nerve involvement.

In most patients the lesion that follows injury is a neuropraxia which rapidly recovers, but occasionally there is an axonotmesis, particularly when the fracture is complicated by dislocation, which usually causes severe traction on the nerve. Neurotmesis may follow open fractures.

LATE LOCAL COMPLICATIONS

1 Involving bone

(a) Avascular necrosis
This condition nearly always affects some fragments of a comminuted fracture,

particularly when these are completely separated from all the surrounding tissues. It is also a specific complication of certain fractures, including subcapital fractures of the head of the femur, fractures of the neck of the scaphoid, and fracture dislocation of the head of the humerus; less commonly, also, fractures of the radial head, lunate bone and astragalus.

The fundamental cause of avascular necrosis is interference with the blood supply to the affected bone. Once necrosis has taken place vascular granulation tissue invades the affected marrow and the process of osteoclastic bone resorption begins. In addition, new woven bone is deposited on the dead trabeculae. Despite these organic changes the mechanical properties of the bone are not necessarily immediately affected, and the dead bone may continue to function adequately for weeks, months or even years.

(b) Infection
Infection may follow a compound fracture or open reduction of a closed fracture. The infecting organisms may be either Gram-positive or Gram-negative, more commonly the former, e.g. staphylococcus. If infection is not eradicated there may be delayed union or non-union.

(c) Non-union
This may be defined as a failure of bones to unite within the usual time. Common causes of non-union include infection, inadequate immobilization, avascular necrosis, distraction, or the interposition of soft tissues.

Once there has been failure to unite the bone fragments usually become linked by fibrous tissue. However, consolidation is still possible, even in the presence of infection, if the bone fragments are immobilized. When the bone ends are sclerotic, cancellous or cortical autogenous bone grafts may be necessary to promote union as well as fixation, and even compression.

If non-union is due to inadequate fixation a pseudoarthrosis forms which, again, makes union impossible without the use of bone grafts. In one sense, malunion is a complication of treatment rather than of the fracture itself.

A recent innovation in the treatment of established non-union is the use of a pulsed electromagnetic current introduced by Hass *et al.* in 1980. These workers used 20 hours of a pulsed electromagnetic current daily in cases of established non-union for periods of up to 3 months combined with immobilization. Such electromagnetic fields aim to generate within the bone small intermittent currents similar to those produced by mechanical stress. Whilst the existence of these piezoelectric currents is established their function is not and there is, therefore, considerable controversy about this method of treatment, particularly as non-union usually arises as a fault in the primary care of the fracture.

(d) Post-traumatic osteoporosis
This condition is usually accompanied by muscle atrophy, and its onset is accelerated when the bone is not subjected to functional stress. Immobilization osteoporosis takes longer to recover from than it does to develop. It is preventable by early mobilization or by activity within the splint or plaster.

(e) Sudeck's atrophy
This syndrome is classically found in the hand following a Colles' fracture or a fractured scaphoid. The hand becomes painful and stiff, leading to loss of function. There may be obvious skin changes and the hand takes on a violet colour. Plain X-rays of the affected part usually show severe osteoporosis. Spontaneous improvement takes place over many months.

2 Muscular complications

Myositis ossificans
This condition is found most frequently in young people, in the muscles around the elbow and thigh. The first sign is usually limitation of movement together with increasing pain. Physical examination confirms the reduction in movement and may reveal a tender mass. The physiopathology of myositis ossificans is in doubt because although it follows fractures it rarely follows the trauma associated with operations on bones. One possible explanation is that the haematoma produced by injury forms fibrocartilage which then undergoes metaplastic ossification.

3 Tendon rupture

This complication is seen involving the extensor pollicis longus after Colles' fractures, or crush fractures of the lower end of the radius. The tendon ruptures as it crosses the tubercle on the dorsal surface of the bone.

4 Nerve complications

An ulnar nerve palsy may occasionally follow excessive valgus deformity of the elbow due to fractures of the lateral condyle failing to unite.

5 Joint stiffness

This troublesome complication may be due to several factors. First, the soft tissues of the limb may have been severely damaged by the injury itself or by inappropriate operations following injury. Secondly, the joint may have been injured, or there may have been an effusion into the joint which has caused intra-articular adhesions to form.

EARLY GENERAL COMPLICATIONS FOLLOWING FRACTURES

1 *Shock* (Section 1.1)
Severe injuries of the pelvis or femur may be followed by hypovolaemic shock due to blood loss.

2 Fat embolus

This complication is a significant cause of death following major bony injury. There are two theories of causation: first, the simple mechanistic theory, which assumes that fat droplets are liberated into the venous and lymphatic channels when a bone is broken and that these then find their way into the systemic venous circulation; second, the suggestion that trauma alters the natural emulsion of fat within the blood stream and leads to the formation of larger droplets which then form emboli. Fat emboli usually produce respiratory or neurological signs 2–3 days after injury, and are often associated with petechial haemorrhages over the anterior axillary folds. Tachypnoea associated with dyspnoea, tachycardia and fever are seen, and a plain chest X-ray shows fluffy deposits similar to those observed in pulmonary oedema. The Pao_2 falls due to a diffusion block in the lungs. When the brain is involved, there is restlessness, increasing irritability followed by stupor, coma, shock, and death.

3 *Pulmonary embolus* (Section 1.5)

4 *Tetanus* (Section 5.5)

5 *Gas gangrene* (Section 5.6)

LATE GENERAL COMPLICATIONS

1 *Renal failure* (*see* Section 1.2)

2 Renal calculi

These may form due to a variety of factors the most important of which are recumbency and infection. The former, particularly when associated with immobilization, leads to hypercalciuria, the latter to the deposition of triple phosphate. The stones of recumbency typically develop in the inferior major calyces which are the most dependent in the supine position.

3 Accident neurosis

Following any major injury a certain degree of neuroticism often develops. This usually disappears once full function has returned but in some patients it may persist until all claims against individuals or institutions are settled.

4.6 Fractures of the cervical spine, their complications and treatment

Frequency and causation

The frequency of severe injury to the cervical spine, i.e. those complicated by spinal cord injury, is approximately 20 cases per million of the population. The two common causes are road traffic accidents and sporting injuries. Among the latter diving into a shallow pool and body contact sports such as rugby football and surfing produce the majority of injuries. In some patients in whom a spinal injury occurs cord damage could be avoided by careful movement of the injured person at the scene of the accident, i.e. turning the patient with the head fixed in relationship to the trunk, a manoeuvre which may require as many as four or five persons. If the patient is conscious the preliminary examination should be restricted to discerning whether the limbs can be voluntarily moved and whether pin-prick produces sensation.

Mechanisms of injury

The commonest forces producing injury to the cervical spine are those of flexion and hyperextension, the latter being also known as a deflexion or retroflexion injury. When an extension injury is mistaken for a flexion injury and treated by hyperextension the result may be devastating. In addition to these two forces there is nearly always some associated rotational or axial compression. The latter, common in diving injuries, frequently results in specific injuries to the atlas.

Major factors modifying the effects of cervical injury are the age of the patient which exerts its effect through the strength of bones and the surrounding spinal ligaments and whether the muscles surrounding the cervical spine are 'on guard' at the time of injury.

1 COMPRESSION FRACTURES

(a) Upper cervical vertebrae

These are extremely rare and are usually caused by falling from a height onto the head. At the level of the atlantoaxial joint such an injury may produce severe damage to the ring of the atlas, because the force of the blow is transmitted through the two lateral masses and the ring of bone then breaks at its weakest points.

Immediately following such an injury there is spasm of the neck muscles, flexion and extension are limited, and the patient often prevents movements of the cervical spine by holding the head rigid These fractures are not necessarily associated with a cord lesion and there may, therefore, be a complete absence of neurological physical signs. However, should the atlas be displaced in a forward direction, instantaneous death may follow if the transverse ligament bracing the odontoid process is torn. If, however, this ligament remains intact, it holds the odontoid to the arch, which minimizes cord damage. To demonstrate a lesion of the atlas the patient should be X-rayed through the open mouth.

(b) Compression fractures affecting the lower cervical spine

Wedging or comminution of the vertebral bodies may occur whether the neck is flexed or extended at the time of the injury. If a large anterior–inferior fragment is produced the remainder of the vertebral body and the disc material is pushed backwards into the spinal canal. In other cases severe compression may burst the vertebral bodies and damage the discs with the result that the bony fragments are thrust into the anterior surface of the cord.

2 HYPEREXTENSION, OTHERWISE KNOWN AS HYPERDEFLEXION OR RETROFLEXION INJURIES

In this type of injury the posterior elements of the spine are so crowded together as to cause a fracture of the articular facets and these, acting as a fulcrum, cause rupture of the anterior longitudinal ligament. Once the latter has occurred the vertebral body comes to rest in a position of anterior displacement with the result that the injury may be mistakenly considered to have been caused by excessive flexion. However, a careful examination of the head for bruising over the forehead or severe facial injuries accompanied by a lateral X-ray which demonstrates fractures of the laminae, pedicles or bases of the adjacent spinous processes, all point to the correct diagnosis.

The accompanying neurological deficit following this type of injury is extremely variable.

Such injuries are treated with the neck held in flexion and with frequent radiological examination.

3 FLEXION, OTHERWISE KNOWN AS HYPERANTEFLEXION INJURIES

When the ligamentous complex of the neck remains intact only relatively minor compression fractures of the vertebral body may occur. When the applied forces are greater an anterior marginal fracture may be produced but this is not a serious injury and immobilization in a collar is usually adequate.

When, in addition to flexion, a rotational force is added, ligamentous tearing allows partial or complete dislocation of one or both articular facets. When bilateral facet dislocation occurs only the anterior longitudinal ligament will remain intact. A partial subluxation is usually associated with minimal neurological impairment but when bilateral facet dislocation occurs a complete tetraplegia normally results.

Radiology of flexion rotation injury

Correct interpretation of lateral and oblique X-rays of the spine is of great importance because, if the forward displacement of one vertebral body on another is less than half a diameter, it indicates that there has been a unilateral facet dislocation, whereas greater displacement indicates a bilateral dislocation.

When no bony injury is seen on the lateral and oblique radiographs it must be assumed that there has been a momentary subluxation followed by spontaneous reduction. This type of injury may become obvious only when the neck is X-rayed in flexion, although a careful scrutiny of a routine lateral film may show that the interarticular facets are not parallel.

Clinical features of a cervical injury

Any conscious patient admitted following an accident which might have given rise to a cervical injury should be regarded as suspect if a complaint of neck pain is made, particularly if following the injury the patient complains of tingling in the feet or hands. Some conscious patients may walk into the A and E department holding the head supported by the hands. Incomplete cord injuries may be associated with stiffness rather than paralysis of the limbs. The diagnosis of tetraplegia should not be difficult to make but on two occasions in the author's clinical experience such an injury has been admitted—head injury, hysteria.

General examination

The aim of a general examination of the patient is to determine the severity and distribution of associated injuries and in addition carefully examine the head and face to ascertain the position of bruising, lacerations or areas of tenderness which may give a clue as to the mechanism of the spinal injury.

Neurological examination

The aims of a thorough clinical neurological examination are to:

1 establish the presence or absence of a cord lesion;
2 establish whether this is complete or incomplete;
3 establish the nature and extent of any root involvement.

These features are established by an examination of:

1 the sensory system;
2 movement;
3 the presence or absence of reflexes, superficial and deep.

1 *Sensation*
This is assessed by reference to the response to light touch, pin-prick, vibration and joint position sense.

Sensation should be tested by proceeding from innervated to denervated areas marking the denervated areas with a skin pencil to indicate the level of the cord lesion or an involved nerve root.

The following points of reference are useful to remember:

(a) the occipital area of the scalp is supplied by C2;
(b) the front of the neck by C3;
(c) the shoulders C5;
(d) the outer aspect of the forearm, thumb, index and middle finger C6;
(e) the fourth and fifth finger C7;
(f) the ulnar border of the hand and forearm C8;

When examining the remainder of the body of particular importance are the anal skin reflex, the 'anal wink' and the bulbocavernosus reflex, the latter. being elicited by squeezing the glans penis or clitoris whilst noting the contraction of the anal sphincter on the gloved finger. Both these reflexes are cord mediated and are absent in the stage of spinal shock which normally lasts for 48 hours. If both these reflexes return in the absence of any sensation the cord lesion can be judged complete.

2 Motor examination

The following are key movements indicating the level of the lesion:

(a) deltoid and biceps C5;
(b) extensors of the wrist C6;
(c) triceps, pronator teres and flexor carpi radialis C7;
(d) finger flexors C8;
(e) intrinsic muscles of the hand T1.

3 Reflex examination

In the stage of spinal shock deep tendon, superficial and the cremasteric reflexes are seldom present but their early return after 24–48 hours is a hopeful sign.

Five main neurological lesions associated with cervical injuries have been identified:

(a) incomplete lesions in which partial preservation of motor and sensory function is present. Should a rapid improvement occur in the first week near normal function may return.
(b) anterior cord syndrome which presents a similar clinical picture to that produced by thrombosis of the anterior spinal artery. In this syndrome there is complete paralysis below the level of the lesion with loss of pain and temperature sensation but sparing of deep pressure sensation, two point discrimination, joint position and vibration sense.
(c) posterior cord syndrome. This syndrome is most frequently associated with hyperextension injuries and fractures of the posterior elements of the spinal column. There is no loss of muscle power but there is loss of deep pressure sensation, deep pain and proprioception.

(d) Brown–Séquard syndrome. This syndrome may follow a stab wound of the neck or more commonly a fracture of the lateral mass. Motor loss, impairment of joint position sense, two point discrimination and vibration sense occur on the side of the injury accompanied by loss of pain and temperature sensation on the opposite side. These sensory losses are accompanied by minimal motor loss.
(e) central cord syndrome. This is the commonest of incomplete cord lesions and although it may occur following any cervical fracture it is more usual after hyperextension injuries involving the spondylitic spines of older patients. It is caused by haemorrhage into the central grey matter with varying degrees of involvement of the white matter. Classically a flaccid paralysis of the upper limbs occurs accompanied by a spastic paralysis or paresis of the lower limbs.

Radiological diagnosis

The following views of the cervical spine are required: anteroposterior, oblique and lateral.

Special types of injury
(a) Fractures of the atlas or odontoid—anteroposterior views through the open mouth.
(b) Fractures in the C5–6–7 region—to obtain a clear radiological view it may be necessary to depress the shoulders.
(c) Suspected posterior spinal ligament injury—X-ray in slight flexion in order to demonstrate the flexion-induced displacement.
(d) Suspected extension injury—radiographs in extension may be necessary.

TREATMENT OF CERVICAL INJURIES

The treatment of cervical fractures remains very much a matter of opinion. Some surgeons adopt a conservative approach; the most conservative of all would never operate. Others adopt a radical approach, fusing the spine in all cases and performing an open reduction, if this is necessary.

Between these two extremes is the area in which most orthopaedic surgeons operate, adopting a conservative approach for some patients and a more radical approach for others. Few surgeons, for example, fuse or reduce the spine by operative techniques in the presence of neurological signs within the first 24 hours of injury, for no one has yet proved that early operation promotes recovery. Furthermore, when there is no improvement in the neurological defect within 24 hours it is highly probable that the spinal cord injury is permanent.

The great improvement in survival of those patients who sustain severe spinal cord injury is due more to improved medical care in the general sense than to advances in surgical technique.

Treatment of complete cord lesion

When the cord lesion is complete, management of the patient is dominated by a desire to avoid complications. These include:

1. pressure sores, avoided by 2-hourly turning and careful attention to the skin;
2. pulmonary complications, avoided by frequent chest physiotherapy;
3. contractures, avoided by regular passive movements through a full range of all joints in the paralysed limb;
4. urinary tract infection.

The proper management of the bladder is of great importance. In the past, urinary tract infection associated with pyelonephritis was the commonest cause of death following cervical injuries.

Opinions on the management of the bladder differ and the place of urethral catheterization is extremely controversial. If a catheter is used in the stage of spinal shock, should it be passed intermittently or should it be permanent?

An alternative is to use a small suprapubic plastic catheter: a paediatric peritoneal dialysing catheter has been found adequate. This is inserted and the bladder allowed to drain at night, but in the daytime the catheter is clipped and released at 2-hourly intervals. The suprapubic catheter can be removed when the residual urine has fallen to less than 100 ml, which is usually within 3 weeks, by which time a true automatic bladder has been established. No antibiotics need be given unless the patient develops signs and symptoms of infection.

Specific fractures

1 *Compression fractures*

In the absence of a cord lesion, compression fractures may be treated by continuous skeletal traction for 6 weeks followed by a polythene collar until interbody fusion takes place. If the cord has been damaged, the patient is put on traction and the spine slowly distracted so that the damaged intervertebral space is widened to a limit of not more than twice the width of the normal. Persistent neurological symptoms and signs are an indication in some quarters, especially in the United States, for surgical decompression of the disc space.
Technique of decompression. The spine is approached through an anterolateral cervical incision. The damaged area is located and the disc is removed from between the shattered vertebra; the posterior vertebral ligament is then divided so that the epidural space can be explored and any prolapsed disc tissue removed.

If the cartilaginous end-plates are intact they are removed and a graft is inserted. The neck is completely immobilized for 6 weeks, after which a protective collar must be worn.

2 *Fracture dislocations*

Fracture dislocations of the cervical spine are unstable and, therefore, are frequently associated with cord damage.

The immediate treatment of such an injury is to institute skull traction. The leather sling which gained purchase from the jaw and occiput, originally used for this purpose, has now been replaced by a variety of metal devices for procuring skeletal traction. These include the Halo device, Crutchfield tongs, the Blackburn caliper and many others. Once the device is *in situ*, in the adult, traction should begin with weights of between 15 and 20 lb. This is gradually increased, and when radiographs show the articular processes are in accurate apposition, the weight is reduced to between 10 and 12 lb.

If the X-ray has shown a unilateral dislocation of a facet, gentle manipulation without an anaesthetic may be tried, tilting the neck away from the affected side. When there has been bilateral dislocation of the articular facets a straight pull of 20 lb is used at first. At intervals, the X-rays are repeated and, if necessary, traction is increased. Once reduced, the traction force is reduced to 10 lb and the neck is kept in slight extension.

If reduction cannot be achieved solely by traction, gentle manipulation under anaesthesia may be tried, and if this also fails an open reduction and fusion is required.

When there has been a severe flexion injury the posterior spinal ligament is destroyed, leaving the neck unstable, liable to cause persistent pain, and to undergo early degeneration. Because of this, fusion is nearly always required.

If an early operation is performed for 'locked' facets, a posterior fusion is nearly always carried out. However, if the operation is delayed, an anterior fusion is probably the method of choice.

3 *Extension injuries*

These do not require traction and are usually treated by immobilization in slight flexion for 3 months in a collar.

5 Soft Tissue Injury

5.1 Management of head injuries
5.2 Diagnosis, complications and treatment of chest injuries
5.3 Treatment of blunt injuries to the abdomen
5.4 Principles involved in the treatment of nerve and tendon injuries, particularly in the hand and wrist
5.5 Aetiology, symptomatology and treatment of tetanus
5.6 Aetiology and management of anaerobic infections

5.1 Management of head injuries

In Western communities the commonest cause of a head injury is a road traffic accident, but in areas of high alcohol consumption there is a condition known as the moving pavement syndrome which is due to drunkenness.

MECHANISMS CAUSING HEAD INJURY

1. The commonest mechanism is one brought about by the application of acceleration, deceleration and rotational forces. The significant aspect of this type of injury is that the subsequent brain damage is not necessarily limited to the point of impact. When the various forces are sufficiently severe the brain directly opposite to the point of primary impact is also damaged, the contrecoup injury.

    Rotational forces applied to the head set up shearing stresses within the brain and between the brain and its coverings, leading to neuronal and vascular damage.

    This type of injury is often associated with 'whiplash' injuries to the cervical spine so that many surgeons refer to the injury as a combined pathology, and speak of it as the craniocervical injury.
2. The static crash. This injury is rare but tends to affect certain occupational groups such as miners, printers and railwaymen.
3. Penetrating injuries. These are rare in civilian life because the majority are caused by missiles. The damage to the brain may be much less than would appear from the external wound, unless an explosive or high velocity bullet has been used. The latter causes a negative pressure wave in its wake which produces extremely severe brain damage.

MAJOR CLINICAL FEATURES OF EACH TYPE OF INJURY

1 *The rotational or acceleration/deceleration injury*

This type of injury, if severe enough, is always associated with loss of consciousness, the degree and duration of which is proportional to the severity of the injury. In addition, there may be severe damage to the cervical spine and, often, varying degrees of injury to the face, involving fractures of the mandible, maxilla, or zygomatic arches.

The most severe facial injury, known as the Forte 3, results in separation of the maxillary and malar bones from the base of the skull. This always produces flattening of the face, but if the suture lines separate, the face is also lengthened, whereas if the suture lines are impacted the face is shortened.

Such extensive injuries are frequently associated with airway obstruction which leads to deterioration of the cerebral condition by provoking cerebral oedema.

2 *The crush injury*

Static crush injuries, if severe, may lead to instantaneous death. In lesser injuries, however, the brain does not move until the compression forces have shattered the skull into splinters, and because of this immediate loss of consciousness does not necessarily follow. As the skull is shattered, fracture lines extend from the vault to the base of the skull, finally involving the various foramina or sinuses. The clinical result is the possible development of multiple cranial nerve lesions together with rhinorrhoea and/or otorrhoea.

3 *Penetrating wounds*

The clinical picture depends upon the instrument used, the site injured, and the magnitude of the cerebral damage. A stab wound of the head may, for example, lead to little disturbance, but should it penetrate the brain stem, there may be single or multiple cranial nerve lesions associated with upper motor neurone lesions involving the extremities.

Massive injury such as that associated with high velocity missiles is nearly always followed by death.

PATHOLOGY OF HEAD INJURIES

Open and closed

Clinically it is very important to distinguish between closed and compound or open injuries of the head because if open injuries become infected brain tissue is at risk. Compound injuries include all those that communicate directly with the exterior or indirectly via the paranasal sinuses or the ear.

Primary brain stem injury

In the majority of head injuries the moderate shearing stresses applied to the brain and its coverings do no more than produce bleeding in small vessels and some neuronal chromatolysis with axonal degeneration. In this situation there may be only a transient period of unconsciousness which may be succeeded by amnesia for the moment of violence and for a variable period prior to the injury. This period is known as retrograde to distinguish it from the amnesia for events following the accident during which, for the most part, the patient is unconscious. When, however, the shearing forces have been sufficient to tear vessels, there may be cerebral oedema, infarction and areas of permanent damage. In these circumstances the depth and duration of unconsciousness increase. Such patients may be comatose, quadrispastic, have stertorous respiration, and pinpoint pupils.

Secondary brain stem injury

The term secondary brain stem injury implies that an event has followed the initial injury which has produced an increase in the volume of the contents of the skull. This most frequently is bleeding, which may be extradural, subdural, or intracerebral. Alternatively, there may be cerebral oedema associated with only slight superficial damage on the surface of the brain. Nevertheless, secondary changes occur only with severe injuries.

When the 'space-occupying' lesion develops, the brain is displaced and, since the skull itself is rigid, movement can take place only in the following directions:

1. the medial aspect of the cerebral hemisphere is pushed downwards and medially beneath the falx cerebri;
2. the temporal lobe is displaced downwards through the tentorium cerebelli, which causes pressure on and elongation of the third oculomotor nerve which is finally paralysed, resulting in a fixed dilated pupil on the side of the lesion;
3. herniation of the lower cerebellum through the foramen magnum produces 'coning'. As this increases in severity the medulla is compressed, producing bradycardia and periodic respiration.

Clinical management

In the absence of an open wound which would require careful débridement the clinical management of a patient suffering from a head injury depends upon:

1. the frequent and regular observation and recording of certain clinical parameters which may be deranged in varying degrees. The derangement can be recorded by reference to a given scale, one in common use is the Glasgow Coma Scale which has been subjected to various modifications according to the individual users.

    The various parameters which are observed and which are evaluated on a sliding scale include:
    (*a*) alertness,
    (*b*) emotional response,
    (*c*) speech,

(d) the degree of confusion,
(e) obedience to command,
(f) eyes,
(g) ability to feed,
(h) continence,
(i) depth and rate of respiration,
(j) spontaneous motor activity,
(k) natural posture,
(l) motor response on the unaffected side,
(m) motor response on the paretic side,
(n) pupils,
(o) blood pressure.

As regards the pupils any head injury, even those not necessarily of great severity, may produce a temporary derangement of the pupils of the eyes. If, however, repeated observations confirm the presence of a dilated pupil not reacting to light, it is highly suggestive of a secondary brain stem injury on the ipsilateral side. This sign is even more valuable if it is associated with external signs of damage on the same side as the pupillary changes.

A rising blood pressure suggests increasing cerebral compression. Similarly, a fall in the pulse rate, respiratory rate or hyperpyrexia all indicate brain stem damage. The position can, however, be confused by the presence of haemorrhage elsewhere or by pulmonary problems caused, for example, by a crushed chest.

2 the personal views of the team responsible for the management of severe head injuries. It must be appreciated, as will be described below, that there is considerable disagreement between different groups as to what represents optimum management.

In addition to a complete neurological examination followed by repeated frequent assessment, all head injuries must be carefully examined to exclude associated injury. Particular attention should be paid to possible airway obstruction or associated chest injury since both conditions aggravate hypoxia and hypercarbia, the latter being particularly important since it induces cerebral vasodilatation and in consequence increases intracranial pressure.

Diagnosis of a secondary brain stem lesion

The clinical diagnosis of a secondary brain stem lesion is made on the evidence of a deteriorating conscious level in a patient usually developing lateralizing signs.

Extradural haematoma
In the classical syndrome associated with an extradural haematoma the patient does not usually lose consciousness at the time of the initial injury or, having lost consciousness, rapidly regains it only to deteriorate slowly after a symptom-free interval. This so-called lucid interval is, however, present in

only 30 per cent of patients who develop this complication. Extradural haematoma is rare in infants and older people.

Acute subdural haematoma
The signs of an acute subdural haematoma usually appear within hours, the mortality of this complication being higher than most other complications of a closed head injury. Subdural haematomata arise from the cortical veins torn as they traverse the subdural space but they are commonly associated with severe brain contusion or lacerations which complicates the diagnostic problem and subsequent management. Furthermore, subdural bleeding is not infrequently bilateral. Symptoms may develop when a layer of blood between 0.5 and 1 cm thick covers the brain.

Intracerebral haemorrhage
This complication follows a severe head injury and is attended by a poor prognosis because it is frequently not amenable to surgery.

Cerebral oedema
This is always a manifestation of a severe head injury. It appears shortly after the injury and results in a patient whose conscious level rapidly deteriorates. If the oedema is unilateral, lateralizing signs will be present whereas if it is generalized its development will be associated with signs of increasing pressure without the presence of lateralizing signs.

INVESTIGATIONS

1 *Plain X-ray of the skull*
It is customary to perform plain X-rays of the skull in all head injuries, and if injury to the neck is suspected the cervical spine should also be included. The information obtained from a plain X-ray of the skull is considerable. It includes:

(*a*) the presence or absence of a fracture line or lines. It is particularly important to note the position of such lines and the involvement or otherwise of the paranasal sinuses. If the fracture appears depressed this is of considerable importance in management.
(*b*) the position of the pineal body. If this is calcified, a lesion on one side of the brain may produce a shift.
(*c*) the presence or absence of an aerocele. This lesion can only appear if the dura mater has been torn at the time of the initial injury and the fracture line communicates with a paranasal air sinus.

When signs of a secondary brain stem injury develop, the following additional investigations may be helpful.

2 *Echoencephalography*
This is a useful non-invasive technique indicating the presence or absence of a

shift of the midline structures. The result can, however, be normal even in the presence of gross intracerebral disturbance so long as the changes are bilateral, e.g. in diffuse oedema or bilateral subdural haematoma.

3 Computerized axial tomography
This investigation is increasingly being used in those hospitals in which a scanning device is available, a scan being extremely valuable in distinguishing between the three major complications of a head injury, i.e. a subdural haematoma, intracerebral haemorrhage and cerebral oedema.

It must, however, be clearly stated that if this diagnostic aid is not available it should not deter the surgeon from performing exploratory burr holes in the presence of advancing physical signs indicating increasing compression.

4 Contrast radiology
This mode of investigation is rarely used in an acute head injury because it is not only time consuming but the patient may be totally uncooperative.

5 Intracranial pressure monitoring
This investigation is linked to the availability of a scanning device since although changes in the intracranial pressure can now be measured, to establish the cause of such changes requires this type of investigation.

The measurement may be made in several different ways:

(a) by the insertion of ventricular catheters. These are introduced via a burr hole and also permit the drainage of CSF if this is appropriate. However, the ventricles may be displaced and their location technically difficult to find.
(b) by extradural catheters. These are also introduced via a burr hole but recording may be difficult due to their compression.
(c) metallic devices. These are snugly screwed into a small burr hole and can be used for either extradural or subdural pressure recording and may be left in position for not longer than 10 days.

Whichever monitoring system is used the catheter is normally connected to an external pressure transducer. The normal intracranial pressure is approximately 10 mmHg and any rise may indicate any one of the complications referred to above.

OPERATIVE TREATMENT

When bleeding is suspected because of a deteriorating conscious level or the development of lateralizing signs, even if its presence cannot be confirmed by investigation, the skull should be explored by burr holes. In general, the first burr hole should be made over the site of any external injury or radiologically demonstrable fracture. If no such injury is present, temporal, frontal and occipital burr holes should be performed.

The whole head should be prepared and draped. The temporal burr hole should be made 2.5 cm above the zygoma and 1.5–2.0 cm in front of the ear, the frontal burr hole in line with the pupil and 2.5 cm within the hairline, and the parietal burr hole over the point of maximum convexity of the skull.

Possible findings
An extradural clot is exposed as soon as the burr penetrates the inner table. If this space is dry, a bluish tense dura indicates the presence of subdural bleeding. If there is no discoloration but the dura is tense, there is either an intracerebral clot or cerebral oedema. To distinguish these two conditions the brain tissue should be explored with a brain needle.

Cerebral oedema
If the diagnosis of cerebral oedema has been made an attempt is commonly made to reduce the rise in intracranial pressure. In some centres this would be attempted by the use of mannitol and in others by the administration of frusemide. If mannitol is used it is administered intermittently intravenously in a 20 per cent solution giving 0.5–1 g/kg. Attention is paid to the plasma osmolality which should not be allowed to rise above 320 mosmol/l since if this occurs there is a considerable risk of renal damage or increasing cerebral oedema.

The use of dexamethasone 10 mg every 6 hours has proved of considerable value in the treatment of cerebral oedema associated with cerebral tumours but it does not appear to be effective in reducing the rising intracranial pressure associated with the severe oedema of a head injury.

Some centres also advocate the use of controlled hyperventilation with muscle paralysis and, in addition to measures used to control the intracranial pressure, would also administer hypnotic agents such as the barbiturates in order to reduce cerebral metabolism.

Communicating injuries
The risk of meningitis and/or cerebral abscess in the presence of an open injury is approximately 10 per cent if there are no overt signs, and about 25 per cent if there is rhinorrhoea.

For this reason sulphadiazine 4 g daily in divided doses together with ampicillin 250 mg four times daily, should be given.

Death following a severe head injury

The criteria of brain death are as follows:

1. an unconscious patient;
2. the presence of bilateral fixed dilated pupils;
3. the absence of any spontaneous respiratory effort;
4. an absence of both superficial and deep reflexes;
5. hypothermia;

6 negative calorimetric test. This test is performed by introducing ice cold water into the external ear. A positive reaction is deviation of the eyes to the contralateral side;
7 a flat electroencephalogram.

These observations must be made repeatedly for several hours before assuming that brain death has occurred.

Late complications of a closed head injury

The ultimate result following any head injury is difficult to forecast. However, the duration of post-traumatic amnesia, i.e. the time from the injury until the patient has a clear, continuous memory of events is particularly important. Following severe injuries in which the duration of post-traumatic amnesia extends over several weeks only a relatively small percentage of patients will return to full time employment especially if this involved serious intellectual involvement.

Symptoms which may remain for a considerable period after even a minor head injury include:

1 headaches,
2 anxiety,
3 vertigo.

When specific cranial nerves have been damaged specific symptoms and signs will develop, e.g. damage to the facial nerve causing facial palsy.

5.2 Diagnosis, complications, and treatment of chest injuries

Classification and aetiology

Chest injuries may be grouped into open or closed. Open injuries are generally caused by knife wounds or bullets, and are rare in civilian life. Very severe damage is inflicted by soft-nosed or high-velocity missiles.

Closed injuries are more frequent. They are usually the result of a road traffic accident and, as such, they are frequently only a part of the total injury, which may include craniocervical damage or rupture of the hollow or solid viscera of the abdomen. The severity of a closed chest injury is in part determined by age.

In young people, who normally have very elastic ribs and costochondral cartilages, the chest can undergo severe compression without fracturing the bony skeleton.

Pathological effects

Once the chest wall is open and a communication exists between the environment and the pleural cavity, air passes into and out of the pleural cavity with each inspiratory and expiratory effort. The open wound must be occluded as soon as possible to minimize the resulting pulmonary dysfunction, since if air accumulates in the pleural cavity the lung on the affected side collapses and eventually the mediastinum begins to move from the midline away from the injured side.

The pendulum movement of the mediastinum leads to embarrassment of the cardiac action and once the shift is established the opposite lung also collapses due to the extrinsic pressure of the mediastinum.

An injury caused by a single knife wound although theoretically an open injury is usually rapidly occluded as the tissues covering the rib cage fall together.

One of the most dangerous complications of a chest wound is tension pneumothorax. This develops when air escapes into the pleural cavity from torn or punctured alveoli, bronchioles, a divided bronchus, or is admitted via a chest wound during inspiration, but cannot escape from the pleural cavity in the expiratory phase because the leaking area is either partially or completely sealed off. This valvular effect leads to the increasing accumulation of air under considerable pressure within the pleural cavity. The result may be a rapid deterioration in the patient's condition due to:

1 collapse of the lung on the side of the injury;
2 collapse of the lung on the opposite side due to displacement of the mediastinum;
3 disturbance of venous return and cardiac output due to the mediastinal distortion.

Closed injuries

In young people, in whom the ribs are less likely to fracture, the compression type of injury may produce local or generalized areas of contusion of the lung with interstitial oedema and bleeding, together with rupture of the alveoli, bronchioles or larger air passages. In this type of injury there is often a time lapse between the accident and the onset of respiratory distress.

In older patients, an injury severe enough to fracture one or more ribs may drive the fractured ends through both the parietal and visceral pleura. Surgical emphysema then usually develops in the subcutaneous tissues and possibly, in the mediastinum.

Intercostal vessels or the vessels of the lung may be torn either by the shearing force of the injury itself or by the injured ribs producing either a haemothorax or a haemopneumothorax.

In addition death may rapidly occur when:

1 a great vessel such as the innominate artery is torn. The diagnosis of this disaster can be made by taking note of the rapid collapse of the patient

following the injury, the absence of the distal pulse on the affected side and broadening of the mediastinum on plain X-ray. This injury demands immediate surgical intervention;
2. the heart is ruptured. This is a cause of death in many closed chest injuries which are immediately fatal. If a contusion of the myocardium occurs a friction rub may be heard and an arrhythmia develops. If a myocardial laceration or rupture of a coronary artery occurs cardiac tamponade develops. This produces distended neck veins, shock and cyanosis and must be treated by immediate pericardiocentesis after which open exploration by means of a sternotomy will be required.

Flail chest

When several ribs are broken in two different places or, alternatively, if the anterior angles or costochondral junctions are dislocated on both sides of the sternum, a flail chest develops, the portion of the chest wall lying between the fractures moving paradoxically. Each inspiratory effort is then associated with an inward movement of the detached portion of the rib cage and an outward movement in expiration. Usually, a minimum of four broken ribs is required to produce these conditions. Since a flail chest occurs only after severe injury there is usually considerable damage to the underlying lung tissue, producing contusion, alveolar haemorrhage, and oedema. Each of these changes further increases the degree of respiratory insufficiency which is already severely disturbed by the mechanical dysfunction. Further, as interstitial bleeding and oedema increase, so lung compliance diminishes and secretions accumulate. Functionally, the net result is an increasing need for respiratory effort to maintain respiratory exchange at an adequate level.

In general, the degree of respiratory difficulty and the speed with which respiratory insufficiency develops is dependent upon the pulmonary function prior to the injury and, thus, lesser trauma is always associated with greater physiological disturbance in the ageing patient.

Management

1. The first step in the management of a chest injury is to make sure that the airway is clear. Airway obstruction is particularly likely when the injury has been complicated by craniofacial trauma. In such patients the tongue may fall back and obstruct the airway in the unconscious patient, or severe facial injuries may cause severe nasopharyngeal bleeding and excessive secretions.
2. General examination of the patient to ascertain and quantify associated injuries.
3. Specific examination of the chest together with plain X-rays of the chest. The latter may demonstrate:

   (a) the site and number of fractured ribs;

(*b*) presence or absence of pneumothorax;
   (*c*) presence of haemothorax;
   (*d*) surgical emphysema;
   (*e*) oedema or contusion of the lung itself;
   (*f*) mediastinal shift.
4 *Blood gas analysis.* Monitoring of the blood gases is essential if respiratory function deteriorates.

Treatment of various injuries

(*a*) Injury to one or two ribs

Although this may be regarded as a relatively minor injury it may still be extremely painful and demand the administration of analgesics of intermediate strength. Furthermore, intensive chest physiotherapy may be required particularly in older patients who already suffer from pre-existing pulmonary disease such as chronic bronchitis to prevent the retention of secretion and subsequent pulmonary collapse followed by infection. If the lower ribs are broken on the left side consideration should be given to a concomitant rupture of the spleen; similarly on the right side hepatic injury may occur.

Immobilization of the affected ribs, which in practical terms is impossible, should not be attempted.

If the patient suffers such severe pain that normal blood gas levels cannot be maintained, relief of the pain and improved respiration can be achieved in some patients by continuous thoracic epidural anaesthesia.

(*b*) Injury associated with the development of a tension pneumothorax

The diagnosis of tension pneumothorax is made on the clinical evidence of rapidly increasing respiratory distress, signs of tracheal deviation, absent breath sounds, a hyper-resonant percussion note over the affected side of the chest and a dramatic fall in the blood pressure.

Urgent decompression can be achieved using any available needle or a trocar and cannula. Once the acute emergency is over a catheter is inserted into the pleural cavity through the second interspace in the anterior axillary line. This should be connected to an underwater seal. If the damaged lung continues to leak air the collapsed lung can usually be re-expanded and the leak sealed by applying negative pressure to the drainage bottle.

(*c*) Pneumothorax, not associated with tension, but accompanied by a haemothorax

This condition may demand adequate resuscitation if the patient develops hypovolaemic shock. Once this has been dealt with, two tubes are usually placed in the chest: a small catheter in the anterior extremity of the second intercostal space to deal with the air, and a larger 28 gauge portex tube through the eighth interspace in the midaxillary line to deal with the blood. Both are connected to underwater seals, and negative pressure may be applied if necessary.

The lower tube should be regularly stripped at 15 minute intervals if bleeding continues.

(d) *The flail chest*
Although much effort has been expended on operations designed to fix the ribs by some form of external or internal splintage, the method of 'pneumatic fixation', originally described by Avery in 1956, remains popular. This method calls for a tracheostomy or the passage of a cuffed endotracheal tube, the use of sedation and/or paralysis, and, lastly, positive pressure ventilation.

Indications for this method of treatment include a rising $Paco_2$: a level above 45 mmHg (6.0 kPa) is unacceptable in the very young whereas a level in the region of 55 mmHg (7.3 kPa) may be acceptable after middle age providing no further elevation occurs. Attention should also be paid to the Pao_2 which is normally about 100 mmHg (13.3 kPa). If this falls to a level in the region of 50 mmHg (6.7 kPa) oxygen should be administered. However, the Fio_2 should be kept below 50 per cent to avoid further damage to the lungs by oxygen intoxication.

If it is impossible to maintain the blood gases at near normal levels by the administration of oxygen by nasal catheters or mask and the unaided respiratory efforts of the patient, consideration should be given to either intubation or tracheostomy. A modern plastic cuffed tube can be introduced and kept *in situ* for about one week so long as the cuff is deflated at intervals. After this period a tracheostomy, see p. 35, should be considered if the patient is unable to maintain the blood gases at near normal levels.

In order to ventilate the patient it is always necessary to sedate him. This can be achieved by a combination of opiates and benzodiazepam. With this drug combination the patient is usually calm and cooperative. If paralysis is required this is achieved by the use of tubocurarine the effect of which lasts for between 20 and 40 minutes.

The efficiency of mechanical respiration can be gauged by the changing values of the blood gases. Even when maintaining mechanical respiration the Pao_2 may remain low because of arteriovenous shunting even when the patient is ventilated with 50 per cent oxygen. To boost an unacceptably low Pao_2 in the face of an adequate Fio_2 a positive end-expiratory pressure may be required.

(e) *Compression injuries leading to pulmonary contusion*
These injuries, found in younger patients in the absence of rib fractures, may become obvious only some 24–48 hours after injury. The first clinical evidence is usually the development of tachypnoea and the finding of wet râles on physical examination. Because the underlying lung is contused haemoptysis and excessive tracheobronchial secretion occur.

Lung function is seriously disturbed, compliance is diminished, respiratory resistance increases, pulmonary diffusion is reduced, and there is arteriovenous shunting. Little can be done in these circumstances apart from supporting pulmonary function by ventilation, as described in section (*d*) above.

Penetrating wounds

1 An open wound should immediately be closed by an occlusive dressing, after which the patient should be moved to the theatre and wound cleansing carried out.
2 A haemothorax should initially be treated by tube drainage. When the source of haemorrhage is from the lung parenchyma, bleeding usually stops spontaneously after re-expansion of the lung because the pulmonary circulation is a low pressure system. If severe blood loss continues it suggests that the intercostal vessels or a major intrathoracic vessel has been injured. Immediate thoracotomy would then be required.

5.3 Treatment of blunt injuries to the abdomen

Although this discussion is chiefly concerned with the problem of blunt injuries to the abdomen it is important to recognize that abdominal trauma is associated with additional injuries in nearly three-quarters of all patients. This is because one of the commonest causes of abdominal injury is the road traffic accident, during which the four major systems, i.e. craniospinal, chest, abdomen and skeletal, may all sustain severe damage.

This type of injury accounts for nearly half the deaths between the ages of 15 and 29 years in highly developed Western societies. All the major systems are interlinked, and each, when injured, may exert adverse effects on the others. Thus, when the chest is so badly damaged that hypoxia and hypoxaemia follow, there is a detrimental effect on the brain, particularly if this organ has also been injured; partially damaged brain cells, which might have recovered if fully oxygenated, die and there is also considerable evidence that hypoxia hastens the onset of cerebral oedema or makes established oedema worse. Alternatively, severe haemorrhage leading to hypovolaemic shock, particularly in the presence of hypoxaemia, may finally result in organic renal damage, i.e. cortical necrosis or tubular necrosis in kidneys that were previously normal.

Essential steps in management

1 *Ensure an adequate airway*
A patient injured just after a heavy meal may vomit, producing a mechanical block to the airway by vomitus, the tongue may cause obstruction, particularly if the jaw is broken, and respiration may be hampered by an associated chest injury.

Although the airway may be free, the associated chest injury may have led to gross and increasing pulmonary dysfunction which may necessitate the passage of a cuffed endotracheal tube, or a tracheostomy, together with positive pressure ventilation.

2 Resuscitation

The second commonest cause of death following an abdominal injury is haemorrhage, which, if massive, e.g. from a torn aorta, produces either immediate or almost immediate death from cardiac failure, or delayed death due to indirect effects such as renal or respiratory failure.

Even closed fractures may lead to the loss of large volumes of blood: e.g. a fractured pelvis may cause the loss of 3–4.5 litres, a fractured humerus 1–2.5 litres. Clinical examination and an assessment of the associated injuries allows approximate estimation of the 'expected' blood loss. If this is then replaced and there is no satisfactory haemodynamic response it is reasonable to assume, in the absence of severe brain or chest injury, that there is internal bleeding.

When difficulties are encountered in resuscitation, a central venous pressure line (Section 1.3) should be inserted or, if available, the Swan–Ganz flow-directed balloon-tipped pulmonary arterial catheter which, when 'wedged' into the pulmonary artery, reflects left atrial pressure and the function of the left ventricle. In the 'free' unstabilized position it still permits a reasonable assessment of left ventricular function. Blood used in an emergency should be of the patient's own group, or, if available, Group O Rhesus negative. If plasma substitutes are given, e.g. dextran, blood for grouping and cross-matching should be taken before they are administered.

Initial attempts to resuscitate the patient should be followed by frequent observations of the pulse rate, blood pressure, central venous pressure, left atrial pressure, the state of consciousness, and the pupil size and reaction. If the patient is breathing by means of a respirator, a record must be kept of the rate, tidal volume, inspired oxygen concentration, and the peak pressure. If the patient is ill enough to require intensive care, a catheter will usually be passed and the urine volume monitored in this way.

Specific signs of abdominal injury

Certain external signs may be present when the abdomen has been injured. Thus, the presence of tyre marks or extensive bruising on one or other side of the chest or upper abdomen may suggest that the liver or spleen, or both, have been injured. Similar marks across the centre of the abdomen are often associated with injuries of the bowel or mesentery.

Plain radiographs of the abdomen may show fractures of the lower rib cage or free air within the peritoneal cavity.

One remaining problem is to distinguish between the pain and tenderness of an injury that involves only the abdominal parietes and one that involves an internal viscus. In most cases the diagnosis of intraperitoneal haemorrhage is obvious because resuscitation fails to have the desired effect in the presence of a normal chest X-ray. Alternatively, when a patient does not initially require resuscitation, an unexpected elevation of the pulse rate may occur accompanied by a fall in the haemoglobin concentration.

Peritoneal lavage

When an intra-abdominal injury is suspected but there is an absence of physical signs despite a suspicious history, an abdominal paracentesis followed by peritoneal lavage is indicated.

Abdominal paracentesis as a diagnostic procedure was first described in 1926 by Neuof and Cohen. Various investigators reported, however, that simple aspiration was positive in fewer than 20 per cent of patients if there was less than 200 ml of blood in the peritoneal cavity. The rate of positive taps increased to about 80 per cent when there was 500 ml. The technique was improved in 1965 by Root, who described the additional use of peritoneal lavage. Investigations in the cadaver show that this method makes it possible to detect less than 50 ml of blood in the peritoneal cavity.

Method

Lavage takes approximately 20 minutes to perform. A multiperforated polythene tube is introduced into the peritoneal cavity via a trocar inserted through a small incision in the subumbilical position, and 20 ml/kg of lactated Ringer's solution, to a maximum of 1000 ml, is allowed to flow into the abdominal cavity by gravity alone. The empty bottle is placed on the floor and the fluid drains from the abdomen. Whereas a paracentesis is considered positive only if at least 0.1 ml of non-clotting blood is obtained, the results of peritoneal lavage can be judged by the visual appearance of the fluid alone. In experienced hands, this method yields no false positive results. It is obvious, however, that not all serious blunt injuries are associated with intraperitoneal haemorrhage; e.g. retroperitoneal injuries to the pancreas or kidneys, which may cause profound hypovolaemic shock, may be associated with a negative paracentesis. However, these injuries are rarely followed by the catastrophic consequences which may result from, say, a delayed rupture of the spleen.

SPECIFIC INJURIES

Hepatic injuries

These are sustained in approximately 15–20 per cent of blunt injuries to the abdomen. Grit, burns or bruises on the right upper abdomen and lower right chest may be found, possibly in an older patient with fractured ribs on the right. In children the chest is so elastic that any degree of intra-abdominal catastrophe is possible without the ribs necessarily breaking.

Abdominal tenderness and rigidity may exist, and both may spread if intra-abdominal bleeding and bile leakage continue. Severe haemorrhage is, of course, associated with hypovolaemic shock.

Classification of severity

Liver injuries may be classified according to their severity into the following three groups:

1   simple superficial lacerations;

2 deep lacerations of the liver parenchyma;
3 severe injuries in which the hepatic veins are torn or avulsed as they converge into the cava.

In any large series 85 per cent of liver injuries fall into Group 1 and are not of themselves associated with any mortality, approximately 10 per cent fall into Group 2 and may be associated with some mortality due either to infection or secondary haemorrhage and approximately 5 per cent fall into Group 3 in which group a mortality rate due to the liver injury itself of over 50 per cent may occur. Occasionally the liver remains intact but the common duct is avulsed from the porta.

Treatment

1 *Minor injuries.* When laparotomy reveals one or more superficial lacerations of the liver bleeding will nearly always have ceased by the time the patient is submitted to surgery. Assuming that there is no other injury a drain should be put down to the area of liver damage which should be left undisturbed for a few days. If bleeding is continuing when the abdomen is explored the liver wound should be sutured by the use of interlocking horizontal mattress sutures, inserting each suture approximately 2 cm from the edge of the wound. Special absorbable tampons through which the stitches can be inserted are now generally available which diminish the danger of the individual stitches 'cutting out'.

2 *Group 2 injuries.* Such an injury will be associated with severe bleeding which can be temporarily stopped by compressing the affected lobe between both hands. Unfortunately, although this manoeuvre will stop the bleeding if it is from the liver alone and, therefore, allow the patient to be resuscitated, as soon as the pressure is released bleeding recommences. However, before proceeding further an attempt must be made to distinguish this type of injury from a Group 3 injury. This can sometimes be achieved by compressing the vessels, i.e. the hepatic artery and portal vein in the free edge of the lesser omentum, a manoeuvre first described by Pringle in 1908. If bleeding continues after the application of an atraumatic vascular clamp across these vessels it suggests that the retrohepatic vena cava or hepatic veins themselves have been damaged.

Assuming that this manoeuvre does appreciably reduce the amount of bleeding what further operative procedure should be performed? The alternatives are as follows:

(*a*) obviously avascular liver tissue can be removed and the bare area packed. This method is subject to the following disadvantages:
   (i) a pack does not necessarily control the bleeding;
   (ii) there may be a fatal haemorrhage when the pack is removed;
   (iii) the pack itself may produce pressure necrosis;
   (iv) secretions and exudate have difficulty in draining and severe intrahepatic or subphrenic infection may occur;
   (v) biliary fistulae commonly develop.
(*b*) the obviously devitalized liver tissue on either side of a major laceration is removed after which the 'fissure' is packed by an omental flap which is

fashioned from the greater omentum, supplied by the right gastroepiploic artery and drained by the right gastroepiploic vein. This 'pack' is inserted into the laceration and the edges of the liver are loosely brought together by liver stitches as described. The protagonists of this method claim that by using an omental pack the dead space of the wound is eliminated and that tamponade produced by the pack controls minor venous bleeding.

The critics of this measure suggest that one may be leaving *in situ* a devitalized mass of liver.

(c) on the basis of these criticisms it can be argued that the correct treatment is to remove that part of the liver lying lateral to the major laceration using the finger fracture technique to divide the liver tissue which was first described by Lin. This method leaves undivided vessels intact and these can then be ligated as they are exposed. Vessels already divided by the traumatic episode must be transfixed if possible in the substance of the liver. Following removal of the liver tissue it is occasionally possible to aid haemostasis by suturing the deperitonealized undersurface of the diaphragm onto the raw area of the liver.

3 *Group 3 injuries.* Fortunately complex liver injuries with laceration of the lobar branches of the portal vein, the retrohepatic vena cava or the hepatic veins are relatively rare, except after gunshot wounds when gross disruption of the liver may occur particularly if this viscus is penetrated by a high velocity bullet, since the kinetic energy of such a body is chiefly governed by its speed according to the formula:

$$E = \frac{mv_2}{2}$$

Several approaches to this type of injury have been tried but the overall mortality remains in the order of 50–70 per cent.

The performance of an anatomical lobectomy does not appear to lower the mortality. In this regard it should be noted that the original division of the liver into right and left lobes was by reference to the attachment of the falciform ligament and the fissures for the ligamentation teres and venosum. However, Hjortsjö showed on the basis of the segmental branching of the bile ducts, hepatic artery and portal vein within the liver that the functional division of the liver into its two major lobes is considerably to the right of these attachments. On the superior surface of the liver there is no superficial marking to indicate this division but on the inferior surface this boundary is indicated by a line extending from the gall bladder fossa towards the inferior vena cava. The plane between the two lobes forms an angle of about 35 degrees with the vertical plane and 20 degrees with the sagittal plane.

The chief difficulty in this type of injury is to control the haemorrhage. In order to gain access to a severe injury the abdominal incision should be converted into a thoracoabdominal approach by dividing the costal margin or alternatively, the incision may be extended upwards in the midline and a sternotomy performed by means of a Sarn's saw. Protagonists of the latter method make the point that when the pericardium and diaphragm are divided the inferior vena cava is easily exposed above the level of entry of the hepatic veins after which the subhepatic cava can be isolated and controlled. In the author's *very limited* experience total control of the suprahepatic cava, however, so reduces the venous return to the heart that the patient collapses forthwith and the anaesthetist demands the restoration of some blood flow.

If a classical thoracoabdominal approach is made division of the right triangular ligament allows the liver to be rotated. If the bleeding is coming from the right hepatic vein it will often be controlled by this manoeuvre alone after which the tear in the vein can be identified and sutured or ligated, whichever is most appropriate, after which the damaged liver tissue itself must be removed as described above.

In order to maintain venous return various authors have described the insertion of temporary caval shunts but these appear to be associated with no reduction in mortality perhaps because when this manoeuvre is deemed necessary other complications defeat the surgeon.

One of the great difficulties facing the surgeon when dealing with class 3 injuries of the liver is undoubtedly the torrential haemorrhage which accompanies them. The massive transfusions required result in the platelets and coagulation factors becoming diluted, stored blood being deficient in these elements. In addition, because the liver is damaged the synthesis of other clotting factors such as Factors V and VIII may be totally inadequate to secure haemostasis. Once the volume of transfused blood exceeds 12–14 units, a prolonged bleeding time is frequent and a haemorrhagic state develops. To correct the thrombocytopenia one unit of fresh blood should be given for each 4–5 units of bank blood, and if there is already an abnormality, platelet concentrates are necessary. Another complication following massive bleeding is the development of disseminated intravascular coagulation, in which the circulating blood becomes a suspension of cells in serum deficient in Factors VIII, V, II and platelets, all factors consumed during coagulation.

Splenic injury

Rupture of the spleen following blunt injuries to the abdomen is more common if the spleen is already abnormal, in particular the malarial spleen is especially prone to rupture following relatively mild trauma, but the leukaemic spleen or the spleen involved in infectious mononucleosis is also more liable to rupture than the normal organ.

The majority of splenic injuries consist of lacerations which run across the convex outer surface but occasionally the spleen is totally shattered or completely avulsed from its pedicle.

The clinical diagnosis should be suspected when the patient develops signs of internal haemorrhage associated with fractures of the left lower ribs. Abdominal rigidity will develop which will extend either slowly or rapidly down the left side according to the severity of the injury. Referred pain in the left shoulder will occur and on occasions the patient will be tender on rectal examination.

In a minority of patients abdominal signs never develop, although a persistently high pulse rate together with a mild pyrexia and a low haemoglobin should alert the surgeon to this diagnosis. It is in this type of case in which the condition is unrecognized that a massive delayed haemorrhage may occur. This complication is said to occur in about 10 per cent of patients in whom the rupture is unrecognized, usually within 16 days of the original injury.

Various theories have been advanced to explain the condition. One theory is that if the diagnosis is not made the omentum walls off the laceration and so prevents further bleeding, but this does not explain why a patient may develop such a dramatic haemorrhage some days later. A second, more plausible, theory is that there is delayed haemorrhage only when the original rupture is associated with a small laceration of the tail of the pancreas. Under these circumstances the membrane enclosing the haematoma is presumed to be gradually digested away by the pancreatic enzymes until, finally, it gives way and produces the final haemorrhage.

Treatment

In the majority of patients the treatment of a ruptured spleen is splenectomy, this is particularly indicated if associated lesions are present or the operator is relatively inexperienced.

There are, however, numerous papers in the surgical literature which now advocate a more conservative approach. Conservation of splenic tissue if possible is undoubtedly desirable, since there is now clear evidence that particularly in childhood fulminating infection is more common following splenectomy for trauma or for the treatment of hereditary spherocytosis. Unfortunately, there are no large series reported in which this approach has been used. Certainly it should only be carried out by an experienced surgeon since the spleen must be completely mobilized so that it can be brought out of the abdomen and inspected in its entirety. If a laceration is present this is sutured using oxfibrin buffers in exactly the same fashion as a laceration of the liver is sutured. When either the upper or lower pole has been partially avulsed the remnants are dissected free. Since the capsule will not itself hold sutures stitches are placed through the splenic parenchyma again buttressed by oxfibrin buffers.

More recently further reports have appeared in the literature suggesting that splenic tissue can be successfully transplanted into the omentum. Intra-abdominal adhesions are reduced to a minimum if this is done. In the rat, autogenous spleen tissue 'takes' in approximately three-quarters of the animals in whom omental implantation is attempted.

Small bowel injury

The small bowel usually ruptures at or near fixed points, i.e. at the duodeno-jejunal flexure or the terminal ileum. The diagnosis of small tears is often delayed for 2 or 3 days until the development of, or the changing physical signs indicate, a spreading peritonitis. Larger lacerations of the bowel are possible, particularly at the duodenojejunal flexure, and may be complete transections. This injury is always associated with free air in the abdomen and the rapid development of a spreading peritonitis.

Treatment
This consists of laparotomy and suture of the injured bowel. Such injuries are nearly always associated with mesenteric lacerations which, if large, give rise to the signs of intraperitoneal haemorrhage. They should be treated by ligation of the injured vessels and, if necessary, resection of the devascularized bowel.

Renal injury

This is usually produced by blows on the flanks or across the lumbar region. A severe blow liable to be complicated by renal injury is frequently accompanied by fractures of the transverse processes of the lumbar vertebra.

The commonest presenting symptom is haematuria which is likely to occur in all patients except those in whom the kidney has been completely avulsed from its pedicle. In addition if a severe corticomedullary injury has occurred a gradually increasing swelling develops in the loin which will be followed by visible bruising. This swelling is chiefly due to extravasated blood but in addition so long as the renal vessels are intact there will also be some blood.

When a renal lesion is suspected an intravenous pyelogram should, if possible, be performed as soon as the patient has been resuscitated. The essential information achieved is as follows:

1. the presence of a normally functioning kidney on the contralateral side. The author has seen a child in whom a solitary damaged kidney had been removed.
2. on the side of the injury:
   (*a*) functional impairment, total or partial;
   (*b*) presence of intrarenal or extrarenal extravasation;
   (*c*) presence or absence of a psoas shadow.

Classification of renal injuries
Group 1 *Renal contusion.* This injury is associated with haematuria which rapidly diminishes and usually disappears within five days. The IVP may show no change or a generalized diminution of function. No mass develops in the flank. Such an injury can be treated conservatively.
Group 2 *Corticomedullary laceration.* This type of lesion may or may not be associated with extravasation. It is associated with gross haematuria and continued bleeding into the perinephric tissues may lead to an increasing mass in the loins.

Treatment of this group of injuries still remains a matter for debate.

(*a*) Some surgeons maintain that when intravenous pyelography shows only the presence of intrarenal extravasation exploration is unnecessary, whereas if extrarenal extravasation is present exploration is mandatory. At operation the damaged kidney should be repaired, either pole being removed and the damaged calyx sutured after which the polar tissue can be trimmed so that the renal tissue can be opposed.

(*b*) Other surgeons argue that even if dye is seen to extravasate from the kidney the patient can be treated conservatively so long as an increasing swelling does not develop in the loin. It is in this group that a pararenal pseudohydronephrosis may slowly develop due to the extravasated blood and urine slowly occluding the pelviureteric junction.

Group 3 The shattered kidney. This condition, in which the kidney is completely disintegrated, is always associated with severe haematuria and an expanding mass in the loin. Exploration is essential and nephrectomy required.

Group 4 The avulsed kidney. This may not be associated with haematuria because urine secretion ceases immediately after the injury. Furthermore, although a mass may form in the loin because of the initial haemorrhage this may not continue to expand since the renal artery and vein rapidly constrict and spontaneous haemorrhage ceases. An intravenous pyelogram will show no function on the affected side and nephrectomy is required. This type of injury seldom occurs in isolation.

In general, in the absence of devastating haemorrhage the majority of renal injuries can be treated conservatively. In one series of 77 patients only 5 were explored.

Injury to the pancreas

Traumatic lesions of the pancreas caused by blunt injury to the abdomen seldom occur in isolation. A common mechanism of injury is the road traffic accident in which the driver is brought into sharp contact with the steering wheel.

It is not uncommon for pancreatic injury to be missed because there may be no dramatic features to suggest its presence when the abdomen is opened. However, if a haematoma is present in the root of the transverse mesocolon, in the periduodenal area or at the duodenojejunal flexure it should be explored. When a haematoma is present in the periduodenal area an extensive Kocher's manoeuvre should be performed so that both the anterior and posterior aspects of the head of the pancreas can be inspected. If the haematoma is in the base of the mesocolon access to the pancreas can be best obtained through the gastrocolic omentum whilst if the haematoma is in the region of the tail of the pancreas the spleen should be mobilized and brought forwards.

When the pancreatic injury appears trivial and little or no secretion from it occurs following the injection of secretin all that is required is a drain to the area.

If, however, a severe laceration of the left half of the pancreas has occurred the simplest and safest procedure is to perform a distal pancreatectomy which usually demands a simultaneous splenectomy. The major pancreatic duct is ligated and the edges of the wound oversewn, a large drain should be brought out into the flank in such a position that if a pancreatic fistula develops the efflux can be readily controlled by an adhesive appliance.

When the laceration involves the head or the right side of the pancreas the problem becomes more difficult and the correct solution a matter for debate. The following solutions have been proposed:

1. pancreaticoduodenectomy. This is a formidable operation carrying a high mortality in the already severely injured patient. It is of course followed by insulin dependent diabetes and exocrine enzyme deficiency;
2. extended distal resection. This can be extended to the left lateral border of the portal vein;
3. if the injury is actually in the head of the pancreas an internal Roux loop can be constructed bringing the free end of the loop up to the head of the pancreas and suturing it around the site of the injury. This is made easier when the duodenum is also lacerated since at least one edge of the circumference of the loop can be sutured in the manner of an intestinal anastomosis. The jejunum distal to the duodenojejunal fistula is then anastomosed end to side into the Roux loop to complete the operation. The author has no personal experience of this method and cannot, therefore, comment on its efficacy.

5.4 Principles involved in the treatment of nerve and tendon injuries, particularly in the hand and wrist

Factors influencing the results of tendon repair include:

1. the site of injury;
2. the tendons involved;
3. the presence of associated injury which may involve:
   (a) tissues covering the tendon;
   (b) nerves;
   (c) joints;
4. the extent of damage to the tendon itself, and the type of injury, whether cut or crushed, whether clean or contaminated;
5. the length of time between injury and treatment;
6. the age, attitude and occupation of the patient;
7. the skill and experience of the surgeon.

Injuries to the flexor tendons in the palm and fingers do less well than injuries to tendons in other parts of the hand. The tendons at the wrist, abductor pollicis longus, the digital extensors, the flexors in the forearm, and the extensors on the back of the hand all do well after repair and produce a good functional result.

Technique of tendon repair

1 Exposure

When exploring the fingers or palm, longitudinal incisions should *not* be made over the midline of the fingers or in the palm. Instead incisions in the finger should be made in the midlateral position and if extensive exposure is required this should be achieved by Z plasties. In the palm skin incisions should follow the skin creases.

2 Repair

Tendons have a blood supply chiefly via the vincula longi and brevia and will heal well if they are handled with care, the ends precisely opposed and the suture line protected from strain. Mishandling is liable to produce adhesions and consequently restricted movement.

(*a*) *Flexor tendons*. These are now normally sutured with a square suture tied within the circumference of the cut ends together with a continuous circumferential suture, both of 6/0 monofilament material in the fingers, 4/0 and 6/0 respectively in the palm.

(*b*) *Extensor tendons*. These tendons are sometimes too flat to be repaired in this manner and so simple interrupted sutures are used.

Following suture the tendons require 3 weeks' complete immobilization in the most relaxed position which can be achieved. Thus when the flexor tendons of the digits have been divided both the fingers and wrists must be held in the flexed position for this period after which 3 weeks of supervised active movements are required following which passive stretching is permitted. Ideally the wrist should be flexed, with the metacarpophalangeal joints held in 90 degrees of flexion and the fingers moderately flexed. Rehabilitation can be tedious and both the splint maker and the physiotherapist play a vital role.

Free tendon grafts

This is primarily required when tendon substance has been lost although in some sites, an extensor pollicis longus tendon transfer achieves an equal or significantly better result.

If it is felt that the immediate insertion of a free tendon graft is inappropriate at the time of the initial surgical exploration of the wound a silicone rod should be introduced into the flexor tendon sheath after excising the damaged tendon. This acts as a spacer preventing the sheath from contracting. Prior to attempting a free tendon graft the joints must be fully mobilized by passive movements after which tendon grafting can be attempted. The palmaris longus tendon, present in 80 per cent of the population, provides a tendon length of between 10 and 15 cm. If this is absent the plantaris or extensor digitorum brevis from the dorsum of the foot is used.

Rehabilitation is as for primary tendon repair.

Tendon injuries on the palmar aspect of the hand and wrist

It is useful to divide the hand into topographical zones, since this will define the problems associated with the anatomy in each area which will affect not only the treatment but also the prognosis of tendon injuries.

Various classifications are available. As many as seven zones have been described. In practice, however, there are three zones which need to be distinguished.

Distal zone
This extends from the distal insertion of the deep flexor tendon into the base of the terminal phalanx, proximally to the midpoint of the middle segment of the finger. In this zone, only the profundus tendon is divided.

Middle zone
This area was previously referred to as 'no man's land', a term no longer useful. It extends from the middle of the middle segment of the finger to the distal palmar crease, and injuries in this zone may divide both superficialis and profundus tendons within the fibrous flexor sheath.

Proximal zone
This extends from the distal palmar crease to the wrist crease and includes the carpal tunnel.

Since writing the first edition the consensus of opinion with regard to management of hand injuries has undergone a fundamental change. It is now considered, assuming that the surgeon is sufficiently experienced, that regardless of the zone of injury *all* the damaged tendons should be repaired. If the surgeon is relatively inexperienced there is a case for delayed repair when the injury involves the middle zone in which disastrous results may follow inadequate attempts to repair both tendons.

When nerves and digital vessels are also damaged it is important, by the use of the operating microscope, to repair these structures at the same time, although sometimes the collateral circulation of blood is sufficient to render vascular surgery unnecessary.

Nerve injuries

Seddon classified the severity of a peripheral nerve injury as follows:

1 *neuropraxia*. This is often caused by ischaemia, compression, or a blow. The axons remain in continuity and recovery is spontaneous and complete.
2 *axonotmesis*. Most commonly caused by crushing, the axons are disrupted within intact sheaths but the nerve trunk remains in continuity and, therefore, each axon grows down its own tunnel and recovery is eventually complete.
3 *neurotmesis*. This implies total disruption of the nerve. There can be no recovery without repair and some axonal confusion is inevitable; recovery is slow and may be incomplete.

This classification although useful is somewhat artificial since in practice there is often a mixture, particularly of lesions 1 and 2.

Technique of nerve repair
Primary suture is normally performed in the following conditions:

1. the wound is fresh and expected to heal promptly; the clean incised wound;
2. skin defect, if any, is easily closed;
3. the nerve is sharply cut across;
4. the nerve ends can be brought together easily;
5. the ends are lying in healthy tissue.

Thus in nearly all cases in which the nerve has been damaged by a lacerating injury primary repair should always be attempted. Only if there is widespread destruction of the nerve making the gap too large to close without tension, or if the general condition of the patient precludes surgery, should nerve repair be deferred.

The results of primary repair are improved by performing the suture using some form of magnification. The most important single factor inimical to nerve healing is tension at the suture line and if the gap is too large, the ends of the divided nerve should be anchored locally and a delayed nerve graft used after healing of the wound has been achieved.

In the acute injury, identification of the correct opposing ends of each separate motor or sensory bundle of nerve fibres is quite possible under the operating microscope. Thus, precise orientation is possible and will inevitably improve results. This is not the case with secondary repair, as the neuromata at the cut ends need to be excised and the exact matching is lost but electrical stimulation of the cut nerve ends in a conscious patient, operated upon under a brachial plexus block, can be used to locate the corresponding bundles if they are not visually obvious.

Nerve repair produces satisfactory functional sensation but this is never entirely normal. The recovery of motor function and muscle bulk, particularly in the small muscles of the hand, is much less predictable, and it is for this reason that an ulnar nerve lesion is particularly serious.

Nerve grafts
Secondary operations performed when large gaps lie between the severed ends are probably best closed by cable grafts constructed from the sural nerve using an operating microscope to obtain correct alignment.

Tests of functional recovery of nervous continuity
1. *Tinel's sign.* Percussion over the advancing edge of the regrowing nerve fibres produces a characteristic tingling sensation. The rate of advance approximates to 1 mm per day after a lag of 10 days which follows the injury.
2. *Sweat test.* The presence of sweating can be demonstrated by a hand print on ninhydrin-impregnated paper. Sweat is absent in denervated skin but recovery is unpredictable and correlates poorly with the quality of sensory recovery.
3. *When light touch returns*, it is called protective sensation, but more precise testing, using two-point discrimination or distinguishing between differing materials can be used to expose incomplete recovery.

4 *Electromyography.* This indicates that the nerve is recovering function some weeks before clinical tests become positive; action potentials can be demonstrated in a recovering nerve before any increased muscle strength can be detected.

5.5 Aetiology, symptomatology and treatment of tetanus

Aetiology
Tetanus is now a rare disease and an even rarer cause of death in Western countries and could be completely eliminated throughout the world if every individual was actively immunized with tetanus toxoid in childhood.

It is caused by an anaerobic terminal spore-bearing Gram-positive rod, the *Clostridium tetani* which is found in the gut of man and animals, particularly herbivores and in cultivated soil. The organism is non-invasive but produces a most powerful exotoxin known as tetanospasmin, the potency of which is surpassed only by the exotoxin of *Cl. botulinum*.

Using isotopically-labelled toxin it has been shown that the toxin, which is avidly taken up by the gangliosides in the CNS, either travels directly up the peripheral nerves from the wound, producing initially at least local tetanus, or enters the blood stream and then ascends the peripheral nerves to the spinal cord and medulla. Taken up by the presynaptic terminals of inhibiting spinal interneurones the toxin prevents the release of inhibitory transmitters with the result that an excessive discharge occurs from the alpha and gamma motor neurones thus producing the spasms typical of tetanus. In addition, the toxin also affects the sympathetic nerve cells in the lateral horn of the spinal cord producing sympathetic overactivity.

Because the transit of the toxin is slow the first effects are usually seen in muscles which possess short motor neurones, i.e. the head and neck muscles, producing the classic symptoms of trismus and neck rigidity and it is only later that the muscles of the trunk and limbs are affected.

Symptomatology
In many patients presenting with overt tetanus no apparent wound is present although the patient may give a history of a minor penetrating wound within the period of incubation which varies between 3 and 21 days. Usually, prior to the development of actual muscular spasm the patient complains of stiffness of the neck and dysphagia and symptoms may precede spasm by as much as 10 days. The shorter this interval the more severe the disease is likely to be.

In the vast majority of patients the presenting features are trismus and dysphagia. Other possible presenting symptoms are neck and back rigidity, cephalic tetanus (i.e. cranial nerve palsies), local tetanus (i.e. symptoms and signs limited to one particular group of muscles) and rarely abdominal pain.

As the condition worsens so the major problem becomes hypertonicity of the somatic muscles which go into intermittent spasms either spontaneously or in response to some trivial stimulus. In severe forms of the disease opisthotonus develops and the patient may be unable to breathe, hypoxaemia and cyanosis developing. During such a spasm, gastric contents may be regurgitated and aspirated and the patient may die of respiratory failure, although this is rare.

Prophylaxis
Active immunization. Individuals whose occupations or pleasures may expose them to an increased risk of this disease, e.g. farmers, soldiers, or children, should be actively immunized. In infants, active immunization can begin between 3 and 6 months of age when it is given as diphtheria, tetanus and pertussis vaccine. A reinforcing dose is then given at the age of 5 years when school begins and a further dose in early adult life.

In adults, three doses of toxoid are usually given either subcutaneously or intramuscularly at intervals of 6 weeks and 6 months. The individual dose varies between 0.5 and 1 ml. After three doses the antibody titre is high enough to protect the individual for between 5 and 10 years and, thereafter, booster doses should be given at intervals.

Treatment of a wounded individual

The treatment of a patient in whom wounding has occurred whether the wound is open or healed is surgical toilet after which treatment chiefly depends upon two factors:

1 the state of immunity of the wounded patient;
2 the philosophy of the attending surgeon.

1 The importance of immunity
If the wound is less than 6 hours old when first seen a patient who has received a complete course of tetanus toxoid and has also received a booster dose within 5 years needs no further treatment.

If, however, a booster dose has not been given within the past 10 years one dose of toxoid should be given. If the patient has not completed a full course of toxoid injections or the immune status is unknown a complete course of toxoid should be administered.

With all other wounds if no booster dose has been given for 10 years one dose of toxoid should be administered together with human tetanus immunoglobulin. The substitution of human for equine immunoglobulin has virtually eliminated the risk of an anaphylactic reaction.

When the patient has never been immunized there remains some controversy, one group maintaining that the patient should receive human tetanus immunoglublin together with a complete course of toxoid whereas the opposing school rely on immediate débridement of the wound together with adequate doses of benzylpenicillin (1 million units i.m.) (300 mg i.m.) 6-hourly for one week.

However, this argument reached its peak prior to the introduction of human tetanus immunoglobulin. When only equine antitoxin was available it was established that approximately 12 per cent of patients were sensitive and that one death occurred every 200 000 injections. The reduction in adverse reactions using human antitoxin appears to have put an end to this particular controversy since it has certainly been shown in the experimental animal that antitoxin is superior to penicillin if the administration of the latter is delayed for only a few hours.

Human tetanus immunoglobulin BP marketed as Hamatet by Welcome is purified immunoglobulin obtained from the sera of healthy human donors known to have high levels of tetanus antitoxin following active immunization with tetanus vaccine. One dose of human antitoxin provides adequate blood levels, i.e. over 0.01 iu per ml of serum, for about 4 weeks since there is no risk of early immune elimination unless there is a history of anaphylaxis resulting from a previous dose of human gammaglobulin. The advised dose is 1 ml given by intramuscular injection which contains 250 iu of antitoxin.

Having received antitetanus serum the patient should immediately begin a course of active immunization using toxoid.

Treatment of the established disease

This depends on the severity of the disease but it must never be assumed that because a patient presents with mild symptoms and few signs that the condition will remain stable. Rapid deterioration ending in death may occur in any patient suffering from tetanus although it is generally acknowledged that the shorter the incubation period the more severe the disease is likely to be and similarly the shorter the interval between the first symptom and the first spasm the more severe the disease (i.e. period of onset bears a direct relationship to the subsequent severity of the disease).

Whatever the degree of severity the disease tends to run a well defined course becoming progressively worse during the first week, reaching a plateau in the second and waning in the third. However, residual stiffness may remain for many weeks.

The following steps should be taken immediately the diagnosis is made.

1   Human tetanus immunoglobulin should be given. There is still no hard and fast rule regarding the dose which varies in different series from 500 to 10 000 iu.
2   Benzylpenicillin or ampicillin should be administered to kill residual organisms.
3   The wound, if present, should be explored and débridement performed.
4   Active immunization with toxoid should be commenced.

Treatment of the mild case

When the patient complains of no dysphagia and has no respiratory embarrassment but merely trismus and a little spasticity, all that is required is adequate sedation with diazepam using 10–30 mg daily in divided doses. Fluids should be administered intravenously for a few days and food withheld. If the disease does not progress in the succeeding days oral feeding can be recommenced and the patient merely observed.

Treatment of the severe case

When the spasms are severe, total paralysis with neuromuscular blocking agents will be required. If this is necessary a tracheostomy must be performed and intermittent partial pressure ventilation will be required. The drugs used include curare if there is associated tachycardia and hypotension or pancuronium if bradycardia and hypotension are present. The dose of either relaxant must be adjusted to abolish spasticity and attenuate the spasms to twitches. The doses of relaxant may be spaced out after 2 weeks and stopped in 3 weeks.

Since tetanus produces no impairment of the level of consciousness sedative and analgesic drugs must be given in order to reduce the mental stress and to damp down autonomic dysfunction. Diazepam is the drug of choice since in large doses it sedates, reduces anxiety, produces amnesia and also because of its muscle relaxant properties it reduces the dose of neuromuscular blockers required. The dose required varies from patient to patient but for the average adult 10 mg every few hours orally will be necessary together with supplementary doses intravenously.

In patients suffering from very severe tetanus a characteristic feature is the development of sympathetic overactivity. This develops from 1 to 4 days after neuromuscular blocking agents have been administered and is characterized by the development of a sustained but labile hypertension, tachycardia, cardiac irregularities, peripheral vasoconstriction, profuse sweating and salivation, pyrexia and ileus. Like the somatic spasms sympathetic overactivity occurs in waves either spontaneously or following a stimulus. At the time of greatest disturbance both the plasma and urinary catecholamine levels are raised above normal levels.

There is, as yet, no complete agreement of the treatment of this particular aspect of tetanus. Heavy sedation with large doses of diazepam is one effective measure and another is the use of adrenergic blocking agents such as propranolol or a combined α and β-blocker in the form of labetalol. The latter drug lowers the blood pressure by blocking α-adrenergic receptors in the peripheral arteries and at the same time concurrently blocks the β-adrenergic receptors notably in the heart. This β-blockage protects the heart from the reflex sympathetic drive normally induced by peripheral dilatation and so the reduction in blood pressure is achieved without cardiac stimulation. As a further alternative the two methods can be combined, i.e. heavy sedation accompanied by small doses of the chosen blocking agent which are gradually increased until the situation is controlled.

In contradistinction to this syndrome patients are occasionally seen suffering from severe tetanus in whom hypotension and bradycardia develops. It has been suggested that this syndrome is due to impairment of the baroreceptors. Whilst these attacks can occur spontaneously they have been described following the severe stimulation produced by endobronchial catheterization.

When hypotension and bradycardia follow stimulation, particularly tracheal suction, the condition can nearly always be avoided by simple measures such as preoxygenation prior to therapy, raising the foot of the bed and raising the arterial carbon dioxide tension.

In all cases of severe tetanus careful control should be kept on the fluid balance, the electrolyte balance and the state of nutrition. Whilst the majority of patients can be adequately sustained by feeding through one of the narrower nasogastric tubes in some severely ill patients parenteral nutrition may occur.

Other than the syndromes described above the common complications associated with severe tetanus are:

1. laryngeal spasm;
2. hyperpyrexia, a temperature rising above 40.5°C (105°F), is an indication for surface cooling;
3. chest infection, bronchopneumonia supervening on areas of collapse;
4. decubitus ulcers;
5. cardiac or respiratory arrest.

5.6 Aetiology and management of anaerobic infections

Anaerobic infections are caused by three main groups of organisms, clostridia bacteroides and the anaerobic or microaerophilic streptococci. The clostridia are responsible for three potentially lethal infections; gas or non-gas forming gangrene, tetanus and botulism. Gas gangrene is rare, it occurs following wounds associated with severe crushing of the tissues, following amputations particularly above the knee and penetrating wounds or surgery involving the large bowel. Tetanus, also rare, is dealt with in Section 5.5. Botulism is caused by *Clostridium botulinum* and is a particularly virulent form of food poisoning.

The bacteroides are Gram-negative strict anaerobes of which three varieties have been recognized, *Bacteroides fragilis, melaninogenicus* and the *Fusobacterium* spp. The first is the most pathogenic but forms a minority of the intestinal species of bacteroides. It causes soft tissue infections alone or in combination with *Bacteroides melaninogenicus*, the *Peptostreptococcus*, or aerobic Gram-negative bacilli.

The anaerobic or microaerophilic streptococci frequently act synergistically with the haemolytic *Staphylococcus aureus* to produce a rare but severe cellulitis sometimes called Melaney's ulceration.

Gas gangrene

Bacteriology
The clostridia are saphrophytes. All are spore-forming obligate anaerobes;

both vegetative and spore forms are widespread in soil, sand and faeces. They are, generally, fastidious anaerobes requiring a low redox potential to grow and to initiate conversion of the spores to vegetative, toxin-producing forms. Their presence in the bowel means that endogenous infections are possible, examples of which are clostridial puerperal sepsis following criminal abortion and gas gangrene of a thigh stump following amputation for arterial insufficiency.

The spores of the clostridia represent a highly resistant resting phase able to germinate when the surrounding conditions are propitious. The spores of *Clostridium botulinum* can withstand a temperature of 100°C for 3–5 hours, a feature that led to the abandonment of simple sterilization by boiling.

In any case of gas gangrene several different species of organism may be found, these include two chief varieties, the saccharolytic varieties which include *Cl. perfringens (welchii)* which is recovered in approximately 80 per cent of patients, *Cl. novyi (oedematiens)* and *Cl. septicum*, and the proteolytic saphrophytes *Cl. sporogenes* and *Cl. histolyticum*.

Each organism produces a plethora of toxins all of which are important in the production of the disease. For example, the lethal action of *Cl. perfringens* is proportional to the rate of production of the alpha toxin which is a necrotizing lecithinase which is responsible for breaking down cell membranes, and in addition collagenases, hyaluronidases, proteases, lipases and a haemolysin are produced. This combination of toxins devitalizes the tissue cells and destroys the local microcirculation thus allowing the infection to spread at an astonishing rate.

The ideal environment for the development and multiplication of clostridia is a reduced oxygen tension such as is found in severely contused or lacerated wounds, particularly when they contain foreign bodies or soil or are already infected. Although there is a high incidence of wound contamination there is a low incidence of actual clinical infection. In some series the contamination incidence is as high as 40 per cent without a single case of overt disease.

Pathology
A wide variety of pathological changes can be produced by clostridial infection. Simple contamination of a wound in which neither significant local or systemic manifestations occur other than a brown seropurulent exudate may occur. This condition is not invasive because the surrounding tissues are basically healthy and the organisms are confined to the necrotic surface tissue. However, this situation can develop into invasive gas gangrene if some further factor decreases the oxidation–reduction potential.

More serious is a clostridial cellulitis and most serious is the development of myositis. Both conditions may be gas forming or non-gas forming, the former representing the more serious form of infection. If gas formation occurs spreading crepitation is observed. In both rapid necrosis of muscle occurs, which is due in part to the necrotizing exotoxins produced by the saccharolytic clostridia and in part to the severe oedema that produces ischaemia. The gas of gas gangrene is at first odourless and is composed mainly of hydrogen and carbon dioxide produced from the muscle carbohydrate by the saccharolytic clostridia. Later, when the dead tissues, now brick-red in colour, are attacked by the proteolytic organism, the muscle changes to greenish-black in colour and the foul odour of hydrogen sulphide develops.

The local process is accompanied by severe toxaemia and progressive haemolytic anaemia due to the circulating exotoxins. Throughout the process of tissue destruction polymorphonuclear leucocytes are few in number while the tissues and the oedema fluid contain large numbers of organisms.

Clinical presentation

If the organisms are confined to the superficial tissues producing a clostridial cellulitis the incubation period between contamination and overt infection may be several days. The dissection occurs above the deep fascia and may spread at an exceptionally rapid rate often producing discoloration of the skin and oedema as well as crepitus. The relative mildness of the ensuing toxaemia distinguishes the condition from a clostridial myositis; nevertheless, this condition can also spread at an alarming rate.

When the infection is deeper and involves muscle the incubation period may be as little as 3 days.

The first symptom is commonly pain in the injured area disproportionate to the severity of the injury. This is followed by increasing oedema and swelling. At a later stage the skin becomes discoloured and vesicles appear from which there is a brown malodorous discharge. If the infection is gas forming crepitus is now found on palpation. At a later stage, as necrosis occurs, the skin becomes black and severe toxaemia associated with a tachycardia which is disproportionate to the degree of pyrexia develops. Jaundice due to haemolysis occurs in approximately a quarter of patients suffering from a clostridial myositis and uraemia occurs in a proportion of patients. This is a serious complication, approximately 50 per cent of the patients dying despite dialysis.

Finally septic shock develops, at which stage, near to death, the organisms may invade the blood stream and produce the classical foamy liver. The time between infection and death may be as short as 1–3 days and if there is very severe muscle damage initially the full clinical picture may develop within 6 hours.

Differential diagnosis

Diffuse clostridial myositis (gas gangrene) is most often confused with other gas-producing infections, which are usually due to mixtures of Gram-negative bacilli and Gram-positive cocci. These mixed infections are not usually as virulent as gas gangrene and respond well to incision and drainage. Crepitant cellulitis should not be confused with clostridial gangrene, since it, too, is well treated by lesser means (see below). Gas in the tissues is not a good differentiating point, since some species (e.g. *Cl. novyi*) do not produce gas, non-clostridial organisms (e.g. *Escherichia coli*) often produce gas, and air can enter tissues through a penetrating wound or from the chest.

The diagnosis must be made early. The cornerstones of diagnosis are the clinical appearance of the wound and presence of large Gram-positive rods in stained smears of exudate or tissue. *Cl. perfringens* in tissue may not exhibit spores, but other clostridia often do.

Prevention
The majority of cases of gas gangrene are preventable if early débridement of a severe wound is performed effectively until a margin of healthy bleeding tissue has been exposed. At the same time parenteral penicillin should be administered 300 mg 4-hourly unless the patient gives a history of sensitivity when lincomycin can be used.

Treatment of the established disease
1 *Antibiotics.* In established disease one of the first steps after persuing general resuscitatory measures is the surgical débridement of the wound combined with adequate antibiotic therapy. If adequate débridement is not performed the risk of a spreading myositis is greatly increased. Penicillin or lincomycin should be administered in large doses.
2 *Gas gangrene antitoxin.* Although antitoxins are now available against the toxins of *Cl. perfringens*, *Cl. novyi*, *Cl. histolyticum* and *Cl. septicum*, these are seldom used in the treatment of the established disease since they are now believed to be of equivocable therapeutic value.
3 *Hyperbaric oxygen.* Various regimens have been described for the use of hyperbaric oxygen in gas gangrene and related infections. One such is repeated treatments of 1½–2 hours at 250 kPa (2.5 atm.) pressure daily. Hyperbaric oxygen may be given in a 'whole body' chamber, which demands that both the patient and the nursing staff are subjected to a hyperbaric environment of some 3 atmospheres, or it can be given in a small chamber which does not involve auxiliaries being exposed to what, in itself, may be a potentially dangerous situation.

By exposing the body to a pressure of 3 atmospheres the amount of oxygen in simple solution in the plasma increases from 0.3 to 4 volumes per cent, and because the partial pressure of the oxygen also rises the rate of diffusion from the plasma into the tissues also increases.

Oxygen probably exerts its beneficial effect by suppressing toxin production, for once this process is halted the disease cycle is broken because spread of the organism stops.

In some patients an immediate improvement follows the initial exposure, in others a steady clinical improvement follows consecutive treatments and in approximately a quarter of patients suffering from clostridial gas forming organisms no improvement can be expected whereas in non-clostridial cases the majority of which are due to anaerobic streptococci the failure rate using this method of treatment rises to approximately 75 per cent.

Although antibiotics should still be given, the customary wide excisions are no longer necessary and incision rather than excision is all that is necessary. In places in which hyperbaric oxygen is available, significantly lower mortality rates have been reported.

Bacteroides infections

This group of strict anaerobes is composed of a large number of non-spore-forming pleomorphic organisms which may be tapered, fusiform, slender rods or branching or rounded bodies. The common members are *Bacteroides fragilis*, *B. funduliformis*, *B. nigrescens* and *B. fusobacterium*. They are normal inhabitants of the respiratory, genital and intestinal tracts and constitute more than 97 per cent of the normal faecal flora. They not only inhabit the large bowel but also the ileum and jejunum, a fact that was not appreciated until anaerobic cultures were made of the small bowel contents. When wound infection follows an intra-abdominal operation, particularly if the bowel has been opened, bacteroides can be cultured if proper precautions, i.e. strict anaerobic cultures, are taken.

The characteristic superficial lesion of the bacteroides group is one of an indolent wound discharging a foul-smelling pus. Septicaemia due to these organisms is rare but has been described.

The bacteroides are sensitive to the antibiotics, lincomycin, clindamycin and metronidazole. The last of these now appears to be the drug of choice and in an established infection can be administered either by the oral route as a suppository, or intravenously. In adults or children over 12 years of age the dose is 400 mg three times a day. This drug has also been used with success as a prophylaxis against infection in colorectal surgery.

Anaerobic and microaerophilic streptococci

These organisms are normal commensals in the vagina and the upper respiratory tract and may be a cause of puerperal sepsis in the former and lung abscess in the latter. They may also cause a cellulitic wound infection or even a true myositis. The classical appearance of this type of wound infection is of small painful ulcers, often beginning at the entry point of a suture, which slowly spread. The ulcerated area becomes surrounded by a rim of gangrenous skin which, in turn, is encircled by a purplish area. This type of lesion is known as Melaney's progressive postoperative synergistic gangrene because this form of gangrene cannot be produced by infection with the *Streptococcus* alone but requires the synergistic action of a *Staphylococcus pyogenes* or *Proteus vulgaris*. A similar condition in the scrotum is called Fournier's gangrene.

As the infection spreads the skin becomes necrotic and black in colour and is finally sloughed from the underlying tissues, usually revealing a mass of liquefying fat.

Treatment
Before the introduction of antibiotics the treatment of this condition was wide excision, removing the affected skin and underlying subcutaneous tissues until the deep aponeuroses were exposed. This form of treatment succeeded because the lesion, although progressive, is indolent in character. Control is now achieved by less radical surgery together with the administration of antibiotics.

Streptococcal myositis

Although a crepitant myositis can be produced by this organism it is exceedingly rare. Unlike true gas gangrene, the clinical course is slow and insidious, and not associated with severe toxaemia. The wound discharge contains large numbers of polymorphonuclear leucocytes and many Gram-positive cocci, in direct contrast to a clostridial myositis in which the discharge contains clostridial rods and few leucocytes.

6 Gastrointestinal Surgery

6.1 Enlargement of the parotid gland: causes and treatment
6.2 Causes and treatment of dysphagia
6.3 Hiatus hernia: symptoms, treatment and complications
6.4 Investigation and treatment of haematemesis, excluding bleeding oesophageal varices
6.5 Management of bleeding oesophageal varices
6.6 Aetiology of gall-stones
6.7 Major complications of gall-stones and their treatment
6.8 Causes of jaundice and the evaluation of diagnostic methods
6.9 Aetiology, diagnosis, complications and treatment of acute pancreatitis
6.10 Diagnosis and management of chronic pancreatitis
6.11 Indications for and complications of splenectomy
6.12 Classification of intestinal obstruction and the general principles of management
6.13 Neonatal intestinal obstruction, excluding anorectal abnormalities
6.14 Surgical causes of malabsorption
6.15 Aetiology, pathology and management of Crohn's disease
6.16 Pathology, clinical course, and treatment of ulcerative colitis
6.17 Aetiology, pathology, clinical presentation and management of diverticular disease
6.18 Pathology and treatment of carcinoma of the rectum
6.19 Congenital deformities of the rectum and anal canal

6.1 Enlargement of the parotid gland: causes and treatment

Enlargement of the parotid gland may be either local or general. When a localized enlargement is found in the parotid region it is nearly always due to a tumour within the gland itself but occasionally some superficial pathology may be present including, for example, a sebaceous cyst of the overlying skin, a swelling of the preauricular lymph node, a haemangioma or a lymphangioma of the overlying tissues. In addition hypertrophy of the masseter can be mistaken for a parotid swelling as also can a dental cyst or a tumour of the facial nerve.

TUMOURS OF THE PAROTID GLAND

It should be noted that similar tumours may occur in all other sites of salivary tissue, i.e. the mouth, palate and submandibular glands. The cell of origin, i.e. the histogenesis of many salivary tumours, remains a matter for debate and furthermore, a precise classification of many of these tumours into benign and malignant forms may be difficult because many tend to grow slowly and their behaviour may be quite difficult to predict on histological grounds.

Pathology

Epithelial tumours of the salivary glands have been classified by the WHO panel into four major groups but since certain tumours cannot be placed into any of these four classes a fifth group has been added labelled, not unnaturally, 'unclassified'.

1 *Pleomorphic adenoma*
This is also known as the 'mixed cell tumour' because it was originally thought that these tumours were composed of both epithelial and connective tissue elements. The most arresting feature is the mucous stroma which may form either cartilage or bone and the second important histological feature is the pleomorphic nature of the cellular component.

The ultrastructure of the epithelial cells found in the tumour indicates that they are of both duct and myoepithelial origin but some cells have features of both types of cells and some are indeterminate, being insufficiently differentiated.

2 *Monomorphic adenoma*
These are benign tumours composed of uniform epithelial cells of only one type. Four different varieties of monomorphic adenoma have been recognized, of which the two which most frequently occur are the adenolymphoma and the oncocytoma.

The adenolymphoma is also variously known as papillary cystadenoma lymphomatosum or Warthin's tumour. This tumour is a distinctive neoplasm consisting of normal lymphoid tissue with germinal centres which contain clefts and cysts lined by a double layered epithelium. It is now accepted that these tumours arise in lymph nodes incorporated within the parotid during its development.

The oncocytoma is composed of large pink cells and is, therefore, also known as the oxyphilic adenoma.

Both the adenolymphoma and the oncocytoma may represent a hyperplastic rather than a neoplastic change since oncocytic changes also occur with advancing age in normal duct epithelium.

3 *Mucoepidermoid tumours*
All these tumours are considered to be malignant although their rate of growth

is variable and their histological appearance gives no indication of their degree of aggression. This type of tumour constitutes between 5 and 10 per cent of all salivary gland tumours and 90 per cent occur in the parotid gland. Macroscopically mucoepidermoid tumours have no capsule. Histologically the tumour consists of small epithelioid cells of variable size which in some areas may exhibit keratin formation. Admixed with these cells are goblet and clear, mucin-producing cells with occasionally, sebaceous cells. All these different cell types form islets or strands within a connective tissue stroma.

4 Acinic-cell tumours

These are rare tumours seldom found in any other tissue than the parotid gland itself. Histologically such tumours are highly cellular with cells arranged in a solid adenocarcinomatous pattern. The majority of the cells have the appearance of the normal serous acinar cells with a finely granular cytoplasm. The aggressiveness of these tumours is exceedingly variable and the histomorphological findings do not help in assessing their prognosis.

5 Carcinoma of the salivary glands

Malignant tumours of the salivary glands are divided into five types:

(a) *adenoid cystic carcinoma*. This tumour was previously known as the cylindroma. It is very malignant and has a typical cribriform histological appearance due to the presence of small cystic spaces arranged in small clusters. These tumours are much commoner in the minor salivary glands than the parotid.
(b) *adenocarcinoma*. These tumours possess a tubular, papillary or undifferentiated pattern.
(c) *squamous carcinoma*. This is a rare tumour confined to the parotid gland itself possessing the same histological structure as squamous carcinoma elsewhere in the body.
(d) *undifferentiated carcinoma*. This is a rare tumour which is so poorly differentiated that it cannot be classified.
(e) *malignant pleomorphic adenoma*. Carcinoma arising in a previously benign pleomorphic adenoma represents not more than 10 per cent of lesions of the mixed cell category.

Clinical presentation of parotid tumours

The majority of parotid tumours, whether benign or malignant, present as painless discrete swellings that frequently have been noted for many years before the patient seeks advice. This is so even when the tumour is frankly malignant such as the adenoid cystic carcinoma. However, four other presenting symptoms and signs may be present when the tumour is malignant:

1 facial nerve palsy. This is particularly common in association with adenoid cystic carcinoma which specifically tends to spread along nerve sheaths and with truly undifferentiated carcinomata.

2   lymphatic metastases. These are particularly common in association with the very rare squamous carcinomata of the parotid.
3   distant blood-borne metastases are observed particularly in adenoid cystic carcinoma and acinic-cell tumours.
4   ulceration of the overlying skin, although this is occasionally seen with large wholly benign tumours such as the pleomorphic adenoma.

Frequency and behaviour of the various tumour types

1   Pleomorphic adenoma
This comprises 90 per cent of all benign tumours of the parotid. However, although this tumour is benign a considerable recurrence rate varying from between 30 and 60 per cent has been reported following simple enucleation. There are three chief causes for this:

(*a*) the tumour may have a multifocal origin;
(*b*) tumour cells may have involved the false capsule which is formed by compression of normal parotid tissue;
(*c*) during enucleation the tumour may become fragmented leading to local reimplantation.

The peak incidence of these tumours is in the fifth decade and prior to presentation the patient nearly always gives a history of a swelling over many years which has been both painless and slow growing.

2   Papillary cystadenoma lymphomatosum
This tumour is predominantly a tumour of males. The peak incidence is in the seventh decade and the tumour may be recognized prior to operation by its cystic nature and the fact that it tends to involve the lower pole of the gland. Such tumours do not appear to recur following simple enucleation.

3   Mucoepidermoid tumours
This tumour accounts for between 5 and 10 per cent of all parotid tumours and although their peak incidence is in the fourth decade they have been reported in childhood. Their clinical behaviour appears to be unrelated to their histological appearance.

4   Adenoid cystic carcinoma
This is the commonest truly malignant tumour of salivary tissue but unlike all other tumours, both benign and malignant it is more common in the minor salivary glands than the parotid itself. The maximum age incidence is in the sixth decade and the tumour may have been present for many years before the patient presents, sometimes with a solitary swelling but otherwise with a swelling associated with a facial palsy, lymph node metastases or blood-borne metastases to the lungs.

5   Adenocarcinoma
These tumours form approximately 5 per cent of all parotid tumours and in

approximately 25 per cent of all cases apart from a diffuse hard swelling in the parotid there is an associated facial palsy.

Treatment

1 *Pleomorphic adenoma*
The tendency of these tumours to recur following simple enucleation has led to alternative methods of treatment being advocated. Which is chosen is determined in large part by the policy adopted by individual surgeons. The following alternatives are available.

(a) *Simple enucleation followed by HER.* This method has been shown in two large series in the UK to be effective in reducing the number of recurrences to practically zero. However, critics of this method would argue that if used in younger patients it leaves a long period for both recurrence and the possibility of radiation induced cancer.

(b) *Total superficial parotidectomy.* To perform a superficial parotidectomy the facial nerve must be identified at the point where it leaves the stylomastoid foramen and traced down along its whole length through the parotid tissue. Since no branches leave it from the posterior aspect, this should be the correct angle of attack. The protagonists of parotidectomy maintain that this technique permits removal of the tumour together with a covering of healthy normal tissue, thus avoiding two of the major causes of recurrence.

The complications of superficial parotidectomy include facial paralysis, dryness of the mouth, salivary fistula, and the auriculotemporal syndrome, which may be distressing. The last consists of gustatory sweating and redness in the cutaneous distribution of the auriculotemporal nerve. One explanation is that divided parasympathetic secreting fibres grow into the sheath of the auriculotemporal bundle so that stimuli that would normally evoke secretion produce sweating.

Critics of total superficial parotidectomy would argue that not only does this operation result in the complications already noted but that it is too extensive for small tumours. Furthermore, although excellent clearance of the tumour may be achieved over nearly all parts of the tumour it is often found that in one part the clearance is minimal, thus still leaving recurrence a possibility.

2 *Limited parotidectomy*
This removes only that part of the gland in which the tumour is situated. Nevertheless, even if this method is adopted a formal identification of the facial nerve must precede resection otherwise partial facial palsy will occur.

Malignant tumours

In the author's experience of malignant tumours of the parotid excision is rarely practical. However, radical excision possibly removing the vertical ramus of the mandible, the temporomandibular joint, the mastoid and the overlying skin is theoretically possible. Radical parotidectomy inevitably means that the facial nerve will be destroyed. In fact, in the case of an adenoid cystic carcinoma it is essential to remove the nerve in its entirety because of this tumour's predilection for infiltrating the nerve sheath.

If the facial nerve is removed in part it may be possible to bridge the gap by means of a nerve graft using the great auricular nerve.

When tumour tissue is left *in situ* then conventional high energy irradiation must be used in an attempt to arrest tumour growth although the overall results leave much to be desired. A further method, neutron irradiation, has been used but again the results are equivocal. The author has only one patient in whom an adenoid cystic carcinoma presented after a history of some 15 years. No facial palsy was present but exploration revealed a clearly inoperable tumour. This was treated by Dr Mary Caterall at the MRC unit at Hammersmith and to date some 3 years after irradiation the tumour appears to be controlled.

GENERALIZED PAROTID ENLARGEMENT

1 Mikulicz syndrome

This condition was originally described by Mikulicz, in 1888, as a benign enlargement of the salivary and lacrimal glands in a middle-aged man. It is, however, now recognized that the disease, though rare, is commonest in middle-aged women and that it is often associated with xerostomia, and keratoconjunctivitis sicca. The histological picture of lymphocytic infiltration of the gland, together with the finding of antibodies reactive to salivary epithelium, suggest that the condition is mediated by immunological mechanisms.

Clinical presentation
The patient presents with gradual enlargement of one or both parotid glands, with or without an associated enlargement of the lacrimal glands. Parotid secretion is much reduced, and the patient may complain of dryness of the mouth and difficulty in swallowing. A similar effect on the lacrimal glands produces conjunctivitis. If the condition progresses, other mucus-secreting glands are affected, leading to dryness of the tracheopharyngeal and laryngeal areas, and to pulmonary infection. When associated with rheumatoid arthritis, the condition becomes Sjøgren's syndrome.

Diagnosis
Intravenous injection of pilocarpine nitrate, 5 mg, will show decreased parotid secretion. Sialography may show the presence of sialectasis and a ^{99m}Tc scan reduced uptake of the isotope. Biopsy will give a typical histological picture of lymphoid infiltration together with ductal obliteration by focal proliferation of the lining and myoepithelial cells.

Treatment

There is no specific treatment for this condition. Dryness of the eyes must be treated by frequent instillation of methylcellulose drops and the wearing of glasses. If this fails to relieve the patient a tarsorrhaphy may be necessary. The dryness of the mouth that produces difficulty in swallowing can be overcome only by taking frequent drinks at meal times. Xerostomia predisposes to tooth decay which, in turn, predisposes to ascending parotitis, hence it is essential that dental caries should be treated. Only when gross enlargement of the gland causes severe deformity should the gland or glands be excised.

2 Acute parotitis

The commonest cause of acute parotitis is mumps. The pathological changes in mumps parotitis are acinar cell necrosis and lymphocytic infiltration of the interstitial tissues. The disease usually follows an incubation period of between 12 and 20 days. Pain develops in the region of one parotid which enlarges and becomes tender. In most patients the condition is bilateral. After 2–3 days the swelling begins to diminish and pain gradually decreases. Associated with parotitis may be a mumps meningitis, pancreatitis, orchitis or encephalitis. No specific treatment is required.

3 Acute suppurative parotitis

This is due to an ascending infection from the mouth, usually in dehydrated postoperative patients, infants, or patients receiving deep X-ray therapy to the face. Once commonplace, it is now rarely seen because of the importance attached to maintaining adequate hydration and performing regular mouth toilet. Usually, only one gland is enlarged. A painful, tender swelling develops in the parotid area and pressure over the duct usually causes pus to discharge into the mouth from the opening of Stenson's duct. As the condition deteriorates the temperature rises and trismus develops, making rehydration by the oral route impossible.

Treatment consists of administering an appropriate antibiotic, e.g. cloxacillin. Irradiation in the postoperative group will often produce resolution if this is done before pus formation. Once an abscess has formed incision and drainage are required.

4 Sialectasis

This produces a recurrent painful swelling of the parotid glands, due to recurrent infection of the dilated acini. The condition is commonly associated with trumpet players and glass blowers. If the former are asked to exhale with the lips tightly pursed and the nose compressed, the gland inflates like a balloon. In severe cases a plain X-ray shows the ducts and acini outlined by air, and sialography shows the ducts and acini grossly dilated.

Treatment
If possible, the patient should refrain from the activity that predisposes to the ascending infection. Any dental condition should be treated to diminish oral infection, and minor degrees of infection can be treated by intermittent administration of the appropriate antibiotic. If the gland is grossly disorganized and both recurrent swelling and pain are causing much inconvenience, a superficial parotidectomy is required.

5 Parotid calculi

Parotid calculi are relatively uncommon particularly in comparison to the frequency of calculi in the submandibular gland. However, the features associated with a parotid calculus are sudden swelling and pain in the gland on the affected side accompanied by a cessation of salivation. A spurt of saliva heralds the relief of symptoms and regression of the swelling. A sialogram showing a stricture of the duct together with proximal dilatation is usually indicative that a calculus has been present even if it cannot be radiologically demonstrated at the time of the investigation. In the presence of the latter radiological findings the duct should be dilated with lacrimal duct dilators.

6.2 Causes and treatment of dysphagia

Definition. The term dysphagia implies difficulty but not pain on swallowing. The difficulty may be intermittent or progressive, and may involve the swallowing of solids rather than liquids, or both. The causes may be classified as follows:

Congenital
(a) Atresia
(b) Stenosis
(c) Dysphagia lusoria

Acquired
Diseases of the wall of the oesophagus
1 Tumours
    Benign
    (a) Lipoma
    (b) Leiomyoma
    Malignant
    (a) Adenocarcinoma
    (b) Squamous carcinoma
2 Strictures
    (a) Due to corrosives

  (b) Due to acid/pepsin regurgitation
3 Neurological
  (a) Infective—
   Diphtheria
   Polioencephalitis
   Syphilitic pachymeningitis
   Bulbar paralysis
   Polyneuritis
  (b) Non-infective—
   Myasthenia gravis
   Thrombosis or bleeding in brain stem
4 Neuromuscular
  (a) Pharyngeal pouch
  (b) Plummer–Vinson–Patterson syndrome
  (c) Diffuse spasm
5 Connective tissue disease: scleroderma
6 Intraluminal obstruction
  (a) FB
  (b) Bolus obstruction
7 Extrinsic pressure
  (a) Pressure by enlarged lymph nodes from any cause
  (b) Dysphagia lusoria, when abnormal vessels become dilated due to atherosclerosis
8 Psychosomatic. Globus hystericus. This condition presents with dysphagia associated with a lump in the throat. Although the majority of sufferers have no organic abnormality they should be investigated since in a minority of patients an organic lesion, most commonly a hiatus hernia, will be found.

 Discussion in this section will be restricted to the diagnosis and treatment of pharyngeal pouch, the Plummer–Vinson syndrome, carcinoma of the oesophagus, benign strictures associated with reflux oesophagitis and achalasia of the cardia.

Pharyngeal pouch, otherwise known as Zenker's pharyngeal diverticulum

Pathology

A pharyngeal pouch is a pulsion diverticulum although there remains considerable disagreement over the causal factor. The following theories have been proposed:

1 failure of the horizontal fibres of the cricopharyngeus to relax during the act of swallowing;
2 premature closure of the cricopharyngeal sphincter during the act of swallowing;
3 hypertonicity of the cricopharyngeal sphincter due to reflex stimulation, possibly because of associated excessive gastro-oesophageal reflux.

Whatever the underlying cause the pouch is formed by an out-pouching of the pharyngeal mucosa and submucosa through the weak area which normally exists between the oblique and horizontal fibres of the cricopharyngeus, otherwise known as Killian's dehiscence.

Symptomatology

This condition is commoner in males than females and classically is more frequently seen in the elderly. In some patients severe dysphagia may occur even though the pouch itself is small and in others small pouches may be incidentally found during the course of a barium swallow in the absence of any symptoms whatsoever. As the pouch enlarges it is displaced sideways, usually protruding to the left side of the neck and a swelling may be observed particularly after eating. The presence of such a high obstruction leads to the spillage of retained fluid or food into the larynx with the result that the patient may develop an irritating cough particularly at night. As the dysphagia increases in severity so weight loss and cachexia follow and in long-standing cases actual pneumonitis develops so that the patient may present with the symptoms and signs of a pulmonary infection.

When the patient suffers from an exceedingly large sac he may be aware of the sac filling during eating or drinking. Apart from dysphagia the main symptoms associated with this condition are regurgitation of food and severe halitosis.

Investigation

The only investigation required for the diagnosis of a pharyngeal pouch is a barium swallow, when the pouch can be seen in nearly every view. If the pouch is large the fundus descends into the superior mediastinum.

Treatment

The correct treatment is excision of the pouch, otherwise the patient is faced with progressive deterioration and, possibly, severe pulmonary complications. The pharynx is approached through a collar incision in the neck at the level of the cricoid cartilage or by an incision along the anterior border of the left sternomastoid.

Following the incision through the deep cervical fascia, the lateral lobe of the thyroid gland is mobilized by division of the middle thyroid veins, if they are present, after which the pouch is gradually dissected free. The essential part of the operation is to divide the sac at the neck and close the defect in two layers. Pharyngeal narrowing is avoided during the reconstruction by passing a large oesophageal tube through the pharynx.

Plummer–Vinson syndrome

This is often termed the Plummer–Vinson–Patterson syndrome because Patterson and Kelly were the first to describe it.

Pathology
The cause of the dysphagia is, at first, spasm of the circular muscle fibres of the upper end of the oesophagus which is later associated with the formation of webs arising from the anterior wall of the cervical oesophagus. The mucosa overlying this area of the oesophagus may be hyperkeratotic, or desquamated and friable. The condition is precancerous being associated with the subsequent development of a postcricoid carcinoma. This condition is always associated with a low serum iron (normal value, 80–160 µg/dl; males 13–31 mmol/l, females 11–29 mmol/l) and a hypochromic microcytic anaemia.

Symptomatology
The main features of this condition are a long-standing dysphagia associated with a sideropenic anaemia and the symptoms thereof.

The syndrome is confined almost exclusively to middle-aged women between 35 and 60 years of age. Glossitis, angular stomatitis, and koilonychia are almost invariably present. The patient complains of progressive dysphagia due to muscular incoordination at the level of the larynx.

Investigations
1 Blood examination reveals a hypochromic microcytic anaemia.
2 Serum iron, low values expected.
3 Barium swallow, reveals an anterior web or pin-hole orifice at the level of the cricoid cartilage.

Treatment
Treatment consists of dilating the web by bougies via an oesophagoscope. At the same time the iron deficiency anaemia should be corrected.

Carcinoma of the oesophagus

Carcinoma of the oesophagus exists throughout the population of the world but epidemiological studies have shown great variations in incidence. Thus, the highest incidence in the male is in the South African Bantu, which is 41 per 100 000 compared to an incidence of 0.6 per 100 000 males in Hungary. In females the highest incidence is again in the Bantu, 36 per 100 000 compared to 3.5 per 100 000 females in the United Kingdom.

Certain aetiological factors have been considered responsible in the Bantu, among which are maize beer-drinking, tobacco smoking or chewing, and malnutrition possibly associated with chronic alcoholism. However, in the Transkei the Bantu women smoke and drink little despite a high incidence of oesophageal cancer.

Rarely, there appears to be a genetic association between the possibly inherited condition of tylosis, thickening of the palms and soles, and the development of carcinoma of the oesophagus in adult life.

Pathology
Carcinoma of the oesophagus may exist at any level, its distribution being in

part determined by the group who report it, since the incidence of upper cervical and hypopharyngeal tumours is always higher in series reported by radiotherapists because radiotherapy has been more commonly used than surgery for this group of tumours.

Approximately half of oesophageal cancers involve the mid third of the viscus, one-quarter the upper third and the remainder the lower third. The disease is approximately four times commoner in men than women, except in the postcricoid region.

Macroscopic appearance. The tumour may be annular, ulcerating, or polypoidal.

Histopathology

Tumours of the upper and middle thirds are usually squamous in type, varying from well differentiated keratinizing to undifferentiated forms. In the lower third the majority are adenocarcinomata which have arisen from the fundal epithelium of the stomach. Submucosal infiltration without obvious macroscopic involvement is commonplace and at the time of death 60 per cent of patients show disseminated disease to regional lymph nodes.

Clinical aspects

Nearly 25 per cent of patients have a history of 6 months or longer before seeking advice. The symptom complexes produced by oesophageal cancer vary from an abnormal sensation behind the sternum to definite dysphagia. Symptoms may also be produced by involvement of adjacent structures. This can happen early because the thin submucosal and muscular layers of the oesophagus provide little resistance to the invasion of neighbouring structures. The dysphagia is mostly related to solid foods, but gradually there is difficulty in swallowing fluids as well. When this stage is reached, there may be overspill into the larynx, with production of pulmonary complications, including lung abscess. As the dysphagia worsens, the nutritional state of the patient suffers and secondary anaemia develops. Diagnosis of carcinoma of the oesophagus is usually made by a barium swallow followed by oesophagoscopy.

Radiological findings

Plain X-rays of the chest may show:

1 enlarged mediastinal lymph nodes;
2 infective complications due to regurgitation.

Barium swallow may show:

1 a stricture failing to relax even after the administration of antispasmodics;
2 increased peristalsis proximal to the stricture and only moderate dilatation;
3 a filling defect with typical shouldering, if barium passes through the stricture a typical 'rat tail' deformity may be seen;
4 oesophageal spasm.

5 one interesting radiological finding is that dilatation of the oesophagus above a malignant obstruction is seldom as marked as that seen above a fibrous stricture of the oesophagus caused by acid/pepsin regurgitation or achalasia.

Oesophagoscopy
This may be performed using either a rigid or fibreoptic flexible instrument. A disadvantage of the former is that a general anaesthetic is required whereas the latter procedure can be carried out under Valium sedation alone. When the former instrument is used a more accurate measurement of the distance of the lesion from the incisor teeth can be obtained and a larger biopsy can be removed. Using a fibreoptic instrument the biopsy material is small in amount and when the lesion is spreading within the submucosa rather than protruding into the lumen the surgeon may have to be content with brushings from the strictured area, an investigation which may give rise to a false negative examination.

Bronchoscopy
This investigation is particularly indicated in the presence of chest symptoms or an abnormal chest X-ray. Direct spread, the presence of a fistula, or carinal deformity due to involvement of the mediastinal lymph nodes may be observed.

Management
Regardless of the method of treatment the overall results are poor. Different series have been reported showing only 2–3 per cent survival over 5 years, a 9 per cent 2-year survival following irradiation, and a 20 per cent survival for 2 years after surgery performed for middle third and lower third tumours. More recently, reports of 20 per cent 5-year survival have been reported using super voltage radiotherapy for the treatment of squamous carcinomata. In general there is a strong argument for irradiating all squamous cell tumours and reserving surgery for adenocarcinoma. Radiotherapy is initially safer than surgery, and following irradiation there may be some improvement in swallowing within 2 weeks. Because of the submucosal spread which is typical of oesophageal tumours the field of irradiation must extend 5 cm above and below the macroscopic limits of the growth. If the tumour has destroyed the whole thickness of the oesophagus, perforation and mediastinitis follow very rapidly, complications which are nearly always fatal.

Preoperative preparation
In the UK the majority of patients suffering from carcinoma of the oesphagus are elderly and already suffering from varying degrees of malnutrition. It is, therefore, essential that an adequate cardiopulmonary assessment is made prior to any surgical manoeuvre. Furthermore, if there has been considerable weight loss, say between 10 and 15 per cent of total body weight a period of preoperative nutritional supplementation is advisable. This may be accomplished either by intubation through the malignant stricture using a fine-bore Silastic catheter which is introduced over a guide wire under radiological

control or a period of parenteral nutrition may be considered using a mixture of synthetic amino acids and 50 per cent dextrose.

Surgery
This is usually reserved for tumours of the middle and lower thirds of the oesophagus although the stomach can be brought out into the neck, allowing relatively high tumours to be excised together with the pharynx.

In the treatment of lower third tumours which are most frequently adenocarcinomata arising from the fundus of the stomach, an accepted exposure is obtained by a left oblique thoracoabdominal incision between the seventh and eighth ribs.

The oesophageal growth is first mobilized, after which the stomach is dissected free and left supplied with blood via the right gastric and gastroepiploic arteries. The upper part of the stomach is then resected and closed, after which an anastomosis is performed within the chest. The wound is closed and an intrathoracic underwater drain is left *in situ*.

Tumours of the middle third are best treated by a three-stage procedure which terminates with the fundus of the stomach being anastomosed to the cervical oesophagus in the neck. Such an anastomosis avoids the problems associated with a mediastinal anastomosis and ensures adequate clearance of the growth. If neoplastic tissue is left *in situ* this should be marked by silver clips to aid the radiotherapist in delineating his fields.

Treatment of the inoperable tumour
If the tumour is inoperable or there is local recurrence leading to renewed dysphagia a tube of the Souttar, Atkinson, Mousseau–Barbin, or Celestin type may be passed. A disadvantage of the Mousseau–Barbin type tube is that a laparotomy is required for its insertion whereas the Souttar or Atkinson type can be directly introduced, after passing a dilator through the growth via a rigid oesophagoscope.

When a tube is *in situ* only semisolid foods can be swallowed; at the first sign of dysphagia the patient should swallow a mouthful of soda water or hydrogen peroxide in an attempt to clear the tube.

One of the greatest trials of the intubated patient is that if the tube enters the stomach free reflux will occur leading to persistent heartburn and 'water brash'. In order to minimize this at night the patient must sleep in a semi-upright position.

Strictures associated with gastro-oesophageal reflux

It was once considered that gastro-oesophageal reflux only occurred in the presence of a Type I, sliding hiatus hernia but the development of newer types of investigation has led to considerable doubts as to the exclusive role of sliding hernia as the cause of reflux. Recent investigators have indeed suggested that there is only a coincidental role between the two conditions and this is supported by the fact that in many patients suffering from the symptoms of reflux no hernia can be demonstrated.

Pathology
When reflux alone is present biopsy of the oesophageal mucosa shows even in the presence of an apparently normal mucosa a widening of the basal cell layer and penetration of the papillae of the lamina propria more than two-thirds of the way through the epithelium to the luminal surface. When naked eye changes in the mucosa are present the classical histological signs of inflammation are present.

When the inflammatory changes extend to involve the submucosa the proliferation of fibrous tissue leads to the development of a stricture, usually short, tapering distally and occurring just above the gastro-oesophageal mucosal junction.

In some patients, a more localized stricture is met with due to healing of a solitary ulcer of the oesophagus, which more truly resembles a peptic ulcer. This type of ulcer is known as the Barrett's ulcer, after the surgeon who first described the condition. Investigation has shown that this type of deep penetrating ulcer is found only in an oesophagus lined by a gastric type of mucosa that does not contain parietal cells. Previous workers thought that this epithelium formed a continuous lining of the oesophagus and extended for a variable distance from the gastro-oesophageal junction.

The origin of this type of mucosa remains in doubt. One theory suggested that the condition was atavistic and congenital whereas another suggests that it arises as a result of metaplasia caused by exposure of the normal oesophageal mucosa to an acid/pepsin environment. In this condition the stricture develops at the squamocolumnar junction and predominantly involves squamous epithelium. Such strictures tend to be short and if a penetrating ulcer is present the stricture may be eccentrically placed and associated with a large inflammatory component.

Clinical aspects
The clinical history of a peptic stricture of the oesophagus is usually diagnostic. A long history of reflux and heartburn precede the insidious development of dysphagia. Even so, dysphagia is not necessarily associated with actual stenosis; both oedema and spasm may produce the symptom.

It may also be noted that as the degree of dysphagia worsens so the severity of heartburn diminishes.

Investigations
Barium swallow and meal. The barium swallow may demonstrate:

1 irregular mucosal folds in the lower oesophagus above a gastric pouch;
2 a smoothly tapering narrowed oesophageal segment running downwards towards the hernial pouch;
3 concentric narrowing of the oesophagus some distance above the oesophago-gastric junction. This appearance suggests a gastric lined oesophagus.

Oesophagoscopy. This investigation is necessary to confirm the presence of oesophagitis and to confirm the benign nature of the stricture. Oesophagitis produces a scarlet-looking mucosa which bleeds easily on contact with a conventional rigid oesophagoscope.

Treatment
Once an organic stricture has developed both active as well as medical treatment are required.

Four methods of treatment are available:

1 intermittent dilatation (bougienage). This method of treatment can be used as a primary method of treatment remembering that as a severe stricture is dilated so reflux together with its symptoms and complications will begin again. However, in some elderly patients dilatation remains the optimal method of treatment so long as it is accompanied by medical means to reduce acid secretion, e.g. H_2 antagonists. Bougienage may be accomplished by tapered mercury-filled rubber Maloney dilators dilating the oesophagus to a diameter of 13 mm, 40 Fr. If the stricture is very tight metal olive-shaped dilators should be passed. If these are passed without the use of a guide wire the great danger is of perforation of the oesophagus;
2 repair of the associated hiatus hernia or an antireflux procedure in the absence of a hernia. Many authorities on this subject have shown that if the oesophagogastric junction is rendered competent the symptoms will be alleviated or eliminated. In part, this can be explained by the reduction in inflammatory oedema in the inflamed area but, possibly, some resolution of the fibrosis also occurs because the intervals between dilatation become gradually longer;
3 excision of the strictured area and replacement with a jejunal or colonic loop. This operation is reserved for severe cases uncontrolled by the measures already described. A loop long enough to provide an intra-abdominal segment is interposed between the oesophagus and the stomach. This assists in preventing oesophageal reflux;
4 the Thal fundic patch. This procedure, like the interposition of a jejunal loop, is rarely used. It consists of incising the stricture in a longitudinal direction and then after mobilizing the fundus of the stomach suturing the serosal surface of the stomach to the gaping opening in the oesophagus.

Achalasia of the cardia

Pathology
This condition is due to a neuromuscular disorder of the lower end of the oesophagus which leads to failure of the lower oesophagus to relax and propagate the normal peristaltic wave initiated by deglutition. Ganglion cells in the myenteric plexus at the lower end of the oesophagus may be deficient and in some patients the extra-oesophageal vagus nerves show Wallerian degeneration. The stagnation of food materials in the oesophagus produces mucosal ulceration and severe oesophagitis.

Once obstruction has developed and there has been decompensation, oesophageal contents may be aspirated into the respiratory passages, producing recurrent bronchopneumonia or lung abscess.

Clinical aspects

The condition is commoner in women and although met with at any age it is commonest in the fourth and fifth decades.

Three stages have been described. First there may be dysphagia associated with retrosternal pain, and the symptoms may be confused with diffuse oesophageal spasm. In the second stage the pain may diminish and the dysphagia may be intermittent. Finally, there is continuous dysphagia associated with retrosternal discomfort, anorexia, and loss of weight. Associated with this stage, also, are the respiratory complications of aspiration.

Investigations

Barium swallow. The precise radiological findings depend upon the stage of the disease. Initially, despite considerable dysphagia, there may be no radiological signs but as the disease advances the oesophagus dilates, becomes flaccid and tapers to its distal end. If the organ has not been washed out prior to the swallow, retained food products are seen in the lumen.

Manometry. This is particularly useful in the presence of symptoms and an absence of physical signs, for in achalasia the normal propagated pressure waves are replaced by a series of waves of lower amplitude, and in the area of the lower oesophageal sphincter there is no relaxation on swallowing.

Oesophagoscopy. This confirms the capacious oesophagus, the presence of food retention, ulceration of the mucosa, and absence of a neoplasm in the area of the radiological narrowing.

Treatment

Two methods of treatment are possible. The first, forceful hydrostatic dilatation of the lower end of the oesophagus, is a method that has little place in modern therapy. The accepted treatment in the absence of contraindication is surgical myotomy or Heller's operation.

This operation consists of division of the oesophageal and gastric muscle in a vertical direction down to the mucosa over a distance of approximately 5 cm. In the past, one of the common complications of this operation was reflux oesophagitis but this can be avoided by dividing the muscle on the lesser curve aspect of the stomach so that the oblique gastric muscle fibres that serve to maintain the acute angle of entry at the oesophagogastric junction are preserved.

Results

A survey of the published results following myotomy shows that approximately 60 per cent of patients obtained complete relief. Transient attacks of dysphagia that remain within acceptable limits are known and a few patients require further operation. The incidence of reflux oesophagitis varies between 3 and 30 per cent, depending on the author, a complication that usually begins within 2 years of operation. Interestingly enough, the radiological signs often remain grossly abnormal even in the presence of clinical improvement.

6.3 Hiatus hernia: symptoms, treatment and complications

The first paper on the subject of hiatus hernia was by Harrington in 1940, followed, in 1951, by Allison, who drew attention to the two types of hernia, the sliding and the paraoesophageal, the former being nearly ten times more common than the latter.

Both are anatomical abnormalities, but whereas the sliding hernia is frequently associated with gastro-oesophageal reflux, the paraoesophageal is subject to the complications of bleeding, ulceration, gastric volvulus, strangulation, perforation, and acute dilatation. Such complications may be sudden and take place in a totally asymptomatic individual. Alternatively, a prodromal period in which the patient complains of dyspnoea and palpitations, particularly in the recumbent position at night, may have preceded the acute complication.

Mechanism of gastro-oesophageal reflux
In a normal individual, reflux is controlled by a variety of mechanisms whose relative importance is open to some doubt. These include:

1 *the lower oesophageal sphincter.* This is a physiological rather than an anatomical concept. Its presence can be demonstrated by manometry studies which disclose a high pressure zone at the lower end of the oesophagus. However, high pressure in this zone does not necessarily equate with gastro-oesophageal competence and, conversely, a low high-pressure zone does not necessarily indicate that reflux is inevitable;
2 *the acute angle of entry of the oesophagus into the stomach.* The importance of this angle has been demonstrated in animals such as the dog, in which division of the oblique fibres passing from the region of the lesser curve over the cardia can be shown to precipitate reflux. In man, the relief of cardiospasm by myotomy on the anterior surface of the oesophagus and stomach also leads to reflux;
3 *the intradiaphragmatic portion of the oesophagus.* This small length of oesophagus is believed to be closed by intra-abdominal pressure. It is maintained in the subdiaphragmatic position by the attachment of the phreno-oesophageal ligament which is stretched and ineffective in the presence of a sliding hernia;
4 *the mucosal rosette.* The bulging of the mucosa into the cardia may produce a valve-like effect when intragastric pressure is raised.

In the past it was considered that a hiatus hernia always accompanied reflux of the gastric contents but it is now recognized that reflux can occur in the absence of any anatomical displacement of the cardia. Thus the prevalence of hiatus hernia has been reported to be no greater among patients with symptomatic reflux than healthy control subjects and in 45 per cent of patients suffering from the symptoms associated with reflux no hernia can be demonstrated.

Symptomatology of reflux
The typical symptoms of gastro-oesophageal reflux are belching, retrosternal burning, and the regurgitation of gastric contents. All are made worse by physical actions which increase the intra-abdominal pressure, such as stooping, and by recumbency. The symptoms are often precipitated by a gain in weight or the presence of a large intra-abdominal tumour such as a fibroid, ovarian cyst or pregnant uterus.

In addition to the classic symptoms already considered reflux oesophagitis may occasionally give rise to a symptomatic iron deficiency anaemia even in the absence of symptoms and occasional nocturnal reflux may result in aspiration and coughing.

Atypical symptoms of reflux include 'indigestion', postprandial fullness, dysphagia and chest pain.

As oesophagitis develops and progresses so the development of a stricture may lead to increasing dysphagia and decreasing reflux symptoms.

Frequency of symptoms
Palmer, in a series of 1000 patients, found that nearly 50 per cent of patients with a radiologically demonstrable hernia had no symptoms even in the presence of oesophagitis, that 9 per cent suffered typical symptoms and that a further 13 per cent suffered such severe chest pain that coronary artery disease had been suspected. Concomitant upper gastrointestinal pathology such as duodenal and gastric ulceration, biliary and pancreatic disease is not uncommon, all or any of which may give rise to symptoms.

Pathological changes associated with reflux
The pathological changes induced by reflux are dependent upon the type of epithelium lining the oesophagus. In the majority of individuals the lower oesophagus is lined by squamous epithelium. The introduction of the flexible fibreoptic oesophagoscope and the performance of more frequent biopsies of the oesophagus in patients complaining of reflux symptoms has led to the finding that prior to the more overt changes of oesophagitis subtle changes take place in the mucosa.

The chief changes include an increasing thickness of the basal cell layer so that it constitutes more than 15 per cent of the total epithelial thickness and penetration of the papillae of the lamina propria more than two-thirds of the way through the epithelium to the luminal surface. These changes are indicative of an increased rate of epithelial cell turnover and are reliable indicators of excessive reflux.

As the condition progresses the continuity of the mucosal lining of the lower oesophagus is interrupted by multiple shallow ulcers and endoscopic biopsies reveal the classical signs of inflammation, i.e. granulation tissue, polymorphonuclear infiltration and granulation tissue.

Further progression leads to an underlying cicatricial fibrosis.

In the 1950s, Barrett drew attention to another type of oesophageal ulceration which, instead of remaining superficial, had all the pathological characteristics of chronic peptic ulceration. This occurs only in an oesophagus lined by a columnar epithelium which resembles the mucosa of the fundus but without parietal cells. The reason for this variation in mucosal type remains in doubt. It may be an atavistic condition caused by a failure to replace the columnar epithelium by squamous, which normally occurs, or, alternatively, it may be acquired; an adaptive change due to the continued presence of acid and pepsin in the lower oesophagus. The latter concept is supported by the finding of similar changes in the oesophagus of patients suffering from reflux. Ulceration in a gastric-lined oesophagus usually involves the entire thickness of the wall, leading to possible perforation or severe bleeding.

Diagnosis
Because a hiatus hernia may be symptomless and another pathology accountable for the symptoms, the first essential in diagnosis is an extremely accurate history. Thereafter a number of investigations are required.

1 *Barium meal.* This investigation will reveal the great majority of sliding herniae, particularly if the radiologist is prepared to examine the patient in a number of different positions, the most important of which is the Trendelenburg position with the stomach already partly filled with barium. If a hernia is still not observed under these conditions it may become so if a patient is asked to increase the intra-abdominal pressure by raising the legs, while at the same time continuing to breathe normally. In an uncomplicated case, a hernia may be mistaken for a large phrenic ampulla which can be induced if swallowing is interrupted by deep inspiration. However, the gastric pouch is recognized by the presence of thick gastric folds which cause transverse indentations in the sac. This pouch lies above the level of the diaphragmatic hiatus in the supine and Trendelenburg positions. If the oesophagus has not been shortened by inflammation, the pouch disappears when the patient assumes the upright position.

Whereas radiology is a satisfactory method of diagnosing the anatomical deformity around the cardia it is *not* an accurate way of diagnosing gastro-oesophageal reflux. The incidence of false negatives is believed to be as high as 60 per cent.

If, however, the oesophagitis is severe, the barium swallow may show lack of mucosal definition and later a 'granular' appearance. A stricture is evident as a narrow segment varying both in length and severity. Usually, it is several centimetres in length and funnel-shaped at its upper end. This distinguishes it from the 'shouldered' defect produced by malignant disease. Further evidence of diffuse oesophageal involvement is the irreducibility of the hernia in the erect position due to shortening of the oesophagus and fixity to the tissues of the posterior mediastinum. When a gastric-lined oesophagus is complicated by the development of a Barrett's ulcer, the ulcer is usually at the junctional zone between the normal oesophagus and the columnar segment. Above the deep crater the oesophagus may be dilated, and distally a gastric pouch can usually be demonstrated. The differential diagnosis of peptic oesophagitis includes a corrosive oesophagitis, early infiltration from a fundal neoplasm, and simple spasm.

2 *Oesophageal pH.* Many investigators have attempted to establish the presence or absence of reflux by monitoring the oesophageal pH. There are many variations in the techniques used and also in the inferences which may be drawn

from the observations made. Some investigators pass an intra-oesophageal pH electrode to about 5 cm proximal to the lower oesophageal high pressure zone and then test for brief episodic reflux by asking the patient to perform a Valsalva manoeuvre, whereas others monitor the pH for several hours.

3 *Bernstein's acid perfusion test.* When the oesophagus is perfused with 0.1 mol/l hydrochloric acid and the symptoms of which the patient complains are reproduced it can be concluded that these symptoms are due to acid reflux. Control perfusions are made with physiological saline.

4 *Oesophagoscopy.* The anticipated changes which may be seen have already been described in the pathological section.

Treatment

It is difficult to establish from the published figures what percentage of hiatus herniae require surgical treatment. Palmer found that only 5 per cent came to operation out of a total of 1000 cases. Among the generally accepted indications for surgery are the following:

1 severe intractable symptoms;
2 oesophagitis producing mucosal ulceration;
3 presence or threat of severe complications such as bleeding or stenosis.

Medical treatment

The majority of patients suffering from herniation and reflux can be adequately controlled by medical means. The chief aspects of medical treatment are:

1 avoidance of stooping, and attempting to sleep in the semi-sitting position.
2 weight reduction;
3 reduction of smoking, a dose correlation has been shown to exist between smoking and reflux and in some patients cessation of smoking produces symptomatic relief;
4 reduction of gastric acidity by the use of simple antacids such as magnesium aluminium hydroxide or by an H_2 antagonist taken at night;
5 the use of alginates such as sodium polymannuronate. This compound forms a viscid gel on the surface of the gastric contents which 'plugs' the cardia and reduces reflux.

Surgical treatment

There is general agreement that any form of repair procedure should not compromise the patient's ability to swallow, vomit, or belch.

The earlier operations such as the Allison procedure were based on an anatomical concept of the problem, whereas later workers have realized that the hernia itself is of little importance compared to the reflux which may follow.

The *Allison operation*, which for so long was the standard procedure, consisted of excision of the peritoneal sac overlying the gastric pouch, reduction of the hernia, which might entail considerable mobilization of the oesophagus, repair of the attenuated gastro-oesophageal ligament and, lastly, reconstruction of the crural sling posterior to the oesophagus.

The first of the newer physiological operations was the *Nissen fundoplication*. This involves plicating the whole circumference of the lower 2–3 inches of the oesophagus into the fundus of the stomach. When completed the oesophagogastric junction resembles an old-fashioned unspillable inkpot. The reconstructed segment may be reduced into the abdomen but regurgitation apparently ceases, even if it remains in the thorax. A criticism levelled at this type of operation is that it is impossible to vomit or regurgitate air. This complication, known as the gas-bloat syndrome, can usually be prevented by performing the wrap around the lower end of the oesophagus after passing a large-bore oesophageal tube or bougie into the stomach and, secondly, making sure that there is no incipient pyloric stenosis.

Another method of achieving a similar result is by the use of the *Belsey procedure* in which a plication is performed leaving a part of the oesophago-gastric junction exposed so that it can distend and allow the retrograde passage of gas or food.

A third approach is that devised by *Collis*, who laid great stress on the length of the intra-abdominal oesophagus, and the acute angle of His. This operation creates an intra-abdominal tube fashioned from the fundus of the stomach, which is then subjected to the closing pressure of the intra-abdominal forces.

Results

It remains impossible from the literature to gauge the relative value of these different operative procedures but between 60 and 80 per cent of those operated upon gain relief. Following the Allison type of repair some writers infer that the operative result depends upon the preoperative function of the lower oesophageal sphincter which, if competent, results in a satisfactory outcome. Nevertheless, many large series using this technique have been reported in which an asymptomatic patient has a recurrent hernia.

Using the other techniques that have been briefly described, success rates of up to 90 per cent have been reported.

Treatment of oesophageal stricture

When there is already stricture formation some form of surgical procedure becomes necessary. The methods described include:

1 *repeated dilatation*. This method is satisfactory if the stricture is so rigid that it remains dilated for some time after the passage of the oesophageal bougies but, unfortunately, dilatation may be necessary at extremely short intervals. This carries the risks of the repeated anaesthetics, and the possibility of tearing the oesophagus. Dilatation may also be indicated if the patient's condition precludes surgical intervention.
2 *surgery designed to prevent further reflux*. It is generally conceded that operations that reduce reflux will often either:
   (a) control the dysphagia by reducing the inflammatory oedema and ulceration;
   (b) improve the condition to such an extent that dilatations are required less frequently.

3 *excision of the stricture and replacement with a jejunal or colonic loop.* This represents the most radical approach of all and is usually reserved for patients whose symptoms cannot be controlled by the methods already described.

6.4 Investigation and treatment of haematemesis, excluding bleeding oesophageal varices

Definition. Haematemesis is the vomiting of blood, which may be bright red if the bleeding is copious and the blood is rapidly expelled from the stomach, or similar to coffee grounds when the haemoglobin has been altered to acid haematin by the gastric acid.

When blood is vomited the source usually lies proximal to the duodenojejunal flexure. Distal to this point melaena occurs.

Aetiology
The two common causes of a haematemesis are chronic duodenal and chronic gastric ulceration which together account for approximately 75 per cent of all cases, bleeding duodenal ulceration being twice as common as a bleeding gastric ulcer. Less common causes of upper gastrointestinal bleeding in descending order of frequency include acute gastric erosions, carcinoma of the stomach, the Mallory–Weiss syndrome, oesophagitis caused by gastric reflux and oesophageal varices.

Rarer still are a miscellaneous group including the blood dyscrasias such as leukaemia, purpura, thrombocytopenia and structural changes such as bleeding from the suture lines, usually when fashioned with non-absorbable materials, anastomotic ulceration, hereditary telangiectasia, ulcerating pancreatic neoplasms and aortoduodenal fistulae following dacron grafts of the aorta itself.

Clinical presentation
The symptoms associated with a haematemesis may be those produced by any form of bleeding, or they may be those of the precipitating cause; for example, a long history of ill health usually precedes bleeding from oesophageal varices caused by cirrhosis, or intermittent dyspepsia bleeding from a chronic duodenal ulcer.

The important points to which special attention should be paid when recording the history are:

1 a history of dyspepsia, when a chronic peptic ulcer will be suspected;
2 a drug history; this is particularly important since several drugs may cause gastric erosions including alcohol, aspirin and the newer 'anti-inflammatory' agents such as phenylbutazone. Recognition that these are the cause of bleeding is important since this is one variety of haemorrhage which should

be treated medically and surgery withheld. However, it should always be remembered that the clinical history may be quite misleading, e.g. a chronic duodenal ulcer may bleed in the total absence of any previous history and the Mallory–Weiss syndrome may develop in the absence of any overt vomiting;
3 age of the patient, since in general the older the patient the more aggressive should be the treatment;
4 first or subsequent bleed, since rebleeding signifies that operation is probably mandatory.

The important points on clinical examination are:

1 the degree of systemic disturbance;
2 stigmata of recognizable disease, e.g. the enlarged spleen and spider naevi associated with cirrhosis, the external evidence of hereditary telangiectasis.

In nearly all major reported series it has been shown that the cause of bleeding can only be established in about 50 per cent of patients from the history and clinical examination alone. It should be remembered, however, that chronic duodenal ulceration is particularly common in cirrhotics and whilst it may be assumed that the source of bleeding is from the oesophageal varices it may well be coming from the associated ulcer.

Therefore, in all patients investigations must be performed to establish, if possible, the precise cause of bleeding but before these are performed the general condition of the patient must be considered and if necessary improved.

The conventional criteria for immediate blood transfusion are:

1 pulse rate faster than 100 per min;
2 systolic blood pressure lower than 100 mmHg or a fall of greater than 50 mm;
3 haemoglobin of less than 9 g/dl.

Since these criteria indicate that the general condition of the patient is unstable, more accurate assessment of the cardiovascular system may be considered necessary. This can be achieved by sequential measurements of either the central venous pressure or the pulmonary artery pressure. Measurement of either is particularly valuable in detecting repeated blood loss, for the CVP will nearly always fall even though the peripheral blood pressure remains steady.

The measurement of the CVP may be considered mandatory in patients suffering from cardiorespiratory disease in order to avoid overtransfusion and the attendant risk of heart failure.

Investigations
1 *Endoscopy.* In the majority of centres fibreoptic endoscopy is now available and is regarded as the first and most important investigation. In approximately 3 per cent of patients the examination may be unsuccessful because of the amount of blood in the stomach or duodenum. Between 10 and 15 per cent of endoscopies fail to diagnose or misdiagnose gastric or duodenal ulceration. Nevertheless, accurate diagnosis is established in over 80 per cent of

patients and some endoscopists would claim an accuracy as high as 96 per cent. Preliminary gastric lavage is considered unnecessary and the majority of patients tolerate this investigation if given 10–20 mg of diazepam intravenously followed by 0.6 mg of atropine.

However, there is general agreement that whilst endoscopy increases diagnostic accuracy it has not affected the number of patients coming to surgery or the overall mortality rate.

2 *Barium meal using double contrast technique.* Radiology provides an accuracy rate of approximately 55 per cent. The problems associated with radiology in the actively bleeding individual are:

(*a*) superficial lesions such as the mucosal tears occurring in the Mallory–Weiss syndrome and the superficial ulcers of acute gastric erosions cannot be identified;
(*b*) a negative finding does not exclude a chronic ulcer since the crater may be filled with clot at the time of the investigation;
(*c*) should a lesion be demonstrated, even then it need not necessarily be the source of bleeding.

Available but seldom used diagnostic measures
1 *Measurement of pH over a period of 24 hours.* When the pH of gastric samples is measured at hourly intervals three distinct patterns of gastric secretion emerge, each with a specific meaning:

(*a*) a high nocturnal acidity (pH 1–2) indicating chronic duodenal ulceration;
(*b*) persistent nocturnal neutralization (pH 5.5) indicating chronic gastric ulceration;
(*c*) persistent achlorhydria (pH consistently more alkaline than 3.5), indicating acute gastric erosions, an effect probably due to back diffusion of acid through the mucosa.

Chandler, who originated this method, claimed an accuracy of about 80 per cent.

2 *Fluorescein string test.* A tape marked with radiopaque strips is passed and its position is verified by screening; 20 ml of a 5 per cent solution of sodium fluorescein is then administered intravenously. Four minutes later the tape is withdrawn and examined for fluorescence with ultraviolet light equipped with a Wood's filter.

3 *Arteriography.* The limitation of this examination is that the bleeding rate must be greater than 0.5 ml/min in order to demonstrate a bleeding point.

4 *Use of ^{51}Cr-labelled red cells.* A radiopaque tube is passed under X-ray control; following its localization, an injection of ^{51}Cr-labelled red cells is given intravenously and aspirates are tested for radioactivity. Although this method has been used in acute blood loss it is more satisfactory when used in patients suffering from chronic gastrointestinal haemorrhage. The method depends on the observation that chromium salts are normally not excreted into the gastrointestinal tract.

General principles of management

The management of upper gastrointestinal haemorrhage demands close cooperation between physician and surgeon. In any series of patients suffering from a haematemesis a *high risk group* can be identified by the following features:

1 *age*. Patients over 50 years of age are more likely to die than those in the younger age groups, the mortality being approximately 2 per cent under 45 years of age, 6 per cent between the ages of 45 and 59 years, 12 per cent between 60 and 69, and 20 per cent over 70;
2 *site of ulceration*. The mortality associated with bleeding gastric ulcers is twice that associated with chronic duodenal ulceration;
3 *recurrent bleeding*. This is particularly dangerous in the elderly or in patients suffering from associated cardiorespiratory disease.

From the above it follows that identification of a solitary ulcer, subacute or chronic in type, may be an absolute indication for surgery, particularly if the patient is over 50 years of age and continues to bleed or has repetitive attacks. Surgery has a further advantage in that recurrent bleeding is unusual, whereas if any patient suffering from chronic peptic ulceration is treated by medical means the incidence of recurrent bleeding within the next 5 years is as high as 20 per cent.

1 Medical management

The mainstay of the medical management of chronic bleeding peptic ulceration is adequate blood replacement, repeated bleeding in the younger patient being treated by repeated transfusion whereas in the older patient the same situation is an indication for immediate surgery. There appears to be reasonable evidence that the H_2 antagonists have little part to play in the management of bleeding from chronic peptic ulcers.

However, there is considerable evidence that H_2 antagonists are of great value in the treatment of acute gastric erosions. It was once thought that the favourable response to this type of therapy was achieved by a reduction in the mucosal blood flow produced by the inhibition of acid and pepsin secretion, an effect which was unlikely to occur when larger blood vessels were eroded. However, this thesis is unproven, certainly in the dog the gastric blood flow is maintained even following the administration of high doses of cimetidine.

2 Surgical management

(a) *Gastric ulceration*. The majority of surgeons would probably still favour the performance of a Billroth I type of gastrectomy when faced with a bleeding gastric ulcer assuming that an adequate gastric pouch is left. However, reports have appeared in the literature suggesting that this condition can be equally well treated by performing a gastrotomy, oversewing the bleeding vessel after taking a four quadrant biopsy to eliminate malignancy, and then performing a vagotomy. If a truncal vagotomy is performed a pyloroplasty is also performed but if a highly selective vagotomy is to be carried out the gastrotomy should be placed along the lesser curve and should not extend within 8 cm of the pylorus so that the nerve supply to the 'antral pump' remains undisturbed.

(b) *Duodenal ulceration.* In the past this condition was most commonly treated by a Polya, Billroth II type of gastrectomy. Unfortunately few young surgeons of today have sufficient experience to deal effectively with a difficult duodenal stump and, therefore, the more commonly practised operation at the present time is truncal vagotomy followed by pyloroplasty and oversewing the bleeding vessel in the base of the ulcer. Two sutures may be required, one superiorly and one at the inferior margin of the ulcer in order to control the gastroduodenal artery, 'the artery of haemorrhage'. If a highly selective vagotomy is performed the bleeding vessel must be approached via a duodenotomy which extends up to but does not divide the pyloric ring.

Any of these procedures may fail due to recurrent bleeding which may arise from:

(i) an anastomosis if one is present or a suture line;
(ii) the development of an erosive gastritis due to 'stress';
(iii) ineffective under-running of the bleeding vessel in an ulcer left *in situ*.

6.5 Management of bleeding oesophageal varices

Frequency
In the United Kingdom bleeding oesophageal varices account for between 3 and 5 per cent of all cases of acute gastrointestinal haemorrhage. In the USA where cirrhosis is a much commoner condition, being ranked fourth as a cause of death in men over 40 years of age, one-third of fatalities follow bleeding and the relative frequency of varices causing severe upper gastrointestinal haemorrhage rises to 10 per cent.

Clinical presentation
The patient is admitted to hospital with an overt haematemesis or if the bleeding is less severe with obvious signs of anaemia and possibly associated encephalopathy. Previous admissions may have already established that the patient is a cirrhotic but even if this diagnosis has already been made and overt signs of severe liver disease are present it should be appreciated that duodenal ulceration is common in this group of patients and that the bleeding may well be arising from this source rather than from established varices. In several large series it has in fact been demonstrated that at least 40 per cent of cirrhotics bleed from lesions other than varices.

Diagnosis
The necessary steps to establish that oesophageal varices are present and that these are the source of the haemorrhage include:

1. the most important investigation is oesophagoscopy and gastroscopy carried out, if available, with fibreoptic equipment. If bleeding has temporarily ceased the varices may be seen on oesophagoscopy as large

tortuous submucosal bluish vessels running longitudinally in the distal oesophagus. The bleeding site may be established either as a clot overlying such a vessel, by visualizing an actual bleeding point, although in some patients the lumen fills with blood so rapidly that the lesion is obscured. The importance of endoscopy lies in the fact that both Mallory–Weiss tears and acute gastric erosions, are particularly common in alcoholics and neither lesion can be detected by barium swallow or meal.

In experienced hands fibreoptic endoscopy achieves an accurate diagnosis in at least 96 per cent of patients and the majority of patients tolerate this investigation well if given 10–20 mg of diazepam by intravenous injection followed by 0.6 mg of atropine;
2 barium swallow and meal. With the increasing use of fibreoptic endoscopy these radiological measures are less frequently used although in about 90 per cent of affected individuals varices can be easily demonstrated by this method. However, as previously stated the demonstration of varices does not necessarily mean that these are the cause of the bleeding.

Assessment following resuscitation of the patient
Apart from establishing the blood group of the patient the serum albumin, serum bilirubin, prothrombin time, blood ammonia, urea and electrolytes must be estimated since each of these investigations has some bearing on the future course of treatment.

Immediate management

1 An intravenous infusion is set up. If the patient is obviously severely ill and hypotensive on admission a central venous pressure line will also be necessary, together with arrangements to monitor the venous pressure, blood pressure, and the pulse rate at half-hourly intervals.
2 An indwelling nasogastric tube is passed, the stomach is aspirated, after which 30 ml of magnesium sulphate are given via the tube, together with 1 g of neomycin every 6 hours.
3 If the prothrombin time is increased, vitamin K is administered by intramuscular injection.
4 Transfusion. The indications for transfusion are those common to any patient who is suffering from bleeding, but in this condition massive transfusions may be necessary and so 10 ml of 10 per cent solution of calcium gluconate should be given with every 1 litre of blood administered. If possible, fresh blood should be used.

If bleeding ceases, the above management is, of course, all that is necessary, but rebleeding is frequent. If this should happen, two conservative measures are available to attempt to bring the situation under control.

1 *The use of vasopressin*
Twenty units of vasopressin given over a period of 10 minutes produces a

transient rise in the mean arterial pressure and a fall in the portal venous pressure lasting for approximately three-quarters to one hour. The fall in portal pressure is the important factor, and this may control the bleeding. Repeated doses may be given and bleeding can be controlled by this method in 50–80 per cent of patients.

Recently, the technique of selective mesenteric arterial infusion of vasopressin has been introduced. Using an arterial catheter placed in the superior mesenteric artery, 0.2 units/ml per min are administered. Almost total success has been claimed for this method which may also be extremely useful immediately prior to a portacaval shunt because it produces collapse of the collateral venous pathways.

Side effects of vasopressin. Abdominal colic, evacuation of the bowels and facial pallor may all follow injection. The most serious side effect is, however, a reduction in cardiac output associated with coronary vasoconstriction. These effects may be sufficient to precipitate anginal attacks and cardiac ischaemia, and deaths following its use have been reported. Vasopressin is, therefore, contraindicated in patients who suffer from angina or whose ECG shows evidence of myocardial infarction.

2 *Oesophageal tamponade*

The Sengstaken–Blakemore tube or one of its modifications is used. This procedure may be successful in a high proportion of patients but it is not without risk.

Method. The tube is passed into the stomach which is then aspirated. The gastric balloon is then inflated with 200–250 ml of air, after which the tube is withdrawn until resistance is encountered. The oesophageal balloon is then inflated to a pressure of 40 mmHg. Nothing is given orally, and if bleeding continues the pressure in the oesophageal balloon is increased to a maximum of 55 mmHg. The oesophageal balloon is deflated at intervals and after a 6-hour clear period the whole is withdrawn.

Dangers associated with the use of balloon compression are:

(a) rupture of the gastric balloon may allow the oesophageal balloon to slide upwards and asphyxiate the patient. To obviate this a pair of scissors should be available to cut across the tube if there is sudden respiratory distress.
(b) aspiration pneumonia. After both balloons are *in situ* and inflated the patient cannot swallow either oral, nasal or pharyngeal secretions, which may well be in excess of 2 l/day. As a result aspiration may occur, particularly if the patient's conscious level is reduced or he/she is confused. The frequency of this complication has been reduced by adding an aspirating tube.
(c) ulceration of the pharynx and/or oesophagus is relatively common following the use of such tubes.

Failure of medical treatment judged by continued or repeated bleeding within 24 hours which occurs in 40 per cent on release of tamponade is an indication for intervention, the magnitude of which is determined by the general condition of the patient and the results of special investigations.

The methods available include the following.

Obliteration of the varices by the injection of sclerosants
Since the first edition of *Tutorials 1* this method of treatment, then not generally accepted, has gained much greater approval. The method was first described by Craford and Frenckner in 1939 but was not introduced into the UK until 1955 by MacBeth. By 1973 Johnson and Rodgers of Belfast, recognizing the high mortality associated with emergency shunt operations, were using sclerosant therapy as their first line of treament of bleeding varices and were able to report their results in 117 patients who received between them 217 injections. They reported control of bleeding in 93 per cent of their patients with a mortality of some 12 per cent, the latter being largely due to hepatic failure. As might be expected the long term survival of individual patients was dependent on the cause of the varices, the majority of patients suffering from an extrahepatic block surviving for long periods whereas the cirrhotics have a continuing mortality despite the arrest of bleeding.

Since that time, modifications of the original technique when only a rigid oesophagoscope was available, have been made. At the present time it is common to pass a flexible sheath with a window cut into its bottom end over a flexible oesophagoscope. The varix then protrudes through the window into the lumen of the sheath and the injection is performed with a needle passed down the biopsy channel of the endoscope. The prolapsed varix is then injected with the sclerosant, STD (sodium tetradecyl sulphate 3 per cent w/v) 3 ml, after which the flexible tube which helps to stop bleeding is then rotated until a further varix is isolated.

A recent controlled trial of this method comparing two groups of patients, one receiving sclerosant therapy and the other medical treatment, showed that the former was more effective in controlling immediate haemorrhage and associated with a much lower incidence of recurrent haemorrhage. Further advantages of sclerosant therapy over emergency shunt surgery are the relatively low mortality of the former as compared to the latter and the avoidance of encephalopathy.

Post mortem examination in patients failing to survive the acute episode show that thrombosis is greater in extent in the superficial than the deep veins. However, repeated haemorrhage is always possible whilst varices persist. In addition mucosal ulceration always occurs in patients who survive for approximately one week. This is commonly associated with 'heartburn' which diminishes as re-epithelialization occurs. However, necrosis of the oesophageal wall may also occur and may lead to perforation of the oesophagus in a small number of patients. Later fibrosis occurs which may be severe enough to produce dysphagia and require oesophageal dilatation.

Other methods which have been described but which are now less commonly used in the majority of centres include the following:

1 *Ligation of the varices*
This is performed via a transthoracic, transoesophageal approach. This

operation was first described by Linton and is an effective method of dealing with the situation in an emergency. Normally, once the patient's condition has stabilized, a portacaval anastomosis is performed.

2 Portoazygos disconnection

This was described by Tanner in 1950. Briefly, this operation consists of the following steps:

(a) the stomach is transected as high as possible in order to interrupt the venous pathways from the stomach to the oesophagus.
(b) all the vasa brevia are divided together with the left gastric vein or veins. The left gastric artery is, however, left untouched so as to preserve the blood supply to the cardiac end of the stomach.
(c) the small proximal gastric stump is anastomosed to the distal stomach.

This operation is also regarded as a temporary expedient to be followed by a portacaval anastomosis where possible.

A modification of this operation based on the principle of isolation of the oesophageal venous circulation from the stomach is the technique of oesophageal transection in which the oesophagus itself is transected after division and ligation of any obvious varices on the surface. The more dangerous aspect of this operation, as compared to the original Tanner procedure, is the risk of oesophageal leakage, which is nearly always fatal. One further disadvantage is that it does nothing to control bleeding from gastric varices.

3 Portacaval or splenorenal shunt

This type of surgery was introduced by Whipple in 1945. Either operation may be performed during or after the cessation of bleeding. However, there is a considerable difference in mortality between emergency and elective shunts. In emergency, mortality rates as high as 20–50 per cent have been reported whereas in elective shunts, assuming that a careful choice has been made, the immediate mortality may be as low as 6 per cent. Controlled trials have established that shunt procedures virtually eliminate the dangers of bleeding but reduce survival, due to a higher death rate from hepatic failure, and increase the morbidity of liver disease by facilitating the development of spontaneous (protein induced) encephalopathy.

Shunt procedures, criteria for selection are:

(a) the patient's general condition should be good;
(b) age below 50 years; neuropsychiatric complications are much more frequent in older patients;
(c) the portal pressure should be elevated;
(d) the portal vein should be radiologically demonstrable;
(e) there should have been repeated bleeding;
(f) hepatic function should be adequate, the serum bilirubin should be less than 1.5 mg/dl (25 μmol/l) and the serum albumin higher than 3 g/dl (30 g/l).

The best candidates for any shunt operation in terms of immediate mortality and immediate postoperative course are those patients suffering from an extrahepatic portal obstruction. In approximately 50 per cent of these patients portal vein thrombosis is secondary to sepsis; umbilical sepsis and osteomyelitis are the commonest foci. The low mortality and immediate good results in this group merely reflect the normal liver function.

If neither the portal nor the splenic veins are available for anastomosis, mesenteric caval shunting can be used, a procedure introduced independently by Marion in 1953 in France, and Clatworthy and his colleagues of the United States. This procedure is most commonly used in children in whom the portal vein is thrombosed, the splenic vein is too small for shunting, or splenectomy has already been performed.

The effects of shunting operations are as follows:

(a) The collateral circulation diminishes and the caput medusa on the abdominal wall may disappear.
(b) The varices of the oesophagus collapse.
(c) Hepatic blood flow is reduced.
(d) The intrasplenic pressure falls by as much as 25 mmHg. A subsequent rise indicates thrombosis of the anastomosis.
(e) There may be temporary jaundice due to the increased bilirubin load caused by the blood transfusion.
(f) Dependent oedema may develop. This is not due to increased pressure in the inferior vena cava but to diminished albumin production by the liver which, in turn, leads to a fall in the colloid osmotic pressure.
(g) Ascites may form or persist if already present, because of failure to relieve the hepatic outflow block. Because of this, hepatic lymph continues to pass through the liver capsule into the peritoneal cavity. An additional factor is the retention of sodium because of secondary aldosteronism. Theoretical considerations suggest that a side-to-side anastomosis would be preferable to an end-to-side in the presence of ascites, but the former operation is followed by a greater frequency of encephalopathy and, except in the terminal stages of liver failure, ascites can always be controlled by a medical regimen.

Complications

Assuming the patient survives operation the major complication is the development of encephalopathy.

The overall incidence of this complication varies in different series, depending on the sensitivity of the investigation and the type of shunt performed. It appears to be more frequent following side-to-side than end-to-side anastomoses, in which the portal vein is completely divided, and it is less common with the smaller splenorenal anastomoses.

Other than the type of shunt, four factors appear to influence the development of encephalopathy:

1 hepatocellular function at the time of and following surgery;
2 the action of the intestinal bacteria on protein;

3 the state of the central nervous system;
4 variations in the nitrogen load.

Encephalopathy is more frequent with advancing age and occurs with greater frequency as the interval following operation increases. Either the brain ages or, alternatively, hepatic function gradually decreases. The disorder may present suddenly as an acute emergency or so insidiously that the early symptoms escape attention.

The precise factor responsible for encephalopathy remains unknown. It is clear that the blood ammonia is raised in hepatic coma and encephalography but the correlation between the concentration of the cation and the degree of mental disturbance is not close. In addition, the terminal picture is complicated by the development of respiratory alkalosis and electrolyte disturbances.

Early symptoms include listlessness, drowsiness, restlessness and apathy. When coma ensues the tendon reflexes are exaggerated, the plantar responses are extensor, muscle twitching and the flapping tremor may develop. When the condition is chronic, there is progressive cerebral degeneration accompanied by intellectual impairment.

Diagnosis
Electroencephalography: changes take place in the alpha rhythm pattern which are non-specific but improved by administration of neomycin.

Treatment
The main aspects of treatment include:

1 withdrawal of protein from the diet or reduction of the intake to 40 g daily;
2 empty bowel by enemata;
3 stop bleeding;
4 oral neomycin to reduce the bacterial breakdown of endogenous protein;
5 correction of electrolyte disturbance;
6 rarely, the performance of total colectomy with an ileorectal reconstruction.

6.6 Aetiology of gall-stones

Gall-stones are found incidentally during routine autopsies in some 20 per cent of the adult white population and it is obvious, therefore, that many must have remained symptomless throughout life. There is some evidence that the incidence of gall-stones in any given population is in some way related to dietary factors among which are a high calorie intake and a diet rich in short chain fatty acids. There is thus a relationship with obesity and there is also a marked familial tendency.

Classification

Gall-stones can be classified into three principal types:

1. pure pigment stones;
2. cholesterol stones;
3. stones of mixed constitution.

To this list must be added the calcium carbonate stone which is associated with calcification of the gall bladder wall and the condition known as 'limey' bile.

The first two varieties are considered to be aseptic formations, a result of derangements of pigment or cholesterol metabolism, whereas the third variety is usually associated with an inflammatory process. Pure pigment or calcium bilirubinate stones are rare, pure cholesterol stones account for about 10 per cent of all stones, and the remainder are 'mixed', but even these contain between 70 and 80 per cent by weight of cholesterol.

Recently, a considerable volume of investigatory work has been carried out in an attempt to understand and localize the precise metabolic derangements associated with stone formation. The stimulus for these investigations has been the frequency of cholelithiasis and its complications in Western society and the desire to find a medical regimen that might either prevent the disease or lead to the dissolution of stones already formed.

Biochemical composition of bile

Biochemical investigations have shown that the three important constituents of bile related to calculous formation are: the bile acids, the phospholipids, and cholesterol. The bile acids, cholic and chenodeoxycholic acid, are synthesized by the liver and represent the end product of cholesterol metabolism. In man, these acids are immediately conjugated with glycine (75 per cent) or taurine (25 per cent) to form the primary bile salts which account for approximately 80 per cent of the solid matter in bile. In addition, bile also contains secondary bile salts, the deoxycholates, which are formed in the intestine during the enterohepatic circulation of bile when bacterial action converts cholic acid into deoxycholic acid and chenodeoxycholic acid into lithocholic acid. Of the two other major fractions in bile, the phospholipids, mainly lecithin, account for about 15 per cent and cholesterol 5 per cent.

The mixed micelle

The present concept regarding the nature of bile is that cholesterol, which is insoluble in water, is held in solution in normal bile because it is taken into micellar solution by the bile salts and the phospholipids. All three classes of compound possess water-soluble hydrophilic groups and water-insoluble (but oil-soluble) hydrophobic groups. When they are presented with a lipid–water interface, those compounds with a large component of hydrophilic groups orientate themselves so that the latter are, in effect, dissolved in the aqueous phase while the bulky lipophilic steroid nucleus is dissolved in the lipid phase.

The highest number of hydrophilic groups is found on the conjugated bile acids because they possess not only the greatest number of hydroxyl groups but also the negatively charged taurine and glycine radicles. Lecithin and cholesterol also organize themselves in a similar fashion, but neither can be actually dissolved in water. Their solution depends on their ability to combine with the bile acids to form the complex aggregates known as the mixed 'micelles', which are polymolecular aggregates comparable to detergents. The stability of such a chemical system depends wholly on the relative concentration of all three lipid classes.

Cholesterol stone formation

An unresolved problem concerning the formation of cholesterol stones is whether the primary disturbance is in the liver cell itself or whether the defect lies elsewhere. Evidence supporting both these views has been discovered.

Certainly extrahepatic factors may have a considerable effect on the composition of bile. Thus, patients suffering from Crohn's disease or who have suffered a massive ileal resection have a two- to threefold increase in the incidence of cholesterol stone formation. This is thought to be because of the disturbance of the enterohepatic circulation of the bile salts due to their reduced absorption.

In man, the normal bile salt pool is small, 3–5 g, and it is turned over approximately six times a day. If reabsorption decreases, only a limited compensatory increase in production is possible, amounting to approximately 20 per cent, after which production fails to keep pace with the loss.

In theory, if the bile salts decrease in quantity the relative concentration in the bile should fall, disturbing cholesterol solubilization and producing a lithogenic bile. In practical terms, as in the clinical conditions sited, it would indeed appear that a lithogenic bile is produced. However, experimental evidence is somewhat conflicting because, in the Rhesus monkey, as the concentration of bile salts falls the phospholipid concentration rises. This change would tend to overcome the adverse effects of the falling bile acid concentration because lecithin associates with the cholesterol fraction to form a liquid crystalline phase.

Cholesterol stones are also common in cirrhosis in which the bile salt pool is also reduced and the biliary concentration of bile salts falls. Since no extrinsic lesion is present, this suggests a primary liver cell defect possibly related to the lipoprotein plasma membrane of the bile canaliculi.

Bile obtained from a gall bladder in which cholesterol stones have formed differs both physically and chemically from normal. Ultracentrifuge studies reveal striking changes in the macromolecules and the cholesterol crystals. Chemically, the bile is oversaturated with cholesterol and the bile salt profile is disturbed.

Secondary factors

1 Stasis

When gall bladder contraction is reduced it is possible that small crystalline deposits may not be flushed from the viscus, allowing more time for the growth of stones. This is probably the reason why cholelithiasis is commoner in women than in men, for each pregnancy, particularly the last trimester, is associated with diminished motility. There is also abundant evidence that truncal vagotomy produces biliary stasis by decreasing the contractility of the gall bladder, and that this operation is associated with an increased incidence of gall-stones. Decreased motility may also enable mucoprotein produced by the epithelial cells of the gall bladder to be retained and trapped in the mucosal niches. Such retained mucoprotein would then increase the viscosity of the bile and form a core and a scaffold upon which crystallization could build up.

2 Infection

In the past, the importance of infection was greatly stressed; Moynihan's dictum was that every gall-stone was a monument to a dead bacterium. However, the importance of infection has been stressed less often of late because gall bladders containing stones are nearly always sterile. However, infection, as in acute cholecystitis, does have two important effects on the biliary tree:

(*a*) mucus production is enhanced and precipitable unconjugated bile acids are formed;
(*b*) infection with *Escherichia coli* increases the β-glucuronidase activity in the bile with the result that bilirubin glucuronide is hydrolysed to free bilirubin, which is then precipitated as calcium bilirubinate, one of the main constituents of 'infective' stones.

Pigment stones

A pure pigment stone is formed only when excessive quantities of bile pigment are produced by red cell breakdown. Pigment stones are believed to represent the precipitation of non-polar unconjugated bilirubin, although it is difficult to demonstrate this substance in the bile, possibly because it is normally selectively reabsorbed by the liver cell membrane.

The greatest incidence of pigment stones occurs in hereditary spherocytosis in which stone formation is twice as common as in other haemolytic states such as sickle cell anaemia or thalassaemia major. A possible explanation of this difference is that the spherocyte contains a normal complement of haemoglobin whereas in sickle cell disease there is a diminished red cell mass and in thalassaemia a reduced amount of haemoglobin per corpuscle.

Medical treatment of gall-stones

The results of the investigations into the formation of cholesterol stones has led directly to the treatment of such stones with a medical regimen. Two chemicals have been shown to be effective in producing dissolution of such stones, chenodeoxycholic acid and ursodeoxycholic acid. To be effective the calculi should be wholly translucent and should not possess a coating of calcium and the gall bladder should be functioning normally, showing normal concentration of dye during the performance of an oral cholecystogram. If adequate doses of chenodeoxycholic acid are administered, the cholesterol saturation index of the bile as obtained by nasoduodenal intubation after the intravenous administration of cholecystokinin can be shown to fall to 0.8 at which point dissolution of 'pure' cholesterol stones begins.

Chenodeoxycholic acid is a normal constituent of human bile, being one of the two main bile acids synthesized by the liver. The probable mechanism of action is that it reduces the output of cholesterol secreted into the bile by inhibiting the enzyme HMG CoA reductase. *In vitro* studies also show that it is a solubilizer of cholesterol monohydrate. It should not be administered to women who may become pregnant, nor to patients with chronic liver disease nor with inflammatory disease of the small intestine or colon.

The only side effect following the administration of this drug is diarrhoea which can be alleviated in most patients by temporarily reducing the dose for a matter of days.

The dose of the drug necessary to produce optimal results is of the order of 10–15 mg/kg of body weight daily. This dose can, however, be reduced by combining its administration with a low cholesterol diet when a dose of 8.5 mg/kg per day given in one dose at bed time has been shown to be effective. However, to be successful the drug may need to be administered for as long as 2 years and there is as yet no data on the recurrence rate following the cessation of such therapy.

6.7 Major complications of gall-stones and their treatment

The major complications of gall-stones are:

1. complications within the gall bladder:
   (*a*) acute cholecystitis
   (*b*) carcinoma of the gall bladder
2. complications within the common duct and liver:
   (*a*) obstructive jaundice
   (*b*) obstructive cholangiohepatitis
   (*c*) biliary cirrhosis
3. complications affecting other viscera:
   (*a*) spontaneous cholecystoduodenal fistula
   (*b*) gall-stone ileus

4 metabolic complications:
   (a) steatorrhoea in the presence of obstructive jaundice
   (b) hepatorenal failure

COMPLICATIONS WITHIN THE GALL BLADDER

Acute cholecystitis

Although acute cholecystitis can occur in the absence of gall-stones, even in these circumstances the disease becomes obstructive at an early stage due to oedema of the cystic duct. The initial description of the sequence of events following the sudden impaction of a stone in the cystic duct or the neck of the gall bladder was made by Rutherford Morrison. Following impaction, the gall bladder becomes distended with mucus, bile and blood due to exudation associated with acute chemical inflammation and transudation secondary to congestion of the gall bladder wall. As the gall bladder becomes distended, so the intraluminal tension interferes with the blood supply to produce necrosis and rupture of the gall bladder wall.

As the chemical phase advances, there is a secondary bacterial infection with coliforms and bacteroides. In the author's personal series of 200 consecutive cases of acute cholecystitis, there was perforation of the gall bladder in 16, but this produced a generalized biliary peritonitis in only 4 patients because, in the remainder, the effects of perforation were masked by the rapid isolation of the gall bladder from the peritoneal cavity by the omentum.

Clinical features
The chief clinical manifestations of acute cholecystitis are pain in the right upper quadrant of the abdomen and a fever that usually rises to between 38 and 39°C. Examination reveals extreme tenderness, rebound tenderness, and rigidity. If the gall bladder perforates before the viscus is sealed from the general peritoneal cavity, the whole abdomen is rigid.

Some observers state that acute obstructive cholecystitis can be distinguished from the non-obstructive variety by the presence of a mass in the former which is not observed in the latter. This is a dubious distinction because the ability to palpate a mass is, in large measure, dependent on the presence or absence of rigidity.

Differential diagnosis
The common conditions from which acute cholecystitis must be distinguished are as follows:

1 *perforated peptic ulcer.* In this condition there is, usually, a previous history of ulcer dyspepsia and only rarely do the signs of peritonitis remain limited to the upper abdomen. In the early stages, there is no fever, and a plain X-ray of the abdomen in the erect position shows air under the diaphragm in 40 per cent of patients.

2 *acute pancreatitis.* This may be difficult to distinguish, but in severe cases there is nearly always severe back pain and hypotension due to plasma loss. Although the serum amylase may be elevated in acute cholecystitis it never reaches the levels seen in acute pancreatitis, i.e. 1000 Somogyi units and above.
3 *miscellaneous conditions.* See Non-surgical causes of acute abdominal pain, Section 1.7.

The investigations required to establish an absolute diagnosis of acute cholecystitis are:

1 *plain X-ray of the abdomen and chest.* The latter is necessary to exclude pneumonic conditions. The former yields evidence supporting the diagnosis in over 60 per cent of patients. The radiological physical signs observed include (*a*) an absence of gas under the diaphragm, (*b*) a soft tissue mass, (*c*) presence of opaque gall-stones, (*d*) gas in the gall bladder itself.
2 *serum amylase.* In acute cholecystitis this is usually less than 500 Somogyi units.
3 *differential white count.* The white count should be elevated with a relative polymorphonuclear leucocytosis.
4 *serum bilirubin.* Jaundice may occur in acute cholecystitis due either to oedema in the region of Hartmann's pouch compressing the common duct, or the presence of concomitant common duct stones.
5 *ultrasonography.* In the presence of calculous cholecystitis this investigation may reveal an increased diameter of the gall bladder, thickening of its wall and lastly, the presence of a calculus.
6 *cholescintigraphy.* This investigation, performed using ^{99m}Tc-HIDA demonstrates blockage of the cystic duct.

Treatment of acute cholecystitis
Much controversy surrounds the question of the treatment of this disease; the major dilemma is whether early or delayed surgery produces the best results.

Du Plessis states that if operation is performed on the basis of clinical diagnosis alone a number of mistakes will be made due to faulty diagnosis. He gives as examples of possible incorrect diagnoses acute pancreatitis, secondary carcinoma of the liver, or primary carcinoma of the gall bladder. It would seem logical to argue that these 'mistakes' are of little ultimate consequence to the patient. He also states that, in approximately 10 per cent of patients suffering from acute cholecystitis, there may be a stone in the common bile duct difficult to diagnose and technically difficult to remove in the presence of acute inflammation. The latter is a more cogent argument. Other authors such as Glenn favour early operation. There is, in fact, no great advantage in rigid adherence to one method or another. Much depends on the skill and experience of the surgeon under whose care the patient is admitted. Those who claim that early operation is time-saving, particularly of hospital beds, are probably wrong, for careful examination of a personal series showed that complications of acute cholecystectomy could delay the discharge of patients for so long that the mean duration of hospital stay became equal to the two separate admissions required to treat the patient conservatively and then readmit for further elective surgery. In the author's series of 200 patients, 100 treated by operation and 100 treated conservatively, 4 patients died in each group. All were over 75 years of age. It became obvious from studying this and other series that acute obstructive cholecystitis is only mortal in the elderly. Of those who died in the author's series, two patients in each group might have been saved by the alternative treatment regimen.

Technical difficulties associated with acute cholecystectomy
Occasionally, operation in the acute stage becomes difficult due to oedema, fibrosis, or distortion of the anatomy. In these circumstances two alternatives exist. First, cholecystectomy can be abandoned and a cholecystostomy alone performed. If this is done all the stones must be removed, otherwise a mucous fistula tends to develop. Alternatively, the cholecystectomy can be performed from the fundus proximally so that, finally, the gall bladder is left attached to the hepatic artery by the cystic artery and the common duct by the cystic duct. If either of these methods is adopted, damage to the common duct should not occur.

Complications of acute cholecystectomy
Apart from damage to the common bile duct itself the chief complications of this operation are:

1 pulmonary atelectasis and embolus;
2 prolonged bile drainage;
3 wound infection.

Conservative management
Conservative management of acute cholecystitis demands bed rest, restricted oral fluids, and analgesics to reduce pain. An appropriate antibiotic is probably helpful but not mandatory.

The abdomen should be repeatedly examined and the abdominal tenderness should be greatly reduced within 48–72 hours. As it does so, an inflammatory mass becomes palpable which should then slowly disappear.

Conservative treatment should be immediately abandoned if there is rapid progression, as opposed to resolution, of the physical signs indicating the development of biliary peritonitis, or increasing systemic disturbance indicating uncontrolled infection.

Occasionally, an acute attack ends in the development of a mucocele of the gall bladder. A large pear-shaped palpable mass develops in the right upper quadrant which at operation is found to contain colourless mucus. If a patient is treated conservatively and the gall bladder is left *in situ* after an acute attack, approximately 30 per cent of patients will suffer further attacks of acute inflammation, suggesting the advisability of interval cholecystectomy.

Carcinoma of the gall bladder

This is infrequent and is rare in the absence of gall-stones. The commoner tumour is an adenocarcinoma, but occasionally, in the presence of gall-stones, squamous metaplasia appears, with the later development of a squamous cell carcinoma. In most patients the disease is inoperable when first seen. The common presenting signs are a mass in the right upper quadrant and obstructive jaundice.

COMPLICATIONS OF STONES WITHIN THE COMMON DUCT

The presence of gall-stones in the common duct does not necessarily lead to the development of jaundice. This is proven by post mortem statistics which show that cholelithiasis is present in 25 per cent of patients dying of intercurrent disease and that stones are found in the common bile duct in 25 per cent of these patients. It is obvious, therefore, that most common duct stones are symptomless. When, however, there are symptoms, the various clinical syndromes that may follow are obstructive jaundice, obstructive cholangiohepatitis, multiple liver abscesses and biliary cirrhosis.

Obstructive jaundice

When obstructive jaundice is due to the presence of stones in the common bile duct it is usually intermittent. The jaundice usually follows an acute attack of abdominal pain, the conjunctivae are noted to be yellow, the urine becomes the colour of cold tea, and the stools putty-coloured. In the absence of gross infection the jaundice commonly fades and disappears within a few days. If there are no contraindications to operation or, alternatively, the jaundice persists, surgical treatment is required. In the absence of jaundice an intravenous cholangiogram may confirm the presence of choledocholithiasis. In the presence of jaundice this investigation is useless. Ultrasonography may be helpful if the common duct is grossly dilated, but this is not an invariable accompaniment of obstructive jaundice due to stones. Furthermore, gall-stones lodged at the lower end of the common bile duct may remain undetected.

Of greater effectiveness is endoscopic retrograde cholangiopancreatography if this is available, performed following a prophylactic dose of a broad spectrum antibiotic to prevent endotoxaemia if the biliary tree is infected, or alternatively, percutaneous transhepatic cholangiography using the skinny-needle technique described by Okuda and others in 1974. Using such a needle the dangers associated with biliary leakage following withdrawal of the needle from the liver are much reduced. When the ducts are dilated they can nearly always be cannulated and the cause of obstruction of the biliary tree established. In a jaundiced patient the prothrombin time should be estimated prior to the investigation and if it is elevated it must be reduced to normal levels by the administration of vitamin K prior to investigation.

Treatment
During routine cholecystectomy an operative cholangiogram should be per-

formed. In many centres this is regarded as a routine procedure performed during every operation whereas in other centres this added investigation would be performed if the common duct is found to be greater than 10 mm in diameter, the accepted upper limit of normal. False positive results may be obtained if the lower end of the duct is in systole at the time the examination is performed and following dilatation of the lower end of the duct by Bake's dilators an abnormal appearance, difficult to interpret, may be seen.

When stones remain in the common duct following cholecystectomy an attempt can be made to relieve the situation by sphincterotomy performed via a fibreoptic endoscope. The chief danger of this procedure is haemorrhage which contributes in greater part to the mortality associated with this condition, approximately 1 per cent.

Cholangiohepatitis

This is caused by a combination of obstruction to the common bile duct, usually by stone, together with infection. The infecting organisms are both aerobic and anaerobic and include the coliforms, of which *Escherichia coli* is the most common, the bacteroides, and the anaerobic streptococci. If the infection is acute, a bacteraemia may develop leading to the onset of chills and fever, mental confusion, dyspnoea, and, possibly, hypotension. The latter usually develops within 10–16 hours of the onset of the disease and may lead to secondary renal failure. Initially, in bacteraemic shock the peripheral skin is warm and dry, but as the condition progresses, peripheral circulatory failure ensues with the development of cold cyanotic limbs. Even in the absence of overt clinical infection, organisms are commonplace in a common duct that contains stones. A further clinical syndrome associated with cholangitis is Charcot's intermittent hepatic fever, a combination of intermittent jaundice, pain and fever.

Route of infection
The precise route by which the biliary tree becomes infected is still open to question. Three alternative hypotheses have been advanced: the haematogenous, lymphatic, and direct intraluminal. Each of these theories has its protagonists and antagonists. When the jaundice rapidly deepens and there is severe fever there is an absolute indication to drain the biliary tree.

The precise operation depends on the anatomical findings at operation; the minimum required is the performance of a cholecystostomy and choledochostomy. In practice, every effort should be made to extract the obstructing stone from the common duct, which will be found to be grossly dilated, thick-walled, hyperaemic, and filled with purulent bile-stained fluid. Prior to, and immediately after drainage, the patient must receive a suitable antimicrobial drug. At the time of the operation, swabs should be taken for the culture of both aerobic and anaerobic organisms and the determination of their sensitivity. At initial microscopic examination *E. coli* cannot by Gram staining be differentiated from any other Gram-negative organism and, therefore, culture and a variety of biochemical tests are necessary. However, the majority of *E. coli* are sensitive to ampicillin and gentamicin or the cephalosporins and these compounds form a suitable starting point for antimicrobial therapy. On theoretical grounds, rifampicin which is concentrated in the bile, should be the ideal agent, but without drainage or the spontaneous relief of obstruction antibiotics cannot actually reach the infected area in high concentration. The development of multiple liver abscesses is an ever-present danger if a conservative policy is adopted, hence the danger of accepting the dictum that Charcot's intermittent hepatic fever is always intermittent. When an abscess forms secondary to cholangitis the clinical condition of the patient deteriorates. The liver itself becomes enlarged, and scattered through it are numerous greenish-yellow areas. Some of these are soft, others solid. If there has been cavitation the pus is deeply bile-stained.

Biliary cirrhosis

Although biliary cirrhosis is more common in association with simple or malignant strictures of the common bile duct it is still occasionally seen in patients who have suffered intermittent obstruction due to stones. There are histological changes around the central bile canaliculi which rupture due to the increased biliary pressure. When an infective element is present a dense concentration of inflammatory cells accumulates in the portal zone which will, in the absence of progressive infection, later be replaced by fibrosis and bile duct proliferation. As the fibrous tissue bands grow in size and coalesce, the lobules are reduced in size. In the later stages, biliary cirrhosis may be difficult to distinguish from portal cirrhosis although foci of liver cell hyperplasia are less conspicuous in the former.

A patient suffering from biliary cirrhosis usually remains in reasonable health, and in the absence of infection physical deterioration is slow to develop. In the late stages of the disease, however, the patient appears very ill, the skin colouration becomes greenish, and there will be portal hypertension and associated hepatic failure. There may be various physical manifestations, which include pruritis, xanthomata, enlargement of the liver and spleen, steatorrhoea, and osteomalacia. Since the hepatic changes may well be reversible, every effort must be made to relieve the obstruction.

COMPLICATIONS AFFECTING OTHER VISCERA

Fistula formation

Acute inflammatory change complicating stones in the gall bladder or common duct may result in adherence of either viscus to the duodenum, with the production of a fistulous tract between the two. Once the acute inflammatory process has resolved the patient may become symptomless. In these circumstances the diagnosis is sometimes made by a plain X-ray of the abdomen which will show air outlining the biliary tree.

Treatment
In general all that is required to deal with a cholecystoduodenal fistula is blunt separation of the two viscera by pressure between the finger and thumb. The gall bladder is removed and the duodenal defect which is never more than a few millimetres in diameter is closed by two layers with catgut.

Gall-stone ileus

Very rarely, a large gall-stone passes from the gall bladder into the duodenum and makes its way down the small bowel. Normally, it impacts in the distal ileum where the lumen of the bowel is narrowest. The obstruction, being of a simple variety, may be present for several days and is associated with intermittent vomiting, small bowel colic, and slowly increasing distension. A preoperative diagnosis may be made if air is present in the biliary tree and a gall-stone can be seen lying in the lumen of the bowel. Treatment consists of resuscitation followed by laparotomy. The stone, if possible, is milked proximally away from the site of impaction and removed through a small enterostomy. The primary condition of the biliary passages may or may not be explored immediately, a decision which depends upon the age, general condition of the patient and the accessibility of the gall bladder which is usually surrounded by adhesions.

METABOLIC COMPLICATIONS

Steatorrhoea

In the presence of obstructive jaundice steatorrhoea occurs because of the absence of bile salts from the intestine. In general, the severity of malabsorption is related to the degree of obstruction, which can be assessed by measuring either the serum bilirubin or the faecal stercobilinogen content.

If the obstruction is of long duration, which is unlikely when the cause is due to stone, there may be nutritional deficiencies due to lack of absorption of the fat-soluble vitamins A, D and K. Lack of vitamin A produces night blindness and hyperkeratosis, lack of vitamin D, osteomalacia with its associated kyphosis and fractures, and lack of vitamin K produces a prolonged prothrombin time associated with spontaneous bruising.

Hepatorenal failure

The mortality of operations performed for the relief of obstructive jaundice is abnormally high, approaching 10 per cent. At least half these patients develop increasing jaundice and progressive renal failure, the hepatorenal syndrome, which is particularly likely if the patient suffers from hypotension during or immediately after operation. It was thought at first that jaundiced patients suffered from a reduced blood volume, but this has been disproved. Current experimental evidence suggests that high circulating levels of bilirubin glucuronide sensitize the cells of the renal tubules to the adverse effects of ischaemia. The glucuronide reaches the tubules after passing through the glomeruli. Such evidence suggests that every effort should be made to avoid hypovolaemic hypotension during operations on the obstructed biliary tree and that renal function should be assisted by the routine use of mannitol infusion daily following surgery.

6.8 Causes of jaundice and the evaluation of diagnostic methods

Definition. Jaundice is caused by the staining of body tissues with bile pigments producing a yellow or yellow-green pigmentation of the sclera and skin. Clinically the condition is recognizable when the pigment level rises in the serum above 40 mmol/l (2.5 mg).

Formation and fate of bilirubin

Approximately 85 per cent of the circulating bilirubin is formed from the breakdown of haemoglobin, and the remainder originates from the haemoproteins of the bone marrow, liver, and kidneys.

When haemoglobin is destroyed, globin is split off from the molecule and iron is removed, leaving the pigment biliverdin, which is then reduced to bilirubin. Nearly 200 mg of unconjugated bilirubin are normally brought to the liver each day, transported in the blood bound to the plasma albumin. Reaching the liver the bilirubin is taken from the plasma into the hepatocyte where in the smooth endoplasmic reticulum it is conjugated with glucuronic acid to form bilirubin diglucuronide, after which it is excreted into the bile canaliculi.

Bile normally contains only conjugated or posthepatic bilirubin which is converted in the small bowel to stercobilinogen by bacterial action. Some stercobilinogen is reabsorbed into the portal circulation, recirculated to the liver to be excreted in the bile, and a small proportion is excreted by the kidneys as urobilinogen.

Aetiology of jaundice
Jaundice may be caused by the accumulation of unconjugated or conjugated bilirubin.

Unconjugated hyperbilirubinaemia is most commonly caused by any condition causing excessive haemolysis. Included in this group would be pernicious anaemia or drug-induced haemolysis associated with compounds such as para-aminosalicylic acid and phenacetin.

A second cause of this condition is Gilbert's syndrome, said to affect 5 per cent of the population. This syndrome is benign, it is associated with normal liver histology and the bilirubin level seldom exceeds 80 mmol/l.

A very rare cause of unconjugated hyperbilirubinaemia is the Crigler–Najjar syndrome in which the bilirubin conjugating enzyme is either absent in the most severe type of the condition which is associated with early death or present in reduced amounts when survival to adult life is possible.

In addition to the above a large number of drugs interfere with the normal metabolic pathway including antibiotics such as novobiocin and rifampicin which interfere with conjugation and the salicylates and sulphonamides which interfere with binding.

It is, therefore, self-evident that in taking the history of any patient suffering from jaundice a careful enquiry should be made as to medicinal agents which have been administered. This applies not only to unconjugated but also to cases of conjugated hyperbilirubinaemia since a variety of drugs affect the excretion of bile, examples of which include chlorpromazine which induces intrahepatic cholestasis and halothane which induces a hepatitis-like reaction.

Conjugated hyperbilirubinaemia

This may be caused by:

1. disorders affecting the bile canaliculi, i.e. the Dubin–Johnson syndrome;
2. disorders affecting the liver cell, i.e. hepatitis, viral, alcoholic or drug-induced, e.g. by oral contraceptives or halothane;
3. intrahepatic cholestasis due to primary biliary cirrhosis;
4. extrahepatic obstruction the causes of which may be classified as follows:
   (a) *malignant*
      (i) carcinoma of the ampulla of Vater;
      (ii) carcinoma of the head of the pancreas;
      (iii) secondary hilar lymph nodes;
      (iv) carcinoma of the common bile duct.
   (b) *benign*
      (i) gall-stones;
      (ii) strictures, either iatrogenic or due to sclerosing cholangitis;
      (iii) intraluminal parasites. These are especially common in Africa, the common offender being the *Ascaris lumbricoides* and in the Far East where *Clonorchis sinesis* is common;
      (iv) pancreatitis, usually mild and transient in acute pancreatitis, occasionally severe and chronic in chronic pancreatitis.

In general, surgery is effective only when the cause of jaundice is extrahepatic.

In the majority of patients careful history taking together with clinical examination will help to establish whether the cause of the jaundice is extrahepatic and, therefore, possibly amenable to surgical interference. Two examples are sufficient to illustrate this point.

1. Jaundice due to gall-stones is frequently preceded by a relatively long history of flatulent dyspepsia terminating in an acute attack of pain rapidly followed by jaundice and possibly fever. Clinical examination will reveal the presence of jaundice and possibly tenderness beneath the right costal margin.
2. Jaundice due to malignant disease of the head of the pancreas is often painless but progressive. In the absence of previous attacks of cholecystitis the gall bladder may be grossly enlarged, Courvoisier's sign.

However, even though the clinical history and examination are exceedingly helpful in establishing the cause of jaundice the use of special investigations is called for:

1. to confirm the clinical diagnosis;
2. in cases of surgical jaundice to establish the correct operative procedure required and whether palliative or radical surgery is appropriate in malignant disease.

Laboratory tests

1 *Serum bilirubin*

Both the conjugated and unconjugated bilirubin levels should be established. The normal total bilirubin level is 16 μmol/l (0.8 mg/dl). An increase above 40 mmol/l is associated as previously stated with overt jaundice. If this is obstructive in type the greater part will be conjugated with glucuronic acid and because this is water-soluble, some will be excreted in the urine, hence the dark urine found in the patient suffering from jaundice.

After some weeks a balance occurs between the rate of production and the rate of excretion and the bilirubin level stabilizes at approximately 300 mmol/l. This is in contradistinction to the situation in hepatocellular disease in which the unconjugated bilirubin is insoluble in water and, therefore, a continuing rise in the total serum bilirubin occurs as the disease progresses for as long as bilirubin is still produced, any fall in the bilirubin indicating improvement.

2 *Enzyme tests*

The three enzymes normally monitored include:

(a) serum glutamine oxalacetic transaminase (SGOT), normal value 10–40 units;
(b) serum glutamine pyruvic transaminase (SGPT), normal value 10–40 units;
(c) lactic dehydrogenase (LDH), normal value 100–350 Berger–Brody units.

These compounds are cellular enzymes that catalyse the process of transamination, the reaction whereby an α-keto acid is converted to an amino acid with the same carbon skeleton. In the presence of tissue damage, particularly of the myocardium or liver, the transaminases escape into the plasma and estimation of the enzyme levels, therefore, serves as an indicator of the severity of such damage. In hepatic jaundice, enzyme levels over 400 units are often encountered, whereas in obstructive or posthepatic jaundice their level is usually below 300 units.

3 Alkaline phosphatase

The value of the alkaline phosphatase in normal adults is between 3 and 13 King–Armstrong units; elevation above this level suggests extrahepatic obstruction. Greater discrimination can be achieved by the use of polyacrylamide disc gel electrophoresis when alkaline phosphatase separates into gut, liver and bone bands. In a jaundiced patient the presence of a gut band suggests an extrahepatic lesion and the distinctive liver band appears when primary liver pathology is present.

4 Urine urobilinogen

The level of urine urobilinogen reflects the amount of bilirubin reaching the intestine. In posthepatic or obstructive jaundice, therefore, because little or no bilirubin enters the gut there is no stercobilin to be reabsorbed, and urobilinogen is absent from the urine. In prehepatic or haemolytic jaundice, in which increased quantities of pigment are excreted into the gut, the amount of urobilinogen present in the urine increases. The normal value is 0–4 mg/24 h (0–6.72 mosmol/24 h).

5 Serum proteins

In a normal adult the total protein is between 63 and 78 g/l. The serum albumin normally comprises 50–65 per cent of the total protein concentration. Depression of albumin formation, usually associated with an increase in the globulin fractions, occurs in all forms of hepatocellular jaundice. The decreased albumin concentration is ultimately one of the factors leading to oedema.

6 Prothrombin time

This is normally between 11 and 14 seconds. In hepatocellular disease the prothrombin time may be prolonged because of the liver's failure to synthesize various clotting factors but it may also be increased in posthepatic jaundice due to the decreased absorption of fat-soluble vitamin K from the small bowel. This is, of course, due to the absence of bile salts.

7 Blood ammonia

The normal range is 0.76–1.36 mg/l (0.05–0.09 mmol/l) of arterial blood. This estimation is usually performed in the presence of stupor or coma. It is then a valuable aid in differentiating hepatic coma from that due to drugs.

8 Serum alphafetoprotein

This protein which is derived from the embryonic liver and yolk sac circulates in the embryo and fetus but persists for only a few weeks after birth. In adult life it reappears in a variety of conditions and so far as hepatic conditions are concerned it makes its reappearance in approximately 30 per cent of patients suffering from hepatocellular carcinoma in the UK.

9 *Full blood count and reticulocyte count*
This investigation is important if it is considered that the possible cause of jaundice is haemolytic, e.g. hereditary spherocytosis.

Radiological investigations

1 *Non-invasive techniques*
(a) *Oral and intravenous cholangiography.* In the jaundiced patient the former is a useless investigation and the latter is also of limited value. However, the use of the latter has been extended by using 50 ml of Biligrafin Forte dissolved in 150 ml of water administered by the intravenous route over an hour.
(b) *Ultrasonography.* Space-occupying lesions within the liver including tumours, cysts and abscesses can all be detected because of the altered echo pattern. However, ultrasonography whilst accurate in the detection of gallstones within the gall bladder is much less effective in detecting stones causing obstruction to the common bile duct. The diagnosis of extrahepatic obstruction depends upon the detection of dilatation of the gall bladder and intra- and extrahepatic ducts above the obstruction and such dilatation is not necessarily present in this condition although it is almost always demonstrable in malignant obstruction. Furthermore, stones lodged at the lower end of the common bile duct are very difficult to visualize and in one reported series only 10 per cent were visualized.
(c) *Computerized axial tomography.* If available this investigatory method will detect even minimal dilatation of the ductal system in the great majority of patients. However, its primary value is in the detection of obstructing lesions, e.g. enlarged metastatic lymph nodes lying outside the common bile duct.
(d) *Radioisotope scanning: ^{99m}Tc–HIDA cholescintigraphy.* A common scanning agent in use at the present time is the iminodiacetic acid derivative labelled with ^{99m}Tc. The advantage of this compound is that it is rapidly extracted from the blood and excreted through the hepatocyte into the bile. An HIDA scan is of limited value in differentiating intrahepatic cholestasis from extrahepatic obstruction. However, tumours, cysts and abscesses of approximately 2 cm or more in diameter can be detected and when widespread hepatocellular disease is present a generalized decrease in hepatic uptake occurs.

2 *Invasive techniques*
(a) *Endoscopic retrograde cholangiopancreatography* (ERCP). With the development of fibreoptic endoscopy cannulation of the ampulla is rapidly becoming a routine investigation in patients suffering from jaundice. The method allows a distinction to be made between extrahepatic obstruction due to carcinoma of the pancreas, common duct stone and biliary strictures.

Because of the possible precipitation of endotoxic shock if the biliary tree is infected a prophylactic dose of a broad spectrum antibiotic should be given prior to the investigation.

(*b*) *Percutaneous transhepatic cholangiography.* This technique is now performed with a narrow bore needle, the skinny-needle technique. The overall success rate in the visualization of dilated intrahepatic ducts can be as high as 98 per cent and in a large percentage of patients even normal ducts can be entered if sufficient passes with the needle are made. This investigation should only be performed if the prothrombin time is normal and if, for example, a totally dilated biliary tree is demonstrated with obstruction at the lower end, indicating carcinoma of the pancreas, the needle can be left *in situ* to decompress the biliary tree and avoid the possible danger of biliary peritonitis.

Liver biopsy

This investigation is useful in distinguishing intrahepatic cholestasis from other causes of extrahepatic obstruction and, occasionally, a secondary metastasis may be inadvertently biopsied.

Techniques
Prior to the biopsy the prothrombin time and platelet count should be estimated. Abnormalities of the prothrombin time should be corrected by the intramuscular injection of vitamin K. A variety of different biopsy needles are available but whichever is used must be inserted into the liver during the apnoeic phase after expiration. The site of skin puncture may be either the midaxillary line at the point of maximum dullness, usually through the eighth or ninth interspace or immediately below the costal margin if the liver is enlarged.

Pleural or right shoulder-tip pain may develop after this manoeuvre but the more serious, and fortunately rare, complications are haemorrhage or biliary peritonitis. The latter is likely if the patient is suffering from obstructive jaundice due to extrahepatic causes.

6.9 Aetiology, diagnosis, complications and treatment of acute pancreatitis

The Marseilles symposium on the Aetiology and Pathology of Pancreatitis agreed that acute pancreatitis should be subdivided into two main types, acute pancreatitis and recurrent acute pancreatitis. The incidence of both conditions is extremely variable. In the United Kingdom it is as low as 5 per 100 000 of the population with the mean age at onset of 50, whereas in the United States the incidence varies from 4 per 100 000 in persons below the age of 30 to 62 per

100 000 of the population in persons over the age of 70 years. It is believed that this variation is accounted for by the greater degree of alcoholism in the latter country.

Aetiology
Most cases of pancreatitis are inexplicable, but certain well-recognized aetiological factors have been identified even though the exact mechanism by which they produce their effect is unknown. They include:

1 gall-stones;
2 alcoholism;
3 hyperparathyroidism;
4 mumps;
5 hereditary lipaemia;
6 postoperatively, after operations interfering with the duodenum;
7 post-traumatic, usually after closed abdominal injury;
8 Aminoaciduria
9 *Mycoplasma pneumoniae* and coxsackie virus B

Of these the two most common are gall-stones and alcoholism. The latter is a common association in France and the United States and in certain areas of the United Kingdom in which alcohol intake appears to be excessive. Although the association between gall-stones and acute pancreatitis is clear, the incidence of gall-stones being as high as 70 per cent in some series of acute pancreatitis, the mechanism by which gall-stones cause pancreatitis remains doubtful. In 1901 Opie described his classic case in which a small gall-stone was found impacted in the ampulla and it was immediately assumed that pancreatitis was caused by the resulting reflux of bile from the common duct into the pancreatic duct, a theory now disproved.

Pathogenesis
For many years the view has been held that the changes observed in acute pancreatic necrosis are due to autodigestion of the gland by its own tryptic enzymes. There now appears to be reasonable doubt as to the validity of this theory on the grounds that:

1 activated pancreatic proteases do not appear to damage living tissue;
2 the passage of bile through a loop of small intestine allowing enterokinase to pass through the pancreas and back into the small intestine through a second anastomosis with almost complete activation of trypsinogen does not produce haemorrhagic pancreatitis;
3 whilst activated trypsin injected into the interlobar spaces gives rise to oedema and intralobular haemorrhage it does not produce necrosis;
4 the intradermal injection of sterile trypsin gives rise to an oedematous wheal but no accompanying cellular necrosis;
5 if trypsinogen was activated in the pancreas to trypsin it might be expected that the blood level of trypsin might be raised and the concentration of trypsin inhibitors would fall but this does not occur.

Experimental evidence now suggests that pancreatic necrosis will only occur if activation of the pancreatic enzymes by enterokinase is accompanied by the presence of cytotoxic-producing bacteria among which would be included the coliform organisms, the clostridia and *Staphylococcus aureus*. All these bacteria are capable of producing a necrotizing lesion if injected alone into the skin.

This situation can be produced in the experimental animal by forming a closed loop of duodenum and then restoring continuity of the gastrointestinal tract by anastomosing the stomach to the jejunum. If this is done acute pancreatic necrosis occurs but if at the same time the duct is ligated no pathological changes occur in the gland.

In the human this series of events could occur if the natural mechanism preventing the reflux of duodenal juice was disrupted. This could and is achieved by sphincterotomy which is occasionally complicated by acute pancreatitis, by a Polya gastrectomy if afferent loop obstruction occurs, when the long arm of a T-tube passes into the duodenum and possibly when a calculus impacts in the lower end of the duct. In the latter case it is not that such impaction leads to the reflux of bile but the disturbance of the normal closing mechanism which allows the reflux of duodenal contents into the pancreatic duct.

Whatever the mechanism the onset of severe pancreatitis leads to the rapid release of a 'toxic broth' into the interstitial tissues of the gland, the peripancreatic tissues and the blood stream. Within the broth are:

1 a variety of proteolytic enzymes including chymotrypsin, carboxypeptidase, elastase and lysolecithin;
2 kallikrein and bradykinin;
3 unidentified short chain peptides which produce myocardial depression and shock lung;
4 endotoxins.

Pathology

It is usual to distinguish three grades of acute pancreatitis, each of increasing severity, according to the pathological changes in the gland; the interstitial or oedematous, haemorrhagic, and gangrenous. In oedematous pancreatitis the gland itself is swollen and oedematous and surrounded by exudate. It has been estimated that between 20 and 30 per cent of the circulating blood volume may leak within 6 hours of the onset of the disease, a finding which has given rise to the expression, the 'pancreatic burn'. In the more severe haemorrhagic and gangrenous varieties of the disease the circulating blood volume is further reduced by pooling of blood in the splanchnic bed.

In haemorrhagic pancreatitis the gland is not only swollen but is also bright red in colour due to bleeding. This may be patchy or involve the whole gland. In this variety of pancreatitis clotting in the small vessels in and around the pancreas may be found, thus impairing the microcirculation. In addition, areas of fat necrosis are found in the region of the pancreas, in the mesocolon and omentum. Although it has always been assumed that this was directly due to the liberation of lipase it is now considered to be due to the combined effects of both lipase and a phospholipase.

In gangrenous pancreatitis tissue necrosis destroys the entire structure of the gland, both exocrine and endocrine, the supporting tissues, and the blood vessels. At the margins of the necrotic areas, collections of polymorphonuclear cells are found but there is now general agreement among pathologists that this is *not* a truly inflammatory lesion and for this reason the term acute pancreatic necrosis is being increasingly used.

Clinical presentation
Acute pancreatitis presents as 'acute' abdomen. In areas in which the incidence is low, the condition may not even be considered and a mistaken diagnosis of perforated duodenal ulcer, acute cholecystitis, or myocardial infarction may be made, the former diagnoses being finally rejected at the time of laparotomy.

The major symptoms include severe pain, often girdle-like in distribution, vomiting, fever, tachycardia, shock and, later, detectable free fluid in the abdomen. Examination discloses a patient, usually with slight fever, who may be slightly jaundiced. The abdomen is usually rigid, especially in the upper quadrants, and rarely discoloured in the loins or around the umbilicus: Cullen and Grey Turner's signs. The patient who is severely shocked and hypotensive may be cyanosed and suffer from air hunger.

The conditions from which acute pancreatitis must be distinguished are perforated gastric ulcer (perforated duodenal ulcer is not usually accompanied by a fall in blood pressure), acute cholecystitis, mesenteric vascular occlusion, myocardial infarction and a dissecting or leaking aneurysm of the aorta. The correct diagnosis will only be made by the clinician if a high degree of clinical suspicion is maintained.

Special investigations

1 *Biochemical*
(a) *Serum amylase.* This is usually elevated above 500 and often to more than 1000 Somogyi units. Only in an occasional patient does the amylase remain normal throughout the course of the disease but the amylase level is not directly related to the severity of the disease. Amylase rather than lipase is measured because the estimation of the former is easier.

Investigation has shown that the initial level of the serum amylase has little if any correlation with the severity of the disease. In the majority of patients suffering from interstitial or oedematous pancreatitis the amylase falls to a normal value within 48 hours of the onset of abdominal pain. This makes retrospective diagnosis by the test virtually impossible.

However, future rises in the amylase, particularly in the presence of additional symptoms and signs, is of considerable diagnostic value.

(b) *Serum calcium.* The normal range of serum calcium is between 2.25 and 2.60 mmol/litre. In acute pancreatic necrosis, enzymes liberated from the pancreas produce fat necrosis in the retroperitoneal fat, omentum and mesentery by the hydrolysis of fat to glycerol and fatty acids, the latter combining with the circulating ionic calcium. As a result the serum calcium falls. If the fall is abrupt, tetany ensues.

In general terms the magnitude of the fall is related to the severity of the disease, and when the level falls by more than 30 per cent, i.e. to a value of 1.75 mmol/l or below, the outlook is usually poor and death probably inevitable.

(c) *Blood sugar.* If the disease is severe, islet function will be disturbed and there will be a temporary rise in the blood sugar.

(d) *Serum bilirubin.* Any swelling of the head of the pancreas is liable to compress the common bile duct, leading to a rise in the serum bilirubin and, possibly, clinical jaundice.

(e) *Serum methaemalbumin.* As necrosis and vascular disruption occur in the pancreas, haemoglobin is liberated into the circulation. In the presence of proteolytic enzymes, haematin is formed, which is bound with albumin to form methaemalbumin. This compound is formed only when free haemoglobin liberated into the plasma by the breakdown of red cells has used up the haptoglobin to which it is normally bound. Methaemalbumin is not usually present in the circulation and its presence in pancreatitis indicates that the pathological changes in the pancreas are haemorrhagic rather than oedematous. A continuing high circulating level of this compound usually signifies the development of complications.

(f) *Plasma fibrinogen level.* The normal fibrinogen level in the plasma is 200–400 mg/dl (2–4 g/l). The fibrinogen level increases in a number of surgical conditions in which there has been tissue injury, including acute pancreatitis. Normally, the value rises towards the end of the first week and in the uncomplicated case falls to normal within 2 weeks. Although the magnitude of the initial elevation bears little relationship to the severity of the disease, an elevation of the fibrinogen level extending into the third and fourth weeks is highly suggestive of complications.

2 Blood counts and sedimentation rate

The total white count is elevated, together with an absolute polymorphonucleocytosis in the early stages of pancreatitis. Persistent leucocytosis or a late rise indicates complications.

The erythrocyte sedimentation rate rises in acute pancreatic necrosis because the condition is associated with tissue necrosis. A persistent rise continuing into the third week is again indicative of complications.

3 Radiological investigation

The place of radiological investigation is initially restricted to plain X-rays of the abdomen in the erect and supine positions. These may show either a single fluid level in the duodenum, the sentinel loop, or, in severe disease, multiple fluid levels in the upper left abdominal quadrant suggesting a more generalized paralytic ileus. Occasionally, opaque gall-stones may be seen, and there may sometimes be a generalized hazy opacity over the abdominal cavity due to a collection of peritoneal fluid. Later, a number of radiological investigations may be required. Particularly important, however, once the disease is quiescent, is a cholecystogram to eliminate or confirm the presence of gall-stones. Other radiological investigations will be referred to when the complications of the disease are discussed.

4 *Computerized axial tomography*
Although this technique is not available in all centres typical changes develop in pancreatitis which may become evident. These include:

(a) thickening of the parietal peritoneum due to oedema;
(b) thickening of the anterior pararenal fascia, eponymously known as Gerota's fascia;
(c) swelling of the pancreas accompanied by blurring of its outline;
(d) decreasing density in the region of the pancreas indicates either early pseudocyst formation or pancreatic necrosis.

5 *Ultrasonography*
This type of investigation is now available in the majority of radiological departments. It is most discriminating in direct contradistinction to CAT scanning when the patient is thin with little or no fat planes. However, it is subject to much greater observer error and is of greatest value in picking up lesions involving the head and body of the pancreas rather than the tail.

6 *Peritoneal tap and lavage*
There is considerable evidence that in many cases of pancreatitis the initial clinical impression as to the severity of the disease is incorrect and that a better indicator of the pathological changes can be obtained by tapping the abdomen. If more than 10 ml of fluid is obtained this denotes serious disease. If the fluid is clear or straw-coloured the condition can be regarded as mild. If, however, it is frankly brown this indicates severe disease. In addition to visual observation the following estimations are of value: the albumin content, above 39g/l indicates severe disease; SGOT, above 10 iu/l indicates severe disease and thirdly, the total protein, above 7.5 g/l indicating severe disease.

Management of acute pancreatitis

The mortality of acute pancreatitis is related to the severity of the disease. If this remains oedematous the mortality is as low as 6 per cent. When, however, the condition progresses to the haemorrhagic or gangrenous stages the mortality in the initial attack may be as high as 50 per cent. The majority of deaths take place within the first 48 hours, indicating that the cause must have been either overwhelming 'toxaemia' or failure to control the hypovolaemic shock, or both.

In part, the hypovolaemia is readily explained in terms of the massive plasma leak that takes place into the pancreas itself and the surrounding tissues. It has been estimated that there may be a 30 per cent loss of plasma volume, the whole being known as the pancreatic burn. However, more subtle changes are at work.

The preliminary measures that must be taken are, therefore, to relieve pain and restore the intravascular volume by plasma or plasma expanders, if necessary controlling the measures taken by repeated measurements of the central venous pressure. In addition, the stomach will be kept empty and the urine output carefully monitored so that incipient renal failure can be recognized.

Supportive measures of possible value
In elderly patients because of the myocardial depressant effect of the 'toxic broth' liberated in acute pancreatic necrosis the patient should be fully digitalized if ECG changes are present.

When the associated ileus is prolonged and it is becoming clear from both clinical and biochemical parameters that the disease is severe total intravenous nutrition should be commenced.

Specific measures of dubious value
A large variety of specific measures have been advocated to control acute pancreatitis.

1 *The administration of aprotinin (Trasylol)*. This drug inhibits the action of kallikrein trypsin and chymotrypsin. It was first introduced into clinical practice in 1958 and at first many reports appeared which suggested that it was highly effective in reducing the initial mortality. In the late 1960s, however, a rather less optimistic view was taken of its use and it was gradually abandoned.

At the present time one is faced with the possible doubtful premise that the drug may perhaps be of use in the middle-aged, non-alcoholic group of patients suffering from this disease.

2 *Corticosteroids*. There is no 'hard' evidence that corticosteroids alter the prognosis of this disease although in general terms it has been shown that corticosteroids assist in maintaining the integrity of the microcirculation in animals suffering from experimental endotoxaemia.

3 *Antibiotics*. The routine use of 'broad' spectrum antibiotics has now been abandoned unless the disease is associated with acute cholecystitis, pulmonary infection or 'shock' lung.

4 *Glucagon*. The use of this drug in the treatment of acute pancreatitis was first suggested in 1973, the theoretical value being to 'rest' the gland. However, an MRC trial performed in the late 1970s showed in a double blind trial no reduction in mortality following the administration of this drug.

5 *Peritoneal lavage*. This was first suggested in 1956 by Wall in Australia. There is no 'hard' evidence to suggest that this manoeuvre reduces the mortality.

6 *Laparotomy*. Many older surgeons were convinced that laparotomy had a definite place in the treatment of pancreatitis. Various series show that laparotomy does not contribute to mortality, but there is no definite evidence that it is particularly beneficial. Those who argue in favour of laparotomy believe that the removal of 'toxic' materials from the abdomen is an important factor in reducing mortality. The recently introduced equivalent of laparotomy is peritoneal dialysis, which is now being increasingly used in the initial stages of the disease.

Future management in the quiescent stage
Once the disease is quiescent, oral and/or intravenous cholangiography should be performed.

The presence of stones in the gall bladder and/or in the common bile duct is an indication for surgery and it is generally agreed that the results are excellent, the majority of patients remaining symptom-free. Another indication for surgery following the acute attack is in those rare cases in which the presence of a parathyroid tumour is established. If alcoholism is related to the acute attack the patient must be encouraged to stop drinking alcoholic beverages because to continue will finally produce chronic pancreatic fibrosis, chronic pain, and both exocrine and endocrine deficiencies.

The ultimate prognosis in the non-alcoholic is good, for the gland returns to normal structure and function so long as necrosis has not occurred.

Complications of acute pancreatitis and their management

1 *Tetany*
The onset of tetany usually occurs within a few days of the onset of the disease and as previously stated a serum calcium below 1.75 mmol/l carries a grave prognosis. However, in the presence of overt symptoms calcium supplements should be given in the form of calcium chloride.

2 *Renal failure*
Because acute pancreatic necrosis is associated with hypovolaemic shock, intravascular haemolysis and unidentified toxic factors, there may be renal tubular or glomerular damage. In the presence of either, the chances of infection are greatly increased. Treatment, as described in Section 1.2, on renal failure, should be instituted.

3 *'Shock lung'*
The development of shock lung will be associated with dyspnoea, cyanosis, decreased Po_2 and diminished lung compliance. Supportive treatment only can be given.

4 *Consumptive coagulopathy and diffuse intravascular coagulation*
Consumptive coagulopathy and rarely diffuse intravascular coagulation may occur, requiring heparinization which in itself may lead to death if large areas of pancreatic tissue have become sequestrated in the region of the splenic vessels.

5 *Postpancreatic mass*
Three pathological lesions may result in a palpable abdominal mass following an acute attack of pancreatitis.

(a) *Pancreatic swelling.* This term is used to describe a condition of the pancreas accompanied by oedema and an inflammatory infiltrate of the pancreas and peripancreatic tissues. The importance of this condition lies in the fact that it will usually spontaneously resolve without surgical intervention. In clinical terms the patient having recovered from the acute attack continues to complain of malaise, nausea and upper abdominal discomfort. A slight fever may be present together with a leucocytosis. Depending on the build of the patient and the degree of abdominal tenderness a mass may or may not be palpable. A definitive diagnosis can be reached by a CAT scan but if this is not available simple clinical observation noting the gradual improvement of the patient eventually leads to the correct diagnosis.

(*b*) *Pancreatic pseudocyst.* A pseudocyst is an accumulation of exudate within the lesser sac which persists after the acute attack has subsided. This condition is usually more easily diagnosed than a multilocular abscess because with the passage of time a mass develops under the left costal margin.

A characteristic feature of pseudocysts is their tendency to vary in size. This is because, for a time at least, a communication may be present between the cyst and a pancreatic duct making spontaneous drainage a distinct possibility. For this reason when the cyst is first apparent it is advisable to wait and see if spontaneous resolution will occur.

The diagnosis is confirmed by ultrasonography and a barium meal produces a typical appearance with the body of the stomach seen to be separated from the spine in oblique views by the distended cyst.

Once a decision to operate has been made the majority of surgeons drain such cysts into the stomach, using the transgastric approach first described by Jedlucka in 1923.

(*c*) *Pancreatic abscess.* This complication only occurs following acute pancreatic necrosis which leads to sloughing of some or all of the pancreas. Colonization of the slough and the surrounding tissues takes place with both aerobic and anaerobic organisms producing the abscess. Clinically the patient, initially severely ill, partially recovers only to develop a high swinging temperature and a marked leucocytosis both of which persist unless adequate surgical drainage is achieved. Once formed the abscess tends to spread within the retroperitoneal tissues as well as into neighbouring organs and blood vessels so that a variety of complications may develop including a massive fatal haematemesis.

Once the diagnosis has been made adequate surgical drainage together with the removal of the necrotic infected pancreatic slough are essential. If this is adequately performed about 75 per cent of patients will survive this, the most serious local complication of acute pancreatitis.

The abdomen should be explored by an anterior transabdominal approach so that the whole abdomen can be examined. All the necrotic pancreas should be removed and the area in which abscess cavities are present should be adequately drained, bringing the drains out onto the surface. Following recovery from the operation an external pancreatic fistula may develop. Fortunately the majority of fistulae close spontaneously and, therefore, they should be treated conservatively. One of the chief aids is the institution of total parenteral nutrition combined with control of the orifice of the fistula so that autodigestion of the skin is reduced to a minimum. Should the fistula fail to close an underlying cause such as retained slough or a pancreatic neoplasm should be suspected.

6 *Duodenal ileus*

This complication usually develops within 14 days of the onset of an acute attack of pancreatitis. A barium meal shows that the stomach empties slowly if at all, the duodenal mucosa is irregular and the duodenal loop widened. In the majority of cases the condition resolves spontaneously but in a minority a gastrojejunostomy may be required.

7 Haematemesis
Severe upper gastrointestinal haemorrhage following an attack of severe pancreatitis may be due to:

(a) multiple gastric erosions in the acute stage of the disease. This condition should be treated by cimetidine;
(b) erosion of a major vessel in patients in whom an 'expanding' pancreatic abscess is present. This condition may be fatal.

8 Burst abdomen
The incidence of abdominal dehiscence, if a laparotomy is performed, is approximately three times higher than the generally accepted level following surgery. The cause is presumably leakage of pancreatic enzymes and the early digestion of catgut stitches in the wound. Wounds should therefore be closed with unabsorbable sutures.

6.10 Diagnosis and management of chronic pancreatitis

Definition. Chronic pancreatitis is a condition in which structural and functional changes are present in the pancreas even in the symptomless patient. Using the Marseilles symposium the condition can be classified into:

1. recurrent chronic pancreatitis;
2. chronic pancreatitis.

The difference between the two groups is clinical rather than pathological since in the recurrent type of the disease the patient suffers from intermittent abdominal pain whereas in the latter variety the pain is constant.

Both types of pancreatitis are rare in most parts of the United Kingdom.

Aetiology

Unlike acute pancreatitis which is associated with an abnormally high incidence of gall-stones chronic pancreatitis is more commonly associated with a high alcohol and high fat intake.

In an experimental animal such as the rat the histological changes associated with chronic pancreatitis can be reproduced if the animal is allowed to drink unrestricted quantities of 20 per cent alcohol and in the same animals if to the high alcohol intake is added a diet rich in fat and protein, the intracanalicular precipitation of protein plugs develops which many investigators think may be the underlying cause of the disease.

Chronic pancreatitis may also develop when the pancreatic duct is blocked either by an inflammatory stricture of the ampulla or occasionally by an underlying carcinoma of the head of the pancreas. A rare cause is hypercalcaemia due to primary or secondary hyperparathyroidism.

Pathology

Macroscopic appearance
A severely diseased gland is so fibrosed that it is often contracted to about half its normal size. The pancreatic margins, so clearly defined in the normal gland are indefinite due to the associated peripancreatic fibrosis. The gland is hard, fixed and may impart a gritty sensation to the palpating fingers highly suggestive of malignant disease.

Histological appearance
Histological examination may show ductal dilatation, cyst formation and periductal and periacinar fibrosis with little derangement of the lobules and acini or there may be pronounced fibrosis accompanied by duct ectasia. In the latter condition there is squamous metaplasia of the lining epithelium together with periductal round cell infiltration. Islet cell destruction is possible and is responsible for diabetes in 5 per cent of the so-called mild cases and 75 per cent in the more severe.

An additional pathological change, rarely seen in the UK, is glandular calcification, the exact significance of which remains unknown since routine radiology of the abdomen sometimes reveals gross pancreatic calcification in the absence of any clinical symptoms.

The cysts seen in chronic pancreatitis may be small but as coalescence occurs so larger cysts are formed which may either remain confined to the organ or burst into the peripancreatic tissues to form pancreatic pseudocysts.

In the early stages of the disease the major ducts may appear normal but as the disease progresses so the ducts may become dilated by the development of strictures, calculi or both.

Clinical presentation

The common presenting symptoms of this disease include:

1. abdominal pain;
2. symptoms due to reduced or absence of exocrine function, i.e. steatorrhoea;
3. symptoms due to endocrine dysfunction, i.e. diabetes;
4. symptoms due to associated disease, i.e.
   (*a*) biliary tract disease;
   (*b*) carcinoma of pancreas;

(c) alcoholism;
(d) narcotic addiction.

1 Pain

The pain of chronic pancreatitis may be continuous, remittent and, occasionally, colicky. It is distinguished from cardiac pain in that it seldom, if ever, radiates to the neck and arms. It may be relieved by sitting up, which may lead to increasing exhaustion if the pain begins in the late evening. When chronic and continuous it can easily be mistaken for ulcer pain but, unlike the latter, it is not relieved by vomiting or alkalis.

The pain may be precipitated by eating or drinking and, apart from the specific metabolic disturbances associated with pancreatitis, e.g. loss of exocrine function which may itself lead to weight loss, patients may literally starve themselves to death in an effort to avoid painful episodes.

2 Steatorrhoea

As increasing deterioration of exocrine function develops steatorrhoea eventually follows and is found in over half the patients. Clinically this condition is recognized by the changing quality of the stools, which become paler, bulkier, loose, and perhaps watery. Such stools are often offensive and may be difficult to flush.

3 Diabetes

The onset of diabetes is usually heralded by the development of thirst and polyuria. This condition is common in the severe cases and less frequent in the milder type.

4 Symptoms due to associated disease

(a) *Gall-stones.* The incidence of gall-stones, and therefore, symptoms due to gall-stones is much rarer in chronic than acute pancreatitis. A review by Berman showed that stones were present only in about a fifth of patients suffering from chronic disease.

(b) *Carcinoma of the pancreas.* Although the two diseases are not commonly associated there are numerous reports in the literature of chronic pancreatitis secondary to carcinoma of the head of the gland.

(c) *Alcoholism.* The published literature makes it clear that pancreatic calcification is commoner in alcoholics suffering from pancreatitis than non-alcoholics. The majority of physicians would also agree that undue amounts of alcohol will often precipitate pain and renewed activity but the converse is not necessarily true and total abstinence may still be associated with attacks of pain.

(d) *Narcotic addiction.* The pain of chronic pancreatitis may be so severe and prolonged that eventually narcotic addiction develops. This is not difficult to believe when one has the opportunity of observing such a patient at first hand.

Investigations

1 Biochemical
(a) *Serum amylase.* So long as functioning exocrine tissue remains the serum

amylase will rise with each attack of severe pain above the upper limit of normal, 200 Somogyi units.

(b) *Pancreatic function studies.* Exocrine function. The duodenum is intubated under X-ray control, after which the pancreas is stimulated by administration of secretin, 1.0 units/kg and pancreozymin, 1.7 units/kg. As the functioning exocrine tissue is destroyed so the total volume, bicarbonate, and enzyme secretion falls. At the time of injection of secretin the patient may develop pain and an elevated serum amylase.

(c) *Glucose tolerance test and plasma insulin level.* Either of these studies may reveal the presence of latent or overt diabetes.

(d) *Investigation of stools.* A simple microscopic examination of the stools may show undigested meat fibres or fat globules. More sophisticated and much more expensive is a fat balance. Using the latter technique a daily excretion of fat in excess of 6 g/day on a diet containing 100 g of fat clearly indicates steatorrhoea.

2 *Radiological investigations*
The following radiological examinations may be of assistance:

(a) *plain X-rays.* These may show pancreatic calcification or gall-stones and, when the patient is complaining of severe pain, a sentinel loop;
(b) *an oral cholecystogram.* Demonstrating loss of biliary function, gall-stones, or both;
(c) *hypotonic duodenography.* This was introduced by Liotta in 1951 and may show deformity of the duodenal mucosa;
(d) *retrograde pancreatography.* This is performed after cannulating the sphincter by using a fibreoptic gastroscope. It may show strictures of the pancreatic duct;
(e) *pancreatic arteriography.* This is a rarely used technique. It makes possible, however, the distinction between chronic pancreatitis and malignant disease due to the different vascular patterns in these two conditions.
(f) *computerized axial tomography.* This investigation which is not generally available may demonstrate a small shrunken pancreas, calcification too ill-defined to be seen on plain radiographs or cyst formation.

3 *Isotope investigation*
Pancreatic scintiscanning is performed using ^{75}Se-selenomethionine which is selectively taken up by functioning pancreatic tissue. A reduced uptake would be expected in severe generalized disease of the pancreas.

Treatment

Essentially the treatment of chronic pancreatitis is medical rather than surgical.

Medical
When alcoholism is a contributing factor every effort must be made to persuade the patient to abstain. Diabetes, if present, should be controlled by insulin, and exocrine deficiencies producing steatorrhoea can be partially alleviated by the

use of pancreatic extracts, the use and dose of which will nearly always require considerable adjustment in the early period.

Surgical
Indications for surgical treatment are nearly always relative rather than absolute. They include:

1. recurrent attacks of pain which are increasing in frequency and severity;
2. continuous pain after meals;
3. marked weight loss due to fear of eating.

The surgical literature reveals that many operations have been proposed and performed in this condition; this itself leads to the conclusion that the majority of surgical manoeuvres are unsatisfactory and, therefore, should not be undertaken before a prolonged period of 'medical' treatment. The surgical techniques available can be divided into those that seek by indirect means to alleviate the condition and those directed at the pancreas itself.

Indirect surgery
1. *Cholecystectomy with or without choledochotomy.* The literature suggests that even relapsing pancreatitis will sometimes respond to cholecystectomy if stones are present in the biliary tree. On the other hand, cholecystectomy should never be performed in the absence of demonstrable gall bladder disease.
2. *Ampullary sphincterotomy.* In 1948, Doubilet and Mulholland published their first article presenting the rationale for this operation and by 1956 they were able to review their results in 319 patients, 190 of whom had been followed up for more than 2 years. They reported an operative mortality of 7 per cent and excellent clinical results in 88 per cent. Prior to the division of the sphincter, radiological studies were used to confirm that the pancreatic and common bile ducts passed through a common channel. This they regarded as an extremely important step before performing sphincterotomy because Doubilet's concept of the aetiology of chronic pancreatitis was that the basic cause was the reflux of bile into the pancreatic duct. Obviously this can happen only if a common channel exists so that spasm or stricture can result in such reflux.

In their series, a higher than average proportion of patients were shown to have such anatomical arrangement. They claimed that sphincterotomy abolished acute attacks or chronic pain and allowed regeneration of the damaged pancreas. However, in 214 patients a diseased gall bladder was also removed and this could, of course, also explain some of their success.

It is interesting that no other surgeons were able to reproduce such good results, that experimental work indicates that fibrosis and stenosis tends to follow sphincterotomy, and thirdly, that any decrease in pressure within the biliary tree after sphincterotomy is only temporary.

3. *Coeliac ganglionectomy.* This operation, either unilateral or bilateral, has been performed by a number of surgeons for the relief of pancreatic pain. The largest reported series is that of Mallet-Guy who reported his results in 42 patients who were followed for a variable period of between 1 and 9 years. He

found that approximately 80 per cent of his patients were relieved of pain although no other surgeon has obtained such a degree of success.

Direct pancreatic surgery
Two rather different types of operation have been described.
1 *Puestow's operation.* The aim of this operation is to retain as much pancreatic tissue as possible and to decompress the gland by opening the duct widely along its anterior surface. The basic concept behind this operation is the belief that sphincterotomy fails due to a multiplicity of strictures along the length of the pancreatic duct. The basic steps of this operation are as follows:

(*a*) The abdomen is opened and the diagnosis confirmed.
(*b*) The spleen is removed and the pancreas is dissected free from the peripancreatic fibrous tissue as far medially as the superior mesenteric vessels.
(*c*) The tail is removed from the gland so that the pancreatic duct can be identified.
(*d*) The duct is now opened along its whole length and a segment of the anterior part of the body is removed.
(*e*) A Roux en Y is fashioned and the jejunal loop is then brought over the pancreas and its serosa is stitched to the peripancreatic tissues.
(*f*) The abdomen is closed.

Puestow described the results in 25 patients: there was 1 death, 2 were not improved and 22 were relieved of pain. The author has also found that this operation gives good results but in about half the patients the pancreas is so shrunken that the operation is not technically possible.

2 *Pancreatectomy.* This operation involves removal of all the remaining pancreatic tissue except for a small cuff of the head lying within the lesser curve of the duodenum. This not only preserves some pancreatic tissue and the common bile duct, but also the superior and inferior pancreaticoduodenal arteries so that necrosis of these various structures is rare.

Fry who has written extensively about this form of surgery in chronic pancreatitis has performed the operation 25 times. A quarter of his patients were narcotic addicts and 14 had had one or more unsuccessful operations. Of the 25 patients, 13 had an excellent result, being free from pain, gaining weight and able to return to work, and the remainder had an indifferent or a poor result. Fry concluded that if the entire head of the pancreas is left recurrent pain is almost inevitable, a conclusion with which most other authors would agree. The natural extension of this procedure would, of course, be total pancreaticoduodenectomy but the mortality rate of this procedure is high and the postoperative condition leaves much to be desired.

Following direct interference with the pancreas it is important to abstain from alcohol, correct the diabetic state and, if possible, control the steatorrhoea.

3 *Miscellaneous procedures*
(*a*) Rarely, chronic pancreatitis is associated with a parathyroid adenoma. Removal of the adenoma then results in total relief so long as the pancreatic pathology has not progressed to complete destruction.

(*b*) Vagotomy and partial gastrectomy have also been advocated but the rationale seems extremely doubtful.

6.11 Indications for and complications of splenectomy

The indications for splenectomy are as follows:

1 Trauma

Accidental rupture
The most common cause of accidental rupture of the spleen is a road traffic accident, the lower left thoracic region and upper abdomen being injured either by direct contact with the steering wheel or alternatively, the strap of the safety belt if this is being worn at the time of the accident. Occasionally the capsule or the hilum may be torn during the course of an operation, e.g. high Polya gastrectomy.

A splenic injury resulting from a road traffic accident may be only a single facet of a multiple injury situation complicated by the development of signs of intraperitoneal haemorrhage, i.e. evidence of haemorrhagic shock, abdominal tenderness or rigidity and possibly bruising or even tyre marks over the lower chest and abdomen. An X-ray of the chest may show fractures of the lower left ribs.

When intraperitoneal haemorrhage is suspected it may be confirmed by peritoneal lavage, a method first described by Gill and his co-workers in 1975. This diagnostic procedure has now almost entirely superseded peritoneal tapping. The method is as follows. The bladder is emptied. A small incision is made 3 cm below the umbilicus and through this a dialysing catheter is introduced into the abdominal cavity. Thereafter 1000 ml of isotonic saline (500 ml in children) is slowly introduced into the abdomen with the patient in a slight Trendelenburg position. After 10 minutes the fluid is syphoned from the abdominal cavity when any blood staining indicates the presence of intra-abdominal haemorrhage. An alternative procedure is to introduce the catheter into the abdomen at the point of maximum tenderness. Few false negative results occur using this method and false positive results are also virtually non-existent in the presence of overt intraperitoneal bleeding.

So far as the spleen itself is concerned three chief injuries are recognized:

1 subcapsular haematoma formation;
2 lacerations with fragmentation;
3 hilar disruption with major vascular damage.

Subcapsular haematoma occurs in some 10–20 per cent of patients sustaining an abdominal injury and in the absence of any other associated intra-abdominal injury is probably unrecognized and undiagnosed in a further group because the physical signs associated with this injury are minimal. The problem with this type of case and also in the patient in whom a minimal capsular rupture has occurred is the development of delayed splenic rupture which may not occur until some 3 weeks after the initial injury when the abrupt development of haemorrhagic shock together with generalized rigidity occurs. In this group of patients immediate laparotomy is required.

The probable mechanism by which so-called delayed rupture occurs is by the slow liquefaction of a subcapsular clot which then by osmosis takes up sufficient fluid to burst the confines of the splenic capsule or the adhesions which have formed around the tear.

Treatment of splenic injuries
As with any situation in which bleeding is a predominant feature resuscitation is required before surgical intervention.

When the physical signs and investigations such as plain radiographs of the abdomen indicate that the spleen has been injured adequate access can be obtained by means of a left paramedian incision; see *Tutorials 3*, page 90. However, in a grossly obese individual with a 'deep' abdomen the operator can expect difficulties, not only in identifying the precise injury which has occurred but also its severity. Occasionally the spleen may have been torn from the splenic vessels at the hilum and be found floating free within the abdomen.

Until recently the great majority of surgeons would have recommended without any reservation whatsoever the operation of splenectomy, taking particular care not to injure the tail of the pancreas or the greater curvature of the stomach, either of which may produce a fatal complication.

However, two observations have led some surgeons to adopt a more conservative approach to splenic injury. These are as follows:

1. following splenectomy in the first 10–14 days the platelet count rises rapidly to levels which threaten the development of intravascular thrombosis. Anticoagulant therapy is indicated if there is a sustained rise above $500\,000/mm^3$.
2. as a late complication the absence of all splenic tissue leads to the danger of overwhelming infection. This danger appears to be greatest in infants under the age of 4 at the time of splenectomy but adults do not appear to be exempt. The major pathogens leading to death are *H. influenzae*, *S. pneumoniae* and the meningococcus. In one series it was found that the greatest danger occurred within the first 2 postoperative years and some authorities recommend the routine use of prophylactic penicillin over this period of time. In addition to bacterial infections malarial infections also appear to be more dangerous in the asplenic individual.

Whilst many series support the above statement contrary evidence has been produced from some centres. For example, in a series of children examined following splenectomy at the Boston Children's Hospital it was found that there appeared to be no added risk of infection in children in whom the spleen was removed for local lesions, trauma or idiopathic thrombocytopenic purpura, a slightly increased risk in patients subjected to splenectomy for idiopathic thrombocytopenic purpura and a considerable risk in children suffering from the Wiskott–Aldrich syndrome in which there is dysgammaglobulinaemia and eczema and in patients with Cooley's anaemia in which the abnormal haemoglobins F and S are found.

When a conservative approach is adopted the bleeding from the torn splenic tissue is controlled either by an omental overlay or a haemostatic agent such as microfibrillar collagen (Avitene). Deeper lacerations require not only this type of treatment but also deep figure of eight sutures and if the tip of the spleen is avulsed this must be removed. Although the author has no personal experience of these methods he has seen three patients in whom a remnant of the spleen has been preserved using these techniques.

A further method of preserving some splenic function is to perform an autotransplantation of slices of splenic tissue into the omentum. This does not appear to the author to be a satisfactory solution since one of the known complications of rupture of the spleen is the condition of splenosis when small implants of splenic cells become adherent to the serosal surface covering the various viscera and produce an intense fibrotic reaction which ultimately leads to intestinal obstruction. The condition grossly resembles endometriosis and is ultimately fatal.

2 Incidental removal

This would include splenectomy as a formal event in the course of an operation.

Until recently, radical surgical treatment of carcinoma of the stomach consisted of removing the stomach, the tail of the pancreas, and the spleen. Now, however, although the spleen may be removed, the tail of the pancreas is left intact in case there should be pancreatic leakage which was a common cause of both morbidity and mortality.

The spleen must be removed if portal hypertension is treated by splenorenal anastomosis. In general, this operation is followed by a lower incidence of encephalopathy than a portacaval shunt but a higher incidence of thrombosis and rebleeding. It has, therefore, been generally abandoned in favour of an end-to-side anastomosis between the divided portal vein and the inferior vena cava.

3 Hypersplenism

The term hypersplenism was introduced in 1907 by Chauffard when describing a patient suffering from hereditary spherocytosis. The condition is now defined as one in which a reduction of one or more of the cellular components of the blood may be reversed by splenectomy.

Classification

Hypersplenism is traditionally classified into primary and secondary types. In the primary type, the spleen enlarges and there is a reduction in some or all of the cellular elements of the peripheral blood in the absence of a demonstrable underlying pathological process. In the secondary type of hypersplenism there are two subgroups:

1. primary splenic disorders associated with secondary haematological effects;
2. primary cellular abnormalities affecting red cells with secondary functional change in the spleen.

The main difference between these two groups is that in primary splenic disorders, e.g. malignant lymphoma, the disease process deforms and alters the splenic anatomy in such a way that an excess of normal cells is diverted into the splenic pulp. In the second group, e.g. hereditary spherocytosis, abnormal red cells are diverted into the pulp by a healthy spleen and there destroyed. One reason for red cell destruction is the dependence of the mature erythrocyte on an adequate supply of glucose to maintain the outer membrane intact. Even in a normal spleen the glucose concentration is only a third of that in the peripheral blood and, therefore, any red cell that is segregated and sequestered is in grave danger of destruction.

The major causes of secondary hypersplenism due to a primary splenic abnormality are:

1. chronic congestive splenomegaly, e.g. cirrhosis;
2. lymphoreticular disease, e.g. chronic lymphatic leukaemia;
3. myeloproliferative disease, e.g. chronic myeloid leukaemia;
4. the reticuloendothelioses, e.g. Gaucher's disease;
5. infections, acute, chronic and tropical;
6. systemic disorders, e.g. rheumatoid arthritis.

Causes of secondary hypersplenism due to a primary cellular abnormality include:

1. congenital causes, e.g. hereditary spherocytosis, thalassaemia, and some cases of genetic red cell enzymopathy such as pyruvate kinase deficiency;
2. acquired, e.g. autoimmune haemolytic anaemia.

Certain types of hypersplenism are uniformly cured by splenectomy although in many patients the treatment of the underlying disorder is of greater importance.

An example of primary hypersplenism cured by splenectomy in the majority of patients is idiopathic thrombocytopenia.

The diagnosis of this condition is made by exclusion, since many different agents, particularly drugs such as aspirin and tolbutamide, may produce a thrombocytopenia. In the absence of any precipitating factor a diagnosis of idiopathic thrombocytopenic purpura is considered if the platelet count is less than $50\,000/mm^3$ ($50 \times 10^9/l$). The disease may be acute or chronic and the most common clinical manifestation is periodic attacks of purpura. The acute form is seen in childhood, and the sex incidence is equal. The chronic form is more common in young adults, and females are more commonly affected than males. The disease is of unknown aetiology but there is possibly an immune factor since platelet-fixing antibodies are found in a high proportion of patients. The acute type commonly undergoes spontaneous remission but corticosteroids are usually given to reduce the risk of intracranial bleeding. Splenectomy, however, provides a permanent remission rate of 80 per cent. Immediately before the operation, if the condition is very severe, a platelet transfusion may be necessary to avoid severe postoperative bleeding.

An example of secondary hypersplenism due to a primary cellular abnormality cured by splenectomy is hereditary spherocytosis, a condition that is inherited as an autosomal dominant and has a wide range of clinical severity. Characteristically, there is acholuric jaundice, often precipitated by strenuous exercise or excessive fatigue. In later life pigment gall-stones form and, occasionally, intractable leg ulcers. This is the most common congenital abnormality of the red cell in Northern Europe. The red cell, usually a biconcave disc, is more spherical than normal due to a loss of surface lipids. The cell membrane is also extremely permeable to the passive influx of Na^+. This forms the basis of the fragility test in which the cells are exposed to decreasing concentrations of sodium chloride. The patient's own red cells labelled with ^{51}Cr have a reduced half-life of 20 days or less.

The abnormal red cells with their 'brittle' membranes are segregated, sequestered, and prematurely destroyed in the pulp cords of the spleen.

Splenectomy in this condition is followed by a return to a normal haemoglobin level, considerable prolongation of red cell survival, and a reduction in the incidence of complications.

The situation is similar in thalassaemia in which there is a congenital defect in haemoglobin synthesis. This condition may occasionally respond to splenectomy.

4 Diagnostic indications

(a) Hodgkin's disease
It has become commonplace in the course of investigating patients suffering from this disease to perform a laparotomy, remove the spleen, perform a liver biopsy, and remove one or more para-aortic lymph nodes. These procedures allow the disease process to be correctly staged and, therefore, give some indication of the correct therapy.

(b) Large abdominal masses
Massive splenomegaly in the absence of other diagnostic symptoms may occur in hydatid disease, degenerative cysts, and the reticuloses, especially lymphosarcoma.

6.12 Classification of intestinal obstruction and the general principles of management

Intestinal obstruction may be classified in a variety of ways:

1 *By duration*
(a) acute
(b) chronic
(c) acute on chronic

Acute obstruction nearly always involves the small bowel, and chronic obstruction, or acute on chronic, the large bowel.

2 *Adynamic and dynamic*
The term 'adynamic' is reserved for patients in whom peristalsis has ceased. True ileus is most frequently caused by pus in the abdomen and, less commonly, by lesions of the spinal cord producing 'spinal shock'. Dynamic ileus implies the presence of a mechanical obstruction leading to excessive peristaltic activity.

The causes of mechanical obstruction may be intraluminal, e.g. a gall-stone ileus, or in the large bowel impacted faeces, mural when the cause is nearly always a neoplasm or extraluminal when the commonest cause is an external hernia or an intraperitoneal band or peritoneal recess bounded by a relatively sharp border, e.g. herniation through the foramen of Winslow into the lesser sac.

However, prolonged mechanical obstruction eventually causes paralysis of the proximal dilated bowel. This is particularly seen in ileal atresia, when the dilated bowel proximal to the atretic segment is incapable of contracting even after the relief of the obstruction.

3 *Simple or strangulating*
The term 'simple' implies that the blood supply to the bowel is intact, whereas in 'strangulating' it is jeopardized. To the practising surgeon this is the most important aspect of obstruction. Strangulating obstruction, if unrelieved, leads to gangrene of the gut, perforation, and peritonitis.

4 *Small or large bowel*
In general, obstruction of the small bowel is more dangerous than in the large because severe early vomiting may lead to a rapid depletion of fluid and electrolytes.

5 *Congenital or acquired*
Congenital causes of obstruction are usually obvious in the neonatal period, i.e. within the first 14 days of life, although babies suffering from Hirschsprung's disease may occasionally go undiagnosed for as long as 3 months.

Malrotation, usually presenting shortly after birth, may also occasionally cause a strangulating obstruction in the adult.

Clinical presentation

The major symptoms of obstruction are as follows:

1 *Pain*
The pain of small bowel obstruction is usually felt in the periumbilical region, whereas obstruction to the large bowel causes a lower abdominal colic, often described by the patient as running across the iliac fossae.

In chronic obstruction the bouts of pain and constipation are often separated, at first, by lengthy intervals which become shorter until finally acute obstruction supervenes. Strangulating obstructions are associated with colic and, in addition, a constant pain due to the presence of the strangulated loop.

2 *Vomiting*
This may be copious and repetitive. The higher the obstruction the earlier is its onset. A patient suffering from low small bowel obstruction is usually vomiting repeatedly within 6 hours.

3 *Constipation and obstipation*

4 *Distension*
This is partly due to gas and in part to retained fluid. The gas content is composed of air which has been swallowed which accounts for the particularly high concentration of nitrogen which may reach 80 per cent of the total volume, gas which has diffused from the blood which accounts for a part of the carbon dioxide present and CH_4 the presence of which is almost entirely due to bacterial fermentation in the large bowel. In addition very variable quantities of hydrogen may also be present due also to bacterial metabolism.

So far as the fluid content of the bowel is concerned this is formed of intestinal secretions. The total potential load of fluid which enters the gastrointestinal tract amounts to between 7 and 8 l/24 hours but of this only about 1.5 l reaches the caecum and then in the ascending colon one further litre is absorbed. When the gut is obstructed reabsorption on the scale referred to above fails to occur and there is an increased secretion of fluid and electrolytes into the lumen of the bowel. These changes occur because as the intestinal secretions accumulate the intraluminal pressure rises and the optimal conditions for absorption are exceeded and secondly, the increase in intraluminal pressure compresses the mucosal veins leading to congestion and oedema and a sharp rise in secretion.

As the intestine dilates so the volume of fluid and gas which it can contain increases as the square of the radius. Thus one metre of undistended bowel approximately 2 cm in diameter can accommodate 300 ml of fluid and air but dilated by only twice this diameter its capacity rises to 1300 ml. It is thus easy to see why a patient suffering from small bowel obstruction, even in the absence of strangulation can become gravely ill due to dehydration.

5 *Perforation*
Progressive distension of the bowel wall leads to diminishing contractility, and as the process continues impairment of viability. Finally, there is mucosal and stercoral ulceration followed by perforation. This cycle of events is always seen in closed loop obstructions, an example of which is large bowel obstruction in the presence of a competent ileocaecal valve. Such obstruction leads to severe fluid and electrolyte imbalance and, probably, greater diffusion of 'toxins' from the bowel into the blood stream. The major effect of diminished viability takes place in the caecum which may perforate as soon as the abdomen is opened and its extrinsic support removed.

Signs of obstruction

1 distension;
2 audible or visible hyperperistalsis;
3 evidence of dehydration, e.g. diminished skin turgor and fall in urine volume;
4 vomiting;
5 failure to pass wind or faeces;
6 peritonism and rebound tenderness in the presence of a strangulated loop.

When faced with suspected obstruction the clinician must ask and answer four questions:

1 Is the obstruction simple or strangulating? If the latter, operative intervention should be carried out without delay.
2 If surgery is required is the patient's general condition satisfactory?
3 What is the level of the obstruction?
4 What is the cause?

The answer to the first question is nearly always solved by careful history taking and physical examination. The second question is related to the degree of dehydration brought about by vomiting or the volume of blood sequestered within a strangulated loop. If the patient is oliguric this is strong confirmatory evidence of dehydration. Slight loss of skin turgor should be treated by the immediate administration of 2 litres of isotonic saline but if signs of impending circulatory collapse and marked oliguria are present 4 litres are normally required. When long segment strangulating obstruction is present, e.g. a small bowel volvulus or mesenteric venous thrombosis, large quantities of blood are lost both into the wall and the lumen of the gut which need replacement prior to surgery.

Level of obstruction
The history may be significant, but additional evidence can also be obtained from plain radiographs of the abdomen taken in the supine and, if possible, the erect position; if this is impossible a lateral film should be taken.

In a normal individual, air/fluid levels may be seen in the stomach, duodenum, the small bowel of a bed-fast patient or a person suffering from jejunal diverticulosis, and in the hepatic and splenic flexures of the large bowel. Apparently excessive air in the absence of distension is meaningless. The radiological signs of obstruction are gas-filled distended loops associated with fluid levels. The dilated loops often form a distinctive pattern due to the arrangement of the circular folds of mucosa. In the upper half of the jejunum these produce a regular and complete cross-hatching; in the lower half of the ileum they are usually absent and the bowel is featureless; in the distended colon, they form an interdigitating incomplete pattern within the lumen of the bowel.

When peritonitis causing ileus precipitates obstruction, the distended loops are often separated by the fluid that lies between them, and the lower half of the abdomen may be hazy or opaque.

The cause of intestinal obstruction
The aetiology of obstruction may be obvious from the clinical history and physical examination. Important and common causes include external herniae, adhesions or bands from previous intra-abdominal surgery, and carcinoma of the large bowel. All require appropriate surgical intervention, particularly in the presence of physical signs indicating that the blood supply to the involved bowel is in jeopardy.

Surgical intervention

Small bowel obstruction

1 The first step in the treatment of a patient suffering from small bowel obstruction is the passage of a nasogastric tube followed by the application of intermittent or continuous suction. It is essential that the stomach is emptied completely since in the presence of severe hypotension due to dehydration the patient may drown in his own vomit whilst still awaiting resuscitation or surgery. Furthermore, if surgery is considered necessary the moment of greatest hazard is immediately prior to endotracheal intubation shortly after the patient is paralysed. At this time vomit may be inhaled producing an aspiration pneumonia which may be fatal in the elderly patient.
2 The second step is determined by the physical state of the patient. In the presence of overt dehydration time should be taken to correct this by the administration of Hartmann's solution or isotonic saline having first taken a sample of blood so that the various electrolyte components can be measured.
3 The third step depends upon the anticipated diagnosis and the response of the patient to the conservative regimen described above. For example, in the presence of multiple laparotomy scars together with a history of recurrent bouts of abdominal pain the best course may be to adopt a conservative regimen considering that the patient is suffering from multiple adhesions rather than a single band.

In some instances such patients are treated by intestinal plication, suturing the small intestinal loops with interrupted serosal sutures into a ladder pattern within the abdominal cavity, or a similar effect can be produced by the Child's Phillips transmesenteric plication method. Neither of these operations has been performed by the author nor is he aware of them having been performed within his own hospitals suggesting that the need for such drastic steps must be extremely rare.

4 When the abdomen is opened or a hernial sac is exposed the following signs indicate the necessity for a gut resection:

   (*a*) loss of the serosal sheen;
   (*b*) obvious perforation of the bowel;
   (*c*) failure of the colour of the gut to change following the application of a warm pack and the administration of oxygen;
   (*d*) obvious lack of pulsation in the mesenteric arteries or thrombosis of the mesenteric veins.

Large bowel obstruction

So far as carcinoma of the large bowel is concerned, approximately a fifth present in this manner, the precise incidence depending somewhat on the site, since obstruction, frequently acute on chronic, is commoner when the tumour involves the left rather than the right colon. Less common causes of large bowel obstruction include diverticulitis, volvulus, and ischaemic colitis. All, except the last-named, may be complicated by perforation or stercoral ulceration. Some patients suffering from large bowel obstruction may require fluid replacement, others require cardiorespiratory resuscitation and all, if requiring surgery, should have the stomach completely emptied before the induction of anaesthesia in order to avoid aspiration.

The operative measures used for the relief of obstructing tumours of the colon include:

1 tumours situated in the caecum, ascending or transverse colon. An immediate right hemicolectomy is as safe as, if not safer than, caecostomy because the latter carries a considerable risk of infection. The mortality of caecostomy in large bowel obstruction may be as high as 50 per cent, whereas the mortality of immediate resection is, in some reported series, lower than 10 per cent;
2 tumours in the descending and sigmoid colon can be treated in several different ways. Probably the best treatment for a carcinoma of the descending colon is a transverse colostomy, delaying formal resection until the bowel has deflated. Tumours of the sigmoid may also be treated in this manner or, if secondary deposits are already palpable in the liver, by a Paul–Mikulicz type of resection.

6.13 Neonatal intestinal obstruction, excluding anorectal abnormalities

Incidence
Based on the World Health Organization statistics, neonatal intestinal abnormalities are approximately eight times less frequent than congenital abnormalities of the central nervous system, which occur in 2–3 per 1000 deliveries. Only two congenital disorders of the gastrointestinal tract are of genetic importance: duodenal atresia, because of its relatively high incidence in Down's syndrome, and fibrocystic disease of the pancreas.

Occasionally, the cause of the obstruction may be obvious on first inspection of the baby, e.g. the anal pit may be absent. More commonly, however, the diagnosis is unsuspected immediately after birth but becomes obvious within 48 hours, when the onset of the following signs leads to investigation.

Signs of neonatal obstruction

1 *Vomiting*
An important sign of obstruction is vomiting, although this may be caused by a variety of other conditions, including infection, birth injuries to the brain, cretinism, or fibrocystic disease. Vomiting is not uncommon in the normal neonate, 50 per cent having at least one vomit during the first 24 hours of extrauterine life. However, vomiting assumes greater significance when it is persistent and bile-stained. In oesophageal atresia vomiting cannot occur, but the baby chokes and becomes cyanosed during feeding.

2 *Constipation*
Another important symptom is failure to pass meconium; 92 per cent of normal infants pass their first meconium stool within 24 hours. Delay beyond 36 hours calls for investigation. It should, however, be noted that in high, small gut obstruction one or more normal meconium stools may be passed even when the obstruction is complete.

3 *Abdominal distension*
The third important sign of obstruction is distension.

Other rare causes include cysts or tumours of the kidney (nephroblastoma), tumours of the nervous system (neuroblastoma), a distended bladder, usually the result of obstruction by congenital urethral valves, and pneumoperitoneum which occasionally exists without an obvious perforation.

4 *Oedema of the abdominal wall*
If the abdominal wall is oedematous, particularly in association with distension, the underlying cause is nearly always a meconium peritonitis due either to perforation of an obstructed bowel or internal strangulation.

Aetiology of obstruction

These were classified by Mason Brown in the following manner:

1. Faults in the passages:
   Congenital
   (a) atresia
   (b) stenosis
   (c) cystic duplication
2. Faults in the powers:
   Congenital
   (a) defects in the myenteric plexus
   (b) pyloric stenosis
   Acquired: paralytic ileus due to peritonitis or maternal drugs
3. Faults in the passenger:
   (a) meconium ileus
   (b) meconium plugs
4. Extrinsic causes:
   Congenital
   (a) adhesions and bands
   (b) annular pancreas
   (c) Meckel's diverticulum
   (d) external or internal herniation
   Acquired: postoperative adhesions

HAZARDS OF NEONATAL OBSTRUCTION

Three hazards face the neonate suffering from intestinal obstruction:

1. electrolyte disturbance;
2. gangrene of the obstructed bowel due to vascular obstruction;
3. inhalation of vomit.

Inhalation of vomit, immediately after birth, is the most dangerous, and if the neonate must be transferred for further investigation and treatment nasogastric suction should be started before the transfer.

Of the various causes, only the commoner will be described in greater detail here.

The atresias

Aetiology
Tandler's theory of failure of vacuolation. This theory was in favour for many years but foundered when it was shown that squamous epithelial cells of skin origin can be found in the gut distal to the atretic segment.

Vascular theory. This was first put forward by Jaboulay and, more recently, Louw of South Africa has produced a great deal of experimental evidence in its support. He showed that destruction of the intestinal vascular network in fetal puppies led to varying degrees of atresia, depending on the size of the vessels destroyed. By varying this he was able to produce single or multiple segments, and diaphragmatic or lengthy defects.

Duodenal atresia

This condition is associated with early vomiting, which may or may not be bile-stained according to the disposition of the common bile duct. In this form of obstruction it is not uncommon for at least one meconium stool to be passed, thereby confusing the clinical diagnosis.

The diagnosis is usually simple and is made on the evidence of plain X-rays of the abdomen. X-rays in recumbency show gross dilatation of the stomach and duodenum; in the erect position, the characteristic double bubble appearance is seen, due to the fluid levels in the distended duodenum and stomach.

Treatment. The operation of choice is duodenoduodenostomy. Unfortunately, the long term prognosis may be poor because approximately 25 per cent of neonates suffering from duodenal atresia are also mongols. In addition, a relatively high proportion suffer from congenital heart disease.

Ileal atresia

This condition is not usually associated with other congenital abnormalities although the bowel in an exomphalos may be atretic.

Presentation. The neonate begins to vomit and, if the obstruction is in the lower ileum, gradual abdominal distension develops. At this stage the diagnosis is fairly simple, erect plain X-rays of the neonate showing multiple fluid-filled dilated loops in the abdomen. Multiple fluid levels also occur in Hirschsprung's disease but a barium enema in the doubtful case shows a microcolon in ileal atresia.

If, however, the condition is unrecognized, the bowel may perforate, leading to a faecal peritonitis. This may be obvious on clinical examination because the abdominal wall frequently becomes oedematous. Plain X-rays of the abdomen at this stage show air in the peritoneal cavity, distended loops of bowel, and a calcified plaque due to the deposition of calcium in the leaking meconium.

Treatment. Once the diagnosis has been made, the treatment following resuscitation is surgical.

Until recently, despite the absence of associated abnormalities, the mortality, even in cases of solitary stricture of the ileum, was of the order of 70 per cent. The high mortality arose from failure to recognize that the distended jejunum proximal to the atretic segment is paralysed by the prolonged distension and a deficient vascular supply: this was both recognized and demonstrated experimentally by Nixon of Great Ormond Street. His work led to radical resections of the distended and hypertrophied loop proximal to the abnormal segment, and to a dramatic reduction in the operative mortality. However, radical resection poses the potential threat of postoperative ileal insufficiency, which is in part overcome by compensatory hypertrophy of the remaining bowel.

However, laparotomy may reveal an inoperable situation due to extensive or multiple lesions in the bowel. Little can be done in these circumstances.

Attention has also been focused, in the operable case, on the type of ileoileal anastomosis that should be performed. Experimental evidence suggests that the ileum should be divided in an oblique fashion and a back-to-back anastomosis performed.

Meconium ileus

This is a relatively rare manifestation of cystic fibrosis. This condition is the most common lethal genetic condition of white infants and is also the most common cause of severe obstructive lung disease in this population group. Cystic fibrosis is inherited as an autosomal recessive condition and affects 1 in every 1600–2000 live births. It was described as a specific entity in the late 1930s and the commonly used diagnostic sweat test was introduced in the early 1950s.

For unknown reasons the serum of sufferers from this condition or heterozygous carriers produces dyskinesia of the beating cilia of explants of the rabbit trachea or oyster gills.

Pathology
The basic pathological defect is one of a widespread disorder of the mucus-secreting glands of the respiratory tract, alimentary tract, pancreas and liver but the underlying physiological disturbance remains to be discovered. When a neonate suffering from cystic fibrosis survives although the lungs appear normal at birth a rapid obstruction of the bronchioles develops due to the tenacious nature of the mucus which is secreted. At first there is no evidence of infection but if the child survives, subsequent pulmonary infection with the staphylococcus, *Haemophilus influenzae* and finally *Pseudomonas aeruginosa* occurs and as the disease progresses hypertrophy and hyperplasia of the mucus glands occurs accompanied by impairment of ciliary function and squamous metaplasia.

If the infant survives the pancreas is found to be small, firm and irregular. Histological examination shows dilatation of the ducts, flattening of their epithelial lining, diffuse fibrosis and enlargement of the acini. At the end stage of the disease the whole pancreas is shrunken and fibrotic although scattered islet cells remain intact. Children who survive die either of pulmonary disease or in a lesser proportion the effects of portal hypertension.

Presentation
Only about 20 per cent of infants suffering from fibrocystic disease present in the neonatal period with signs of small gut obstruction and in this group the disease is severe, nearly all the exocrine glands of the body being affected. A rarer mode of presentation in this severe group is with the low sodium syndrome due to the excessive loss of sodium in the sweat. About 15 per cent

of infants suffering from this disease present somewhat later with rectal prolapse and the remainder attend the paediatrician with a history of recurrent chest infection, diarrhoea and failure to thrive.

Meconium ileus may be complicated by volvulus of the heavy distended loops of bowel and depending on how early in fetal life this occurs the volvulus may progress to gangrene of the bowel followed by perforation and the development of a meconium peritonitis.

Diagnosis

It is now possible to diagnose the condition in the second trimester of pregnancy on the basis of decreased levels of 4-methylumbilliferyl-guanidinobenzoate (MUGB)—reactive arginine ester protease in the amniotic fluid.

In the living noenate, however, in whom the diagnosis is suspected a plain X-ray of the abdomen will reveal distended small bowel loops many of which do not contain fluid levels. Many of the distended loops possess a ground glass appearance due to the admixture of air with the viscid meconium. In addition, particularly in the right iliac fossa, extraintestinal speckled calcification may be observed which is due to leakage of meconium into the peritoneal cavity.

In addition to this radiological evidence quantitative sweat tests can be performed. Screening tests for sweat chloride have been devised which depend upon the intensity of the hand imprint made on a silver nitrate containing paper or agar. The sweat chloride precipitates with the silver and the intensity of the print is roughly proportional to the sweat chloride concentration. In the definitive test sweat is obtained by pilocarpine iontophoresis, a chloride concentration greater than 60 mmol/l (60 mEq/l) is diagnostic, between 50 and 60 suggestive; the sodium concentration is usually 10–20 mmol (mEq) higher.

Treatment

There are two chief methods of treating meconium ileus. The first is merely to resect the long segment of dilated bowel which contains the turgid meconium and then perform an end-to-end anastomosis and the alternative approach adopted by many paediatric surgeons is to resect this loop but then to join the proximal end to the side of the distal loop bringing out the open end of the latter onto the abdominal wall as a temporary iliostomy. Through this pancreatin can be instilled to liquefy the remaining turgid meconium.

Prognosis

The prognosis in this condition is always overshadowed by the eventual development of chronic obstructive lung disease complicated by superimposed antibiotic-resistant infection. However, the gastrointestinal symptoms may antedate the pulmonary picture by months or years although in 75 per cent of infants suffering from meconium ileus pulmonary symptoms are present in the third year of life.

Hirschsprung's disease

This condition was first described in 1886. The precise aetiology and an acceptable method of treatment was only worked out by Swenson in 1948, although many previous observers had noted the absence of ganglion cells in the distal colon without appreciating the significance of the observation.

Pathology
The condition is due to aganglionosis of the bowel which leads to defective contractile activity and hence a lack of forward propulsion of the faecal stream. This defect in the myenteric plexus extends proximally from the anorectal junction. In 75 per cent of infants the defect is restricted to the rectum and sigmoid, in a smaller proportion the whole colon is involved and in rare cases even the small bowel may be affected. In addition to the common lesion affecting the rectum and sigmoid, ultrashort-segment disease has also been described in which only a small part of the lower rectum is abnormal. Short-segment involvement is five times more common in males than in females but the sex incidence appears to be equal in long-segment disease. Recent Japanese workers in this field have suggested that aganglionosis of the bowel arises because of failure of the ganglion cells to migrate distally from the more cranial parts of the alimentary tube during the sixth and seventh weeks of intrauterine life. This hypothesis fits in well with the known anatomical distribution of the disease if one assumes that all the ganglion cells of the bowel are ultimately derived from the vagi.

Presentation
In approximately 40 per cent of infants suffering from Hirschsprung's disease the diagnosis is made within the first 3 months of life and in the remaining 60 per cent within the first year.

When the condition presents in the neonatal period the typical signs of obstruction occur. Somewhat later the infant may begin to suffer from intractable attacks of enterocolitis which are the major cause of death in the untreated infant. This complication occurs most commonly in infants below 3 months of age and in particular suffering from long-segment disease. It is because of this potential danger that early diagnosis is so important.

If the disease is unrecognized the infant will slowly develop gross abdominal distension, severe constipation and fail to thrive. It is unusual for an untreated infant to survive but if this should occur the condition will then have to be distinguished from idiopathic megacolon which normally presents during potty training when the infant becomes constipated, incontinent and distended.

Diagnosis
The condition should be suspected in every case of neonatal obstruction especially if some normal meconium is passed but the abdomen remains distended.

Confirmatory investigations
1 *Plain X-rays of the abdomen.* These may merely show non-specific distention of the small bowel with fluid levels. In short-segment disease the colon also appears to be grossly distended and an important feature is an absence of gas in the pelvis.

2 *Barium enema.* This investigation is of little use in the first few weeks because time is required for the gut proximal to the aganglionic segment to dilate thus producing the typical coning effect at the junctional zone upon which the radiological diagnosis depends.

3 *Rectal manometry.* In a normal infant when the rectum is distended by a balloon the anal pressure falls whereas in Hirschsprung's disease irrespective of the length of the aganglionic segment the converse applies, i.e. distension of the rectum is followed by a rise in the intraluminal pressure in the anal canal.

Typical figures, rounded to the nearest whole figure are as follows:

(a) Normal infant: resting pressures—$7 \pm 4 \, cmH_2O$ in rectum, $14 \pm 6 \, cmH_2O$ in anal canal. Following rectal distension anal canal pressure falls in all infants to an average of $7 \pm 4 \, cmH_2O$.

(b) Infants suffering from Hirschsprung's disease: resting pressures—$12 \pm 4 \, cmH_2O$ in rectum, 19 in anal canal. Following distension the anal canal pressure rises to between $22.5 \pm 14 \, cmH_2O$.

4 *Rectal biopsy.* This is most commonly performed in the neonate by a suction apparatus which results in a dome of mucosa and superficial submucosa 3 mm thick in its thickest part being obtained. This type of biopsy should be taken prior to the administration of any rectal washouts or enemata, otherwise the oedema precipitated by such therapy reduces the depth of the submucosa which is obtained.

A biopsy taken by this method confirms the diagnosis of Hirschsprung's disease when ganglion cells are absent and coarse nerve fibres are seen ramifying in the superficial and deeper parts of the submucosa.

Additional investigations which may be applied to this biopsy material are as follows:

(a) the biopsy may be stained for acetylcholinesterase activity by the method described by Karnovsky and Roots in 1964. In a normally innervated distal colon and rectum enzyme activity is barely discernible in the lamina propria and the muscularis mucosae whereas in Hirschsprung's disease acetylcholinesterase activity can be found in the parasympathetic nerve fibres of both layers.

(b) if a biopsy sample of about 4 mg of tissue can be obtained the acetylcholinesterase activity can be quantitatively measured. In the normal infant the greatest amount found was 10.9×10^{-7} units/g as compared to 63×10^{-7} units in Hirschsprung's disease and no overlap between the two groups of infants was found.

Treatment

Many infants suffering from Hirschsprung's disease can be successfully treated immediately after birth by repeated washouts. If this method is unsatisfactory a colostomy must be made in the transverse colon, leaving the affected segment untouched. At this operation, however, a black silk stitch should be inserted in the wall of the bowel at the junctional zone because the cone appearance gradually disappears after the bowel is decompressed. If there is any doubt at all as to at which point in the bowel the colostomy should be made a series of biopsies should be taken from various points around the colon and examined by the frozen section technique. This is extremely important since it is essential that the colostomy is performed in normal bowel.

Even following the performance of a decompressing colostomy attacks of severe enterocolitis may occur but a much more serious complication is prolapse of the colostomy. Resection of the prolapsed bowel should be avoided since this may so reduce the effective length of the unaffected bowel when the definitive operation is attempted it might be found that the affected gut cannot be resected and the continuity of the bowel restored.

Definitive surgery
Four basic operations have been designed to remove the aganglionic segment and restore the continuity of the bowel.

1. The first of these is Swenson's operation which was modelled upon the older operation described by Maunsell and Weir. Basically the diseased segment is identified by repeated frozen sections if needed and this is then resected. Since the disease always extends distally to the level of the anorectal junction the final stage of the operation must be performed from the perineum after eversion of the anal stump and pulling through the proximal bowel.
2. The retrorectal transanal pull-through operation devised by Duhamel in 1956. This operation is open to the objection that the new rectum consists of an anterior half which is aganglionic and one specific complication due to this anatomical arrangement is the development of an anterior pouch in which faecal masses may accumulate.
3. Endorectal pull-through without primary anastomosis described by Soave in 1963.
4. Endorectal pull-through with primary anastomosis described by Boley in 1964.

The latter two operations involve dividing the rectum at some suitable level and then dissecting out the mucosa after infiltrating the wall of the gut with saline and adrenaline. The muscular layer of the gut is left intact so that no injury can possibly occur to the pelvic floor or the parasympathetic outflow to the bladder.

The mortality rate for any of these operations lies between 1 and 3 per cent in practised hands and some degree of faecal incontinence may occur. However, postoperative enterocolitis for reasons which are totally inexplicable, is somewhat more common following Swenson's operation and the Soave manoeuvre.

6.14 Surgical causes of malabsorption

The causes of malabsorption of greatest interest to the surgeon include:

1. gastric surgery;

2 Crohn's disease of the small intestine;
3 blind loop syndrome, usually the result of:
   (a) previous operations, e.g. side-to-side enteroanastomosis;
   (b) multiple strictures, e.g. Crohn's disease or tuberculosis of the small bowel;
   (c) jejunal diverticulosis;
4 defective bowel motility, e.g. post-irradiation fibrosis;
5 surgical excision of the small bowel;
6 pancreatic disease:
   (a) carcinoma of the head or body;
   (b) chronic pancreatitis;
7 obstructive jaundice.

Less common causes include the Zöllinger–Ellison syndrome and thyrotoxicosis.

Clinical picture
The most characteristic complaint of a patient suffering from malabsorption is the frequent passage of pale, bulky and offensive-smelling motions. Although the basic cause may be progressive, the diarrhoea itself may be intermittent, and even an alteration in the environment, e.g. admission to hospital, may produce an abrupt improvement. The change in the character of the stools is due to their fat content. Gross examination shows the faeces to be greasy, and if they are emulsified on a glass slide with ethyl alcohol and examined under a microscope, fatty acid crystals may be seen. If they are then stained with alcoholic Sudan III, neutral fat in the form of yellow orange globules, is observed.

Investigation of steatorrhoea

Once steatorrhoea has been confirmed by simple tests of the faeces it is necessary to quantify the fat loss and, if possible, establish the cause.

Biochemical investigation

1 *Fat balance*
This is performed by collecting the stools for a period of 3–4 days or, if the patient becomes constipated, for slightly longer. Although the majority of faecal fat is derived from unabsorbed dietary fat, 1–2 g a day still appears in the faeces when a normal individual is placed on a fat-free diet.

The beginning of the test period is usually signalled by a marker such as charcoal or carmine red; alternatively, a continuous marker may be used, administering a non-absorbable material such as phenol red or barium sulphate.

The normal percentage of fat lost in the stools per day is approximately 7 per cent. When the diet contains 50–100 g of fat the upper normal limit of fat in the stools is 6 g/day, and in the majority of patients suffering from steatorrhoea the amount of fat excreted is roughly proportional to the intake.

An alternative method of measuring fat absorption is by oral administration of ^{131}I-labelled triolein.

2 D-*Xylose test*
In the presence of primary intestinal disease there can also be an associated defect of carbohydrate absorption. This can be detected by administration of D-xylose, which is rapidly absorbed from the normal bowel and reaches its peak concentration in the plasma within 1–1.5 hours.

The test is performed by administering 25 g of D-xylose by mouth and measuring the amount excreted in the urine within 5 hours. The normal value varies between 4.7 and 7.5 g; the lower limit of normal is 17 per cent of the total oral dose.

3 *Measurement of the exocrine function of the pancreas*
When primary disease of the pancreas is suspected, an attempt can be made to measure pancreatic exocrine function. The principles of direct testing of pancreatic function are as follows. The duodenum is intubated under radiological control, after which the pancreas is stimulated first by secretin and then by pancreozymin. After the first injection of between 1 and 5 clinical units/kg of secretin, the volume of juice and the bicarbonate concentration are measured, and following the injection of pancreozymin, volume and pancreatic enzyme concentrations are measured.

In about 10 per cent of patients with carcinoma of the body the volume of pancreatic juice excreted is within normal limits but, commonly, the enzyme level is low and the bicarbonate concentration high. In chronic pancreatitis a low volume response is usually obtained with a low bicarbonate and a reduced, but still relatively high, enzyme level.

Radiological investigations

1 *Plain abdominal X-rays*
These may show:

(*a*) pancreatic calcification in the presence of chronic pancreatitis, a disease uncommon in the UK but commoner in France and the United States;
(*b*) multiple air-filled diverticuli of the small bowel;
(*c*) multiple distended loops of small bowel in Crohn's disease.

2 *Hypotonic duodenography with air contrast*
This technique is appropriate for demonstrating irregularities in the wall of the duodenum, deformity and irregularity of the mucosal pattern indicating either carcinoma of the head of the pancreas or chronic pancreatitis.

3 *Pancreatography and retrograde cholangiography*
Cannulation of the ampulla of Vater via a fibreoptic endoscope is indicated if stone or stricture of the common bile duct or primary pancreatic disease is suspected.

4 Small bowel meal

This is performed by duodenal intubation. The method is useful for demonstrating strictures of the small bowel, blind loops, fistulae, or the mucosal changes of Crohn's disease. In conditions such as gluten-sensitive enteropathy, the small bowel is dilated and the contrast media develop an abnormal pattern variously known as flocculation, puddling, fragmentation, or segmentation. In a large variety of small bowel conditions, e.g. jejunal ulceration, gastrocolic fistula and the Zöllinger–Ellison syndrome, the jejunal mucosal folds may be thickened.

Intestinal biopsy

In addition to radiology, a more specific investigation of the small bowel is provided by the use of the Crosby–Kungler capsule which is designed to cut off a mucosal specimen after it has been sucked into the capsule through a side hole. Unfortunately, only one specimen per passage can be obtained. Other capsules such as the Carey capsule allow multiple biopsies to be taken after only one passage.

The mucosal specimen obtained is first examined under a dissecting microscope, after which it is sectioned. The appearances of the biopsy are particularly significant in gluten-sensitive enteropathy in which villous atrophy is present. The microscopic appearances are also diagnostic in cases of lymphatic infiltration and postirradiation damage.

Miscellaneous chemical investigations

Malabsorption of fat is associated with a concomitant loss of other nutrients, certain of which are essential to normal life; among these are vitamin B_{12}, vitamin K, vitamin D, calcium, magnesium, and folic acid. Various methods of investigating these parameters have been introduced and if low values are found in the blood each should be separately investigated.

The major surgical causes of malabsorption will now be discussed in greater detail.

SURGICAL CAUSES OF MALABSORPTION

1 Postgastrectomy malabsorption

This is usually mild and may only be detected by investigation. The magnitude of the disturbance is usually greater following a Polya than a Billroth type of resection. The various explanations offered for malabsorption following gastrectomy are:

(a) poor mixing of foods and enzymes;
(b) reduced pancreatic secretion and a lack of post-prandial coordination in the delivery of pancreatic juice and bile salts;
(c) inactivation of the pancreatic enzymes in the afferent loop;
(d) blind loop effects caused by the afferent loop;

(e) occasionally, when a gastroileal rather than a gastrojejunal anastomosis is accidentally performed.

The degree of steatorrhoea which normally follows partial gastrectomy is probably of little clinical significance. It has been shown, for example, that there is little correlation between it and weight loss even after a total gastrectomy, a more significant factor affecting weight being the diminished food intake due to post-cibal symptoms such as dumping or the small stomach syndrome. When, however, steatorrhoea is severe, there may be secondary manifestations such as vitamin D deficiency resulting occasionally in osteopenia and osteomalacia.

Treatment
Possible treatments of postgastrectomy steatorrhoea include shortening or removing the afferent loop, conversion of a Polya to a Billroth gastrectomy, and the administration of oral pancreatic enzymes.

2 Surgical diseases of the small bowel

(a) *Crohn's disease*
Steatorrhoea occurs in approximately a third of patients suffering from Crohn's disease due to loss of mucosal surface area caused by extensive disease, extensive resection, or the development of internal fistulae, all of which effectively reduce the absorptive capacity of the small bowel and increase bacterial contamination. Any of these factors, either alone or in combination, diminishes the absorption of bile salts and may eventually lead to a reduction of the bile salt pool. The various tests described all show varying degrees of abnormality.
Treatment. There is no evidence that the medical treatment of Crohn's disease reduces the steatorrhoea even though it may reduce the symptoms. If internal fistulae have developed, surgical correction may improve the condition by increasing the effective functional area of the bowel and reducing bacterial contamination.

Extensive resection of the ileum may, however, make the symptoms worse by removing the bowel from which bile salts are absorbed. This leads to increasing diarrhoea, because bile salts entering the colon reduce water reabsorption. The continued loss of bile salts may eventually reduce the bile salt pool to such a degree that the body can no longer compensate by increased synthesis. Interference with fat absorption follows, and steatorrhoea develops.

(b) *Jejunal diverticulosis and blind loops*
These conditions may remain symptomless throughout life; alternatively, there may be recurrent attacks of abdominal pain, borborygmi and malabsorption. The cause of symptoms in these conditions is bacterial contamination. *Escherichia coli*, bifido bacteria and bacteroides proliferate in blind loops or diverticuli and split the conjugated bile salts.

The deconjugated bile acids are toxic to the mucosa and, in addition, the bile salt concentration eventually falls below the critical 'micellular' level, leading to steatorrhoea.

If the bowel is sterilized by administering an appropriate antibiotic, bile salt deconjugation is decreased and the steatorrhoea diminishes. A similar effect can be achieved by oral administration of conjugated bile salts, thus demonstrating the importance of bacterial bile salt deconjugation.

Other subtle changes that take place, apart from the overall reduction in bile salts, include an alteration in the ratio between the taurine and glycine conjugates and in the trihydroxy to the dihydroxy bile acid ratio. These alterations are of considerable clinical importance because the bile acids are not all equally effective at efficient micelle formation.

Treatment. Jejunal diverticulosis is seldom isolated to a particular area of the bowel but, if investigation should prove this to be so, resection is the ideal; otherwise, intermittent treatment with antibiotics may be of assistance. Blind loops, the result of previous surgery, e.g. side-to-side anastomosis, or natural disease should be excised.

(c) Massive resection of the small intestine

The commonest reasons for massive surgical resection of the small bowel are vascular accidents such as mesenteric thrombosis or strangulation by a midgut volvulus. Massive small gut resection is followed by three clinical stages.

(i) the immediate postoperative: this is dominated by a severe loss of fluid and electrolytes, in which hypovolaemia, tetany, magnesium depletion and hypoalbuminuria may all occur;
(ii) the intermediate period: during which the severe, watery diarrhoea diminishes and nutritional problems begin;
(iii) the late stage: when a balance is achieved between the absorptive capacity of the bowel that remains and the degree of physical activity, by which time the total weight loss may be as great as 25–30 kg.

Such severe metabolic disturbance is seen only after resections of more than one-third of the entire bowel and, in general, ileal resections produce greater degrees of metabolic derangement than jejunal. In this stage there may be megaloblastic anaemia, fatty degeneration of the liver, and gastric hypersecretion due to defective inactivation of gastrin.

Treatment. Once the tertiary stage has been reached, treatment consists of vitamin supplementation, the relief of bile salt diarrhoea by the administration of cholestyramine, the substitution of long chain by medium chain triglycerides, the reduction of intestinal motility by codeine phosphate or diphenoxylate hydrochloride and, lastly, the substitution of the lost bile salts by polysorbate 80, which acts as an emulsifying agent. In a few patients the interposition of a reversed intestinal loop may reduce rapid transit of the intestinal contents but there is little information concerning the optimum length for such a loop. If gastric hypersecretion is a problem, vagotomy may be required if the usual medical treatment fails to relieve the symptoms.

In patients in whom the intestinal tract has been so shortened by resection or disease that high output and malabsorption persist despite the medical regimen described total parenteral nutrition may be required either temporarily or permanently.

This mode of nutrition is provided via a catheter placed in the subclavian vein. A variety of catheters exist but the danger in all is the development of infection. This most commonly occurs at the catheter tip and may be asymptomatic, bacteria being found on routine culture of this part of the catheter after its withdrawal. In other patients, however, a clinical infection develops with evidence of a septicaemia accompanied by a swinging temperature. In such cases the blood culture may or may not be positive.

Nutrient materials. The aims of intravenous nutrition are to:

(i) provide sufficient calories to satisfy the energy requirements of the individual;
(ii) provide protein in the form of amino acids so that nitrogen loss does not occur. In a child attention must be drawn to the fact that the child has to grow;
(iii) provide fluid and electrolytes;
(iv) provide trace elements.

In addition to the above any patient who is being sustained on parenteral nutrition alone must receive an adequate supply of all vitamins. These aims are achieved by providing in the adult between 2000 and 3000 kcal/day by means of a mixture of amino acids and 50 per cent dextrose to which a 10 per cent solution of fat is added. The amino acids may be provided as Aminoplex (Geistlich) which is made up in various strengths containing varying quantities of synthetic L-form amino acids and the fat is provided as Intralipid (KabiVitrum) which consists of a mixture of fractionated soya-bean oil, fractionated egg lecithin, glycerol and water.

Fluid, electrolytes, trace elements and vitamins are also given intravenously.

Some patients will be found to be intolerant of such large quantities of dextrose in which case insulin must be added to the intravenous solution.

When permanent total parenteral nutrition is required the catheter is inserted and the affected individual wears a portable pump in order to deliver the fluid into the circulation so that he can remain ambulatory.

(d) Endocrine malabsorption

Zöllinger–Ellison syndrome. Although oversecretion of gastric acid produces in the small bowel irritative changes which of themselves produce diarrhoea, true steatorrhoea has also been recorded. This is probably due to the low intestinal pH, which reduces the action of pancreatic lipase. If the intestinal acidity is reduced by gastric aspiration, the steatorrhoea is temporarily reduced.

Thyrotoxicosis. There may be a moderate increase in the frequency of bowel action together with mild steatorrhoea due to a decreased transit time. Radiological examination and intestinal biopsy show no evidence of organic disease.

(e) Obstructive jaundice
All patients suffering from obstructive jaundice suffer from steatorrhoea due to the absence of bile salts from the intestine, in addition the accumulation of bile salts in the skin results in intractable pruritis. When the obstruction is intrahepatic it may be compatible with a prolonged life and in these circumstances a deficiency of the fat-soluble vitamins A, D and K eventually develops.

Treatment. The treatment is essentially dependent upon the cause. In 'surgical' jaundice an attempt should be made to direct the bile into the gut. When high malignant strictures of the hepatic duct occur or external compression of the duct in the hilar region has occurred the intractable pruritis can be relieved by the use of a variety of stents passed through the strictured area.

When the cause of the jaundice is lower in the biliary tree, e.g. a carcinoma of the head of the pancreas, an attempt should be made to remove the lesion. This will effect access of the bile salts and bile pigments into the gastrointestinal tract but because many surgeons feel that total pancreatectomy is a safer operation than the classical Whipple's procedure pancreatic enzymes must be given orally with the food if the resulting steatorrhoea is to be avoided.

6.15 Aetiology, pathology and management of Crohn's disease

Definition. Crohn's disease has been recognized as a clinical entity since 1932 when it was described by Crohn and his colleagues. In their original description these authors defined the condition as a regional ileitis, acknowledging the inflammatory nature without being able to specify a cause. The position remains the same today except that it is now realized that the disease may affect any part of the gastrointestinal tract from the mouth to the anus.

Aetiology
The following suggestions have been up forward:

1. *Genetic factor.* The evidence in favour of a genetic factor is based on the following:
(a) family aggregations;
(b) the unexpected frequency of the disease in monozygotic but not dizygotic twins;
(c) the frequency of the disease in patients who also suffer from ankylosing spondylitis; in such patients Crohn's disease is 30 times commoner than in the general population.

Even despite the above features the genetic factor involved certainly cannot be one of straightforward Mendelian inheritance.

2. *Food.* Crohn's disease is commoner in Europe than elsewhere and the reported incidence of this condition has also increased in Scotland and

Sweden. The importance of manufactured foods with chemical additives has aroused considerable speculation.

3 *Immunological.* Consideration has been given to possible sensitization to exogenous antigens or to the tissues of the gastrointestinal tract provoking an autoimmune type of response. No clear cut evidence exists, however, and the fact that complement, often an important factor in cell-mediated immunity, is not taken up is regarded as an important negative finding.

However, an immunological basis for the disease would serve to explain the extragastrointestinal manifestations such as uveitis and arthritis which occur in Crohn's disease.

4 *Infective.* The suggestion has frequently been made that the disease is infective, and for many years an intensive search was made for *Mycobacterium tuberculosis*. This was finally abandoned, but recently the theory has been revived by the finding of a comparable disease in animals caused by a mycobacterium. The therapeutic effectiveness of sulphasalazine in Crohn's disease could be explained on an infective basis. Recent work has also suggested that an agent similar to that causing sarcoidosis may be responsible, for in both conditions the Kveim test is positive.

Finally, an RNA virus has recently been isolated from the gastrointestinal mucosa and lymph nodes in patients suffering from both Crohn's disease and ulcerative colitis which cannot be found in normal individuals.

5 *Lymphatic obstruction.* A lesion similar to Crohn's disease can be produced in experimental animals by feeding powdered glass or, alternatively, by injecting iron particles into the mucosa. Either procedure results in a granulomatous lesion.

Pathology
Gross appearance. The disease may be acute, in which case the bowel appears congested and the bowel wall thickened and turgid. In the commoner chronic form the bowel has been likened to an eel in rigor mortis. The affected bowel and its mesentery are thickened, and enlarged mesenteric glands can be seen or palpated in the mesentery.

Although great importance was attached to the latter finding by earlier writers, recent investigations have shown that the nodes are equally enlarged in ulcerative colitis. When the bowel is opened, the wall is seen to be thickened, and oedematous. The lumen is generally narrowed and long narrow linear ulcers run along the mucosa. The ulcers have swollen, overhanging edges of inflamed mucosa. From the ulcers fissures may extend deeply into the wall of the bowel. The changes described give rise to the classic cobblestone appearance observed on X-ray.

One of the most characteristic features of Crohn's disease is the presence of skip lesions, long intervals of apparently normal bowel separating the diseased areas. The bowel proximal to a lesion may be dilated due to the obstructive nature of the diseased portion. Multiple adhesions, internal fistulae, and abscess formation are common.

Microscopically. The chief histopathological feature of Crohn's disease is the formation of non-caseating granulomatous lesions that resemble sarcoidosis. Each is composed of large mononuclear cells and foreign body giant cells.

There is considerable oedema of the mucosa and submucosa. Lymphoid follicles may be seen in the submucosa and deeper layers. The mucosa itself may appear fairly normal, apart from fissures lined by epithelioid cells, but as the ulceration continues the exudate of polymorphonuclear leucocytes, lymphocytes, epithelioid cells and mononuclear cells increases.

Since Crohn's disease can involve the whole of the large bowel it is obvious that one difficulty may be to distinguish this disease from ulcerative colitis. The main distinguishing pathological features upon which reliance can be placed are:

1   presence of the confluent linear ulcers;
2   deep fissures;
3   sarcoid-like granulomata, which appear not only in the bowel wall but also in about half the involved lymph nodes.

Clinical presentation

The symptoms of Crohn's disease are in large measure related to the site of the disease. The frequency of the various sites of involvement as determined by the examination of several large reported series are as follows:

1   terminal ileum and ascending colon 60 per cent;
2   small bowel 20 per cent;
3   large bowel alone 20 per cent.

The disease may occur in childhood but is more common in early adult life. Once the disease is sufficiently severe to produce symptoms they are nearly always progressive.

The common presenting symptoms are:

1   abdominal pain due to intestinal obstruction caused by either oedema or fibrosis of the affected bowel, in which case the pain is intermittent and colicky in nature, or constant abdominal pain due to peritoneal irritation.
2   Diarrhoea due to:
    (*a*) destruction of the mucosa of the terminal ileum leading to defective fat absorption or inability to absorb bile salts. The latter spill over into the colon and produce a typical watery diarrhoea;
    (*b*) internal fistulation, producing blind loops and functional shortening of the bowel;
    (*c*) stricture formation leading to alteration in the bacterial flora of the bowel.
3   when the large bowel alone is involved, particularly when the involvement is total, severe diarrhoea accompanied by blood and mucus is a prominent feature of the disease.
4   weight loss or in childhood disease failure of growth. This is due to malnutrition brought about by loss of the absorptive capacity of the small bowel due to the disease itself, failure of absorption due to bile salt deconjugation by the abnormal intestinal flora, by fear of pain following eating and lastly, loss of protein in the form of mucus.

In addition to these specific symptoms of gastrointestinal disease the following general manifestations of the disease may be present:

1   fever;

2 anaemia, hypoproteinaemia, hypoprothrombinaemia, vitamin deficiency disorders and gross fluid and electrolyte imbalance;
3 polyarthritis of the rheumatoid type especially in childhood;
4 pyoderma gangrenosum;
5 iritis;
6 oral ulceration;
7 finger clubbing.

In addition perianal disease in the form of recurrent abscesses, fissures or fistulae occur in about 15 per cent of all patients and about 90 per cent of those patients in whom the large bowel is involved alone.

As the disease progresses so enterovesical fistulae may develop causing frequency, dysuria and the passage of flatus per urethram.

Physical examination
This may reveal little, but in an advanced case the following signs may be present:

1 a palpable abdominal mass, often in the right iliac fossa;
2 signs of intestinal obstruction;
3 evidence of anaemia, hypoproteinaemia, or vitamin deficiency;
4 cachexia;
5 perianal disease: external fistulae, especially if a previous operation has been performed.

Investigation
1 *Sigmoidoscopy and biopsy.* This may be negative unless the disease is involving the large bowel.
2 Full blood count together with serum iron, vitamin B_{12} and folic acid; 50 per cent of patients have a deficiency in one or all of these factors. In active disease the ESR will be raised above normal.
3 *Radiology.* A barium enema followed by a small bowel meal are usually performed.

The following radiological signs have been described:

(*a*) In non-stenotic lesions, blunting, flattening and thickening of the valvulae conniventes.
(*b*) Fusing of the mucosal folds.
(*c*) Evidence of ulceration, deposition of barium in the linear ulcers leads to the classical cobblestone appearance.
(*d*) Further destruction of the mucosa leads to loss of the cobblestone and replacement with an irregular network of barium.
(*e*) Palpation of the barium-filled loops reveals their lack of pliability, and their rigidity.
(*f*) Stenosis: when the lesions are small in length the radiological appearances are not dissimilar to those produced by multiple tuberculous strictures, when of greater length, the string sign of Kantor is created.
(*g*) Proximal to stenotic areas gas- and fluid-filled distended loops may be seen.

The most valuable radiological physical signs, according to Dyer, are contraction and rigidity of the bowel wall.

4 *Faecal fat.* At least a third of all patients suffering from Crohn's disease have steatorrhoea, and numerous investigators have shown that the degree of malabsorption correlates with the site and extent of the disease. Cooke laid great stress on the presence of steatorrhoea before and after surgery, claiming that a continuation of the steatorrhoea after resection indicated a high recurrence rate. This has since been disproved.

Treatment
The treatment of Crohn's disease is essentially medical until the symptoms of the disease become intolerable or the complications life-threatening. There is, however, little evidence that medical treatment affects the natural history of the disease.

Among the various medical measures applied in Crohn's disease are the following:

1 correction of anaemia and vitamin deficiency states by appropriate means, together with supplementary elemental diets.
2 Drug therapy including:
   (*a*) salazopyrine;
   (*b*) steroids;
   (*c*) anticholinergic drugs such as diphenoxylate to diminish the diarrhoea;
   (*d*) immunosuppressive agents, e.g. azathioprine. Although the author has personally treated several severely ill patients with this drug and seen dramatic relief of symptoms, larger trials report that it is of little positive value.

Symptoms which demand operation include:

1 intractable severe abdominal pain due to intermittent obstruction;
2 uncontrollable diarrhoea.

Complications which may demand operation include:

1 severe bleeding;
2 malnutrition due to the development of either internal or external fistulae;
3 growth retardation in childhood.

Small bowel disease

Two major surgical procedures have been described for the treatment of Crohn's disease involving the distal small bowel; each has a mortality of between 2 and 5 per cent.

1 resection followed by ileotransverse colostomy;
2 a bypass operation leaving the diseased portion of the bowel undisturbed and anastomosing the small bowel proximal to the lesion to the transverse colon.

Examination of published work shows that within the first 5 years after surgery the results of bypass procedures are worse than those following excision, but after this interval the incidence of recurrence becomes the same for both types of surgery; the total incidence of recurrence rises to approximately 60 per cent.

The classic symptoms and signs of recurrent disease are:

1 abdominal colic;
2 diarrhoea;
3 palpable mass;
4 fistula formation, internal or external;
5 exacerbation of perianal symptoms;
6 return of systemic symptoms or signs.

Large bowel disease

Severe uncontrollable large bowel disease must be treated by total proctocolectomy and ileostomy. The recurrence rate following this operation is between 10 and 30 per cent depending on the series reviewed and, as with small bowel disease, recurrence tends to be within 5 years. Recent papers have shown that if a small bowel lesion also requires resection at the time of colectomy it does not increase the frequency of recurrence.

6.16 Pathology, clinical course, and treatment of ulcerative colitis

Aetiology
The aetiology of ulcerative colitis is unknown. A number of factors have, however, at one time or another been incriminated. They include psychological factors, infection, collagen disease and, lastly, autoimmunity.

Recent work has shown that the age-specific incidence of ulcerative colitis is similar from continent to continent, lending support to the hypothesis that it is not due to extrinsic causes because these could reasonably be expected to vary in different localities. There is considerable evidence, however, that the incidence of colitis differs between different races. In communities in which a high degree of diagnostic accuracy can be expected, as in the USA, it has been shown that the incidence of the disease is significantly lower in the black than the white population and a similar distinction can be drawn between the Maori and New Zealanders of European extraction.

Pathology
This disease is a diffuse, non-specific, inflammatory condition of part or the

whole of the large bowel and predominantly affects the mucous membrane. The inflammatory changes nearly always begin distally and extend proximally. If the disease is severe, mucosal ulceration develops and may later be followed by perforation of the bowel.

Immunological studies suggest that total colitis is different from the more restricted forms of the disease, for in the latter, serum immunoglobulin levels remain normal whereas in the former the serum α_2, β and γ globulins and the IgA and IgG concentrations are high.

Unlike Crohn's disease the pathological changes in ulcerative colitis are restricted to the large bowel except in patients with severe disease of the caecum and ascending colon associated with an incompetent ileocaecal valve; in such patients the so-called 'backwash ileitis' may develop.

Macroscopic appearance of the colon

External. The external appearance of the bowel is one of congestion and dilatation of the small blood vessels, an appearance which is always exaggerated when the bowel is rendered ischaemic by ligation of the appropriate blood vessels during resection. The total length of the bowel is often reduced. When there are lymph nodes in the mesentery they are soft and fleshy.

Internal. The internal appearance in the advanced case is one of diffuse ulceration, varying from shallow ulcers involving only the superficial layers of the mucosa to ulcers involving the whole thickness of bowel, exposing the muscle coats and, in extreme cases, perforating the bowel.

A second typical feature of colitis is the development of inflammatory pseudopolyps which appear in about 20 per cent of patients with total involvement of the colon. These are the result of severe inflammatory changes in the islets of mucosa that remain between the ulcers.

Microscopic appearance

The microscopic appearances of the bowel in colitis are dominated by an acute inflammatory process. Oedema, dilated blood vessels, and an inflammatory exudate of polymorphonuclear leucocytes, lymphocytes and plasma cells are found. These changes extend through the submucosa of the bowel if the disease is severe. Secondary infection of the already diseased mucosa produces crypt abscesses in the crypts of Leiberkühn. These burst either onto the surface or into the loose connective tissues of the submucosa. As the disease progresses the surface ulceration becomes confluent and the acute inflammatory cells are replaced by cells more typical of a chronic inflammatory process including lymphocytes, plasma cells, eosinophils and mast cells.

The ulcerated areas of the bowel rapidly become covered by a vascular granulation tissue but when the inflammatory process resolves, either spontaneously or as a result of medication, the granulation tissue is replaced by a mucous membrane which shows a variable degree of atrophic change, a cuboidal type of epithelium replacing the normal columnar epithelium. The muscularis mucosa, which may be destroyed in the acute phase, is replaced by fibrous tissue although excessive fibrosis is not a common feature. Sufficient fibrosis may, however, occur to lead to some thickening of the wall of the bowel and in places narrowing of the lumen.

When total colonic disease has been present for many years malignant changes may occur in areas of atrophic or dysplastic mucosa. The cumulative risk factor is now believed to be much smaller than was at first reported. In the past it was firmly believed that approximately 50 per cent of patients suffering from total involvement for over 10 years developed malignancy but this figure has now been revised downwards to a cumulative risk of 13 per cent after 15 years.

Such tumours arise most commonly in the rectum and descending colon, are frequently multiple and highly undifferentiated.

Clinical presentation

Symptoms
Rectal bleeding, abdominal pain together with severe diarrhoea form the classical triad of symptoms in this disease. In addition, fever, weight loss, joint disorders, erythema nodosum, pyoderma gangrenosum, necrotizing cutaneous vasculitis and severe anaemia may be present.

Physical examination
This may reveal little in the absence of complications. Minor anorectal complications such as fissures and sinuses may be present but these are not as common in ulcerative colitis as they are in Crohn's disease in which their incidence together with more severe anorectal complications has been reported to be as high as 15 per cent. In severe total colonic involvement the patient may be obviously 'toxic', may have lost considerable weight and may be very anaemic. If toxic dilatation of the colon has occurred the abdomen may be grossly distended and when perforation of the bowel follows signs of a spreading peritonitis may be present.

Diagnosis
The initial clinical diagnosis may be confirmed by:
1 *Sigmoidoscopy*. This allows visual examination of the rectum and lower colon to 25 cm but often for technical reasons unless a flexible instrument is used examination beyond 15 cm is frequently impossible. The common visual changes in the rectum are loss of the normal vascular pattern due to oedema and thickening of the mucosa and spontaneous or contact bleeding from the mucosa. Less commonly actual ulceration or pseudopolyps are seen in the distal bowel but if the disease is extensive no upper limit will be seen and blood and mucus will fill the lumen of the instrument from above.

2 *Colonoscopy.* This investigation is somewhat unnecessary in ulcerative colitis since in some 95 per cent of patients the rectum is involved and the diagnosis can, therefore, be made by sigmoidoscopy alone, indeed in severe fulminating colitis this investigation may be positively contraindicated because of the danger of perforating the bowel wall. In chronic colitis of long standing, however, colonoscopy may be of value in permitting the surgeon or physician to take multiple biopsies of areas in which radiological examination suggests malignant changes have taken place.

3 *Double contrast barium enema.* This examination should also be avoided during acute exacerbations of the disease. Its chief value is to establish the extent of the disorder, to monitor the progress of the disease, to exclude malignant change and to distinguish between ulcerative colitis and colonic involvement in patients suffering from Crohn's disease elsewhere in the gastrointestinal tract. The radiological appearances of colitis include absence of haustration, narrowing of the lumen, shortening of the colon, ulceration, pseudopolyposis and the appearances of malignant ulceration. In the presence of deep ulceration the outline of the bowel may be very irregular.

Differential diagnosis

Differential diagnosis includes any cause of bleeding from the large bowel, rectum, or anal canal. Rarer conditions that may mimic colitis are radiation proctitis and ischaemic colitis. In certain areas amoebic colitis is common, and a search for Entamoeba or the Shigella species would be necessary.

Natural history of the disease

The natural history of distal disease has been studied by several groups. In one recorded series it was calculated that the cumulative probability of extension of the disease from the rectum to the descending colon was 12 per cent after 10 years and that the probability of radical surgery indicating that the disease had spread to involve the whole colon was between 3 and 5 per cent.

Complications of colitis

The more serious complications of fulminating total colitis are as follows:

1 *Perforation*

This accounts for approximately one-third of all deaths from severe colitis and it usually occurs during the course of the first attack. The perforation may be sealed by the omentum in which case the signs of general peritonitis will be absent although the patient's general condition deteriorates or it may lead to severe pain and generalized abdominal rigidity. If the patient is on systemic steroid therapy the physical signs associated with peritonitis may be masked even though the patient is acutely ill.

2 'Toxic' dilatation

This complication carries a high mortality, occurring in approximately 3 per cent of all cases of total colonic involvement frequently during the initial attack. The pathogenesis of this complication is an extension of the acute inflammatory process into the deeper layers of the colon leading to neuromuscular paralysis of the affected bowel with subsequent dilatation and loss of peristaltic activity. The condition may be difficult to distinguish clinically from perforation of the bowel. The patient collapses, becomes mentally confused and the abdomen becomes rapidly distended. Plain radiographs of the abdomen reveal gross distension, usually worst in the ascending and transverse colon. Biochemical and haematological tests usually reveal marked fluid depletion, severe hypokalaemia, leucocytosis and marked anaemia. The outlook is serious, the mortality varying between 20 and 40 per cent in reported series', the cause of death usually being perforation.

3 Severe colonic bleeding

This is a relatively rare complication once again occurring in severe disease which is involving the whole of the large bowel. Whereas both perforation and toxic dilatation are absolute indications for immediate operation when bleeding occurs the lost blood should be replaced and the patient carefully observed. If, however, repeated transfusions are required over short periods of time surgery should be considered.

Treatment

The precise treatment of any patient suffering from colitis depends on the severity of disease both in pathological and clinical terms. In general terms since the surgical treatment of colitis carries a not inconsiderable mortality, varying in different series from between 3 and 10 per cent, initially at least unless toxic dilatation or an obvious perforation is present medical management is indicated.

The main lines of treatment are the administration of corticosteroids and salicylazosulphapyridine. The former may be administered both systematically and topically. A common medical regimen is the administration of prednisolone 5 mg orally three times a day and a prednisolone enema (Predsol) at night, possibly every night for 21 days and thereafter every alternate night for 42 days. The dose of prednisolone by mouth can be altered upwards to as much as 60 mg daily in divided doses if the disease is severe and showing little tendency to go into remission and in extremely severe cases the drug can be administered intravenously up to 120 mg being given over a 24-hour period. When the disease is severe enough to warrant the intravenous administration of corticosteroids it is essential to give oral potassium in order to combat the steroid-induced hypokalaemia. This should be given as a fluid preparation by mouth in order to minimize the dangers of small gut ulceration or perforation. In all patients on high doses of steroids a further disaster, i.e. perforation, may occur and, therefore, the abdomen should be examined daily. In addition a stool chart should be kept, the patient monitoring the frequency of the motions, their consistency and their content.

So far as salicylazosulphapyridine is concerned this drug is degraded in the colon by bacterial action to 5-aminosalicyclic acid and sulphapyridine. Any side effects usually occur in patients of slow acetylator phenotype. The dose given depends somewhat on the severity of the disease, in severe disease 1–2 g 6-hourly may be given and once the disease is under control 0.5 g 3 or 4 times a day.

Whereas the continuous administration of corticosteroids has little effect on reducing the relapse rate sulphasalazine (Salazopyrin) appears to diminish the number of relapses in any given patient.

There is also increasing evidence that total bowel rest either by the use of an elemental diet or a temporary period of intravenous feeding may help to induce a remission. However, it has become obvious that patients presenting with total colonic involvement, children and patients over middle age are particularly at risk from their disease, and when the presenting symptoms and the disease are severe, if an early remission is not obtained, surgical treatment should be carried out without delay.

Surgical treatment
The indications for surgical intervention in ulcerative colitis are:

1. failure of medical treatment accompanied by severe disabling diarrhoea and metabolic disturbance;
2. the presence of life-threatening complications;

Major factors which have led to improved results and an improved quality of life following surgery for ulcerative colitis are:

1. closer cooperation between physician and surgeon so that a larger number of patients undergo an elective rather than an emergency operation;
2. the development by Brooke of immediate mucocutaneous suture in the construction of the ileostomy;
3. the development of improved ileostomy appliances.

In general two operations have, until recently, dominated the surgical treatment of this disease.

1. *Total colectomy followed by an ileorectal anastomosis.* This operation is particularly associated with Aylett who stressed the importance of reducing the blood supply to the rectum by dividing the superior haemorrhoidal or inferior mesenteric artery. Later reports lay little stress on this aspect of the operation but suggest that the ultimate result following resection of the large bowel and upper rectum is determined by the state of the rectal mucosa at the time of the operation. If only minimal disease is present in this part of the bowel then the number of satisfactory results is much higher than in those patients in whom severe rectal disease is present. Indeed in a high proportion of the latter group of patients a later rectal excision has to be performed together with a formal ileostomy.
2. *Panproctocolectomy, removing both colon and rectum and establishing a Brooke type of ileostomy in the right iliac fossa.* The complications of ileostomy are numerous, see *Tutorials 2*, p. 160. The overall mortality of this operation performed as an elective procedure may be as low as 3 per cent, the majority of

early deaths being due to the development of intra-abdominal sepsis and pulmonary complications. When this operation is performed in the presence of the complications of the disease, especially toxic dilatation or perforation, the mortality may reach 50 per cent, the majority of deaths being due to uncontrolled sepsis.

A patient in whom an ileostomy is performed must wear an appliance throughout both the day and night since the stoma discharges continually, normally some 300–500 ml of porridge-like material each day, once established.

This has led to a search for methods of controlling the discharge. In 1966 Koch first described the construction of an intra-abdominal reservoir which if made with a valve mechanism produced by intussuscepting a part of the efferent limb into the reservoir holds some 400–600 ml of the ileal contents and can only be emptied by the insertion of a soft rubber tube through the nipple valve. Many complications of this surgical procedure occur and it is not a technique which should be practised outside large units in which experience of the method and its complications can be readily acquired. The late Sir Alan Parks and his associates adopted a somewhat more sophisticated approach by constructing a reservoir from the terminal 50 cm of the ileum and then anastomosing the ileal spout projecting from the reservoir to the anal canal at the level of the dentate line having first divided the rectum some 6–8 cm above this level and then removing the mucosa from this stump, thus preserving sphincteric control over the emptying of the rectum. Patients following this procedure either empty the reservoir spontaneously or by the use of a catheter. However, this operation is also associated with a relatively high incidence of complications, especially pelvic sepsis. Lastly, it should be noted that an attempt is being made by some surgeons to leave a longer segment of rectum denuded of its mucosa and bring the ileum through this, anastomosing it to the anal canal.

Considerable changes in the surgical management of ulcerative colitis can, therefore, be forecast in the future as experience with the more sophisticated surgical procedures becomes more widespread.

6.17 Aetiology, pathology, clinical presentation and management of diverticular disease

Aetiology
Diverticular disease is related to diet. The evidence supporting this statement is the rarity of diverticulosis in the African Bantu living a rural life, and its increasing frequency in this same ethnic group when urbanized and the diet is changed from one containing roughage to one containing refined carbohydrate.

This epidemiological finding has been confirmed in the experimental animal, for rabbits and rats fed on a diet containing white bread, butter, milk, sugar, and added vitamins develop diverticulosis within 4 months. Painter has calculated that this is equivalent to a human on the same diet developing diverticulosis within half a lifetime.

Physiopathological changes
(a) *Pressure changes.* In experimental animals with induced diverticulosis, and man suffering from the naturally occurring disease, significant changes develop in the colonic intraluminal pressures. In both, the intraluminal pressure is consistently above normal, due possibly to the bowel becoming segmented by interhaustral contraction rings. As the taenia contract, the sigmoid shortens, and if the circular muscle contracts simultaneously the sigmoid lumen is radically diminished. As a result, the intraluminal pressure rises and forces the mucosa through the sigmoid wall, especially through the weakest parts where the vessels penetrate the muscle.

(b) *Anatomical changes.* These physiological derangements are associated with hypertrophy of both the circular and the longitudinal muscle coats of the bowel. In the uncomplicated case, the bowel appears somewhat shorter than normal and the diverticula may be clearly seen. Since the diverticula have no muscle coat they cannot empty, which is probably the major cause of the complications of this condition because the inspissated faeces produce mucosal ulceration. This may be followed by infection, leading to the clinical syndrome of diverticulitis, followed later by fibrosis or other more acute complications.

Clinical presentation
The incidence of diverticular disease increases with advancing age and the symptoms resemble those of the irritable colon syndrome. Attacks of left and right iliac fossa pain may accompany irregularities of bowel habit and the occasional passage of mucus. However, the 'irritable' colon is predominantly seen in a younger age group.

Diagnosis
In the presence of minimal symptoms the diagnosis is usually made by the radiologist.

In 1923, Marxer, and later, Marxer and Spriggs, described a condition of the bowel they considered represented a prediverticular situation. A barium enema at this stage shows that the bowel does not dilate and that the mucosal surface has a 'ragged outline'. Other descriptive terms that have been applied to this appearance are the 'saw-edged' or 'saw-toothed' bowel. The precise pathological significance of these changes has never been wholly understood but they are never present without an associated hypertrophy of the colonic muscle. Spriggs and Marxer stated that when such patients are followed, in due course overt diverticulosis develops.

In severer disease, contrast radiology of the colon demonstrates typical diverticula confined to the left colon and sigmoid in approximately 75 per cent of patients, although occasionally they appear only in the right colon or, alternatively, along the entire length of the bowel. The diverticula vary greatly in size, and long after the barium enema has been performed they may remain outlined by the retained barium because of their inability to empty.

Natural history of diverticular disease

The course of diagnosed diverticular disease is both variable and completely unpredictable. Parks and Connel followed a total of 445 patients admitted to Queen's University Hospital, Belfast, and found that two-thirds were suitable for medical treatment and one-third required surgery. The medical regimen consisted of diet and the administration of bulk-producing laxatives. One in four of the patients required readmission and only 25 per cent remained symptom free. However, the symptoms were considered severe in only 5 per cent of the total number. In the majority, the symptoms consisted of only mild, intermittent, aching in the left iliac fossa, together with occasional irregularity of bowel function; 158 of the 445 patients required surgery, the majority at the time of first admission due to some complication. The commonest form of operation was an exploratory laparotomy followed by a colostomy and drainage.

Surgical treatment of the uncomplicated case

In the absence of complications, but in the presence of severe disabling symptoms two separate operative approaches have been advocated. The first and most traditional is resection followed by end-to-end anastomosis. The resection takes the form of a high anterior resection because the disease always stops at the level of the rectosigmoid junction. The proximal line of resection is always open to doubt because the disease is often extensive and, in most patients, some diverticula will be left *in situ*. This leads to the danger of recurrent symptomatic disease but in most recorded series the incidence of this is low, certainly less than 15 per cent.

More recently, in 1964, Reilly proposed that sigmoid diverticulosis should be treated by a longitudinal colonic myotomy, exposing the mucosa over the whole length of the affected segment. This treatment is aimed at diminishing the effects of the muscular hypertrophy. The results of Reilly's operation were recently reviewed by Smith of Edinburgh who found that, following operation, 23 out of a total of 25 patients were symptom free for periods varying from 1 to 2 years. Smith also investigated the intraluminal colonic pressures in these patients after simulation by prostigmine and found that the high pressure present before operation was drastically reduced by myotomy. The operation appears to have a sound physiological basis but the results reported by Smith have not been duplicated elsewhere.

Complications of diverticulitis

Perforation

The most serious complication is perforation, which may lead to either a faecal or a purulent peritonitis. Even today, faecal peritonitis carries a high mortality due to the gross physiological disturbances resulting from the severe endotoxaemia.

Before exploration the patient often requires intensive resuscitation with plasma, corticosteroids, and intravenous antibiotics. Once the general condition of the patient is satisfactory from the anaesthetic point of view a nasogastric tube is inserted and laparotomy performed. Opinion is divided as to the correct surgical procedure following peritoneal toilet and lavage with noxythiolin.

Some surgeons perform a transverse colostomy and also drain the affected area; others merely drain the area of the perforation hoping that if a faecal fistula forms it will heal spontaneously. There is little difference in overall mortality whichever method is used, but if a transverse colostomy is performed a period of many months may elapse before it can be closed without fear of producing a faecal fistula. In this group, a barium enema must be performed before attempting closure. Any extracolonic leak is a contraindication to closure, and even if the enema appears to be satisfactory, there may still be leakage when the colostomy is closed. Such a leak usually heals spontaneously after a few weeks. To avoid this complication many surgeons advocate resection of the diseased bowel before closure of the colostomy, usually about 12 weeks after the acute episode, closing the colostomy about 3 weeks after the resection.

Pericolic abscess
When the perforation is slow to develop a pericolic abscess forms, which in most patients can be treated in the manner of an appendix abscess, with bed rest, antibiotics, and intravenous fluids. Assuming a favourable course the mass slowly resolves. If a mass remains after apparent resolution an associated carcinoma of the colon should be investigated.

Fistula formation
Commoner in males than females, the most frequent fistula is one between the bowel and the bladder. Two classical symptoms develop: the first, and more frequent, is intermittent cystitis, and the second, less common, is the passage of flatus per urethram.

The differential diagnosis includes similar anatomical fistulae due to malignancy or Crohn's disease. The intermittency of the symptoms differentiates fistulae due to diverticulosis from other conditions. In addition, all types are associated with specific radiological and cystoscopic appearances.

Treatment consists of resection of the diseased colon and closure of the bladder, which is usually accomplished with two layers of stitches after freshening the edges of the defect by excising the surrounding fibrous tissue. If, however, the repair is difficult, omentum can be brought down and stitched into the gap. An indwelling urethral catheter must then be left *in situ* for at least 2 weeks.

Haemorrhage
One of the classic complications of diverticulitis is severe rectal bleeding which may occur in the total absence of any previous symptom. It is often severe, the patient passing sufficiently large quantities of bright, fresh, red blood to cause collapse. Despite the fact that diverticulosis accounts for over 90 per cent of

cases of severe large bowel bleeding, all other possible causes—carcinoma, polyps and inflammatory diseases—must be excluded by the appropriate investigations. The treatment is one of ultraconservatism, and if the patient is admitted in hypovolaemic shock the situation is corrected by blood transfusion.

6.18 Pathology and treatment of carcinoma of the rectum

Incidence
The number of deaths from carcinoma of the rectum is approximately 5000 per annum or one-fifth of the total from carcinoma of the bronchus.

Aetiology
1 *Pre-existing villous papilloma.* The evidence for this is based on both clinical and histological observations. Clinically, apparently benign tumours may eventually pursue a malignant course after some years. Histologically, thorough sectioning of an apparently benign lesion often reveals areas of carcinoma *in situ* or frankly invasive cancer. The frequency of malignant change in this type of tumour varies between 6 and 75 per cent according to the different published series.
2 *Familial polyposis.* This condition is inherited as an autosomal dominant and affects males and females in equal numbers. Symptoms of bowel disturbance begin at an average age of 16 years and overt malignancy develops within 15 years, so that most untreated victims die by the time they reach early adult life.
3 *Ulcerative colitis.* The incidence of malignancy in this condition is related to the length of the history. Cancer of the rectum and colon is approximately 20 times higher in patients who have suffered for 20 years as compared to 5 years. However, the risk of cancer is almost exclusively related to those patients suffering from a total colitis; patients suffering from a distal proctitis or proctocolitis appear to have only a slightly increased incidence of malignancy.
4 *Adenomatous rectal polyps.* Satellite polyps are encountered with great frequency in association with carcinoma of the rectum. A problem, therefore, arises in the relationship between the adenomatous polyp and the pathogenesis of rectal cancer. Modern evidence and argument suggests that true invasive cancer only rarely arises from such benign tumours but it has been argued that size is an important factor and that 40 per cent of rectal polyps over 2 cm in diameter are malignant.

Pathology of rectal cancer
Gross appearance. At the time of clinical diagnosis the commonest gross appearance of a rectal cancer is that of an ulcerating lesion with raised everted edges and a sloughing base. Less commonly, the growth may be annular, the lesion completely embracing the lumen. It has been calculated that from its first

macroscopic appearance it takes approximately 2 years for the growth to completely encircle the bowel. Other macroscopic types include the polypoid, mucoid, colloid, and diffusely infiltrating. A pre-existing lesion with malignant potential such as ulcerative colitis or familial polyposis results in the development of multiple tumours but even in the absence of such a lesion, more than one lesion occurs in approximately 3 per cent of all patients.

Histopathology
Rectal tumours are all carcinomata ranging from well differentiated to completely anaplastic. Modified Broder's classifications have been applied to them by such authorities as Dukes. However, if multiple biopsies are taken of any single tumour it will usually be found that the degree of differentiation varies from place to place. This is a feature of some importance since as the tumour becomes increasingly anaplastic so there is a greater tendency to intramural spread and downward extension is of course of great importance in determining the possible level of clearance of the tumour. It appears, therefore, that multiple biopsies should always be taken from any rectal growth. In general, the histological degree of dedifferentiation of rectal tumours bears a direct relationship to the extent of the spread and to the ultimate prognosis.

Spread
Cancer of the rectum spreads in the manner common to all other malignant tumours.

(*a*) Spread along the axis of the bowel as described above is determined by the degree of dedifferentiation. A well differentiated tumour may spread no further than 2 cm in the submucosa whereas a highly dedifferentiated tumour may spread some 4 cm or even more if it is of the rare infiltrating type. Whilst the tumour is spreading circumferentially around the bowel it is also infiltrating outwards involving the muscle of the rectum and finally traversing its whole wall. Once having reached the extraperitoneal structures it continues to progress but anteriorly such progression is delayed by the fascia of Denonvilliers although occasionally direct prostatic invasion is seen. The fascia of Waldeyer also plays a part in restricting the tumour's posterior extension so that direct sacral invasion is also rare.

(*b*) Lymphatic spread has been extensively investigated, particularly by Miles in the 1920s. He found that with both intraperitoneal and extraperitoneal rectal tumours those lymph nodes immediately posterior to the rectum are the first involved and that thereafter the spread is predominantly upwards until finally the para-aortic nodes are involved. Only in low rectal tumours possessing a high degree of malignancy does extensive downward spread occur. Lateral dissemination may occur from intraperitoneal tumours or in those patients in whom upward spread is hindered by complete involvement of the superior haemorrhoidal chain. Lymph node involvement is present in nearly 50 per cent of patients when first seen.

(*c*) Transperitoneal spread. If an extraperitoneal tumour breaches the peritoneum of the pouch of Douglas or rectovaginal pouch, tumour can spread across the peritoneum producing in an advanced state a 'frozen' pelvis, neoplastic replacement of the ovaries or a mass in the omentum.

(d) Venous spread results in the development of secondary deposits primarily in the liver, secondaily in the lungs.

Pathological staging

The original staging of rectal cancers was performed by Dukes, who divided the pathological material into three groups: Group A, a tumour limited to the wall of the rectum. Group B, a tumour extending into the extrarectal tissues but with no lymphatic metastases, and Group C, tumours with demonstrable regional lymph node involvement. Later the C group was subdivided into C_1, lymph nodes present below the level of ligature of the inferior mesenteric vessels, and C_2, lymph nodes reaching above this level.

Symptomatology

The common symptoms of rectal cancer include:

1. bleeding, especially on defaecation;
2. passage of mucus;
3. alteration in bowel habit;
4. early morning 'explosive' motion;
5. continuous rectal discomfort;
6. tenesmus;
7. if the tumour infiltrates the anal canal, fissure-like pain;
8. if there is pelvic infiltration, sciatic pain;
9. occasionally, rectal cancers of the upper third present with acute intestinal obstruction or perforate, causing pelvic peritonitis;
10. occasionally, urinary obstruction.

The diagnosis of rectal cancer is made by a combination of digital examination, sigmoidoscopy, and biopsy.

1 *Digital examination.* This gives some indication of the size of the tumour, its fixation and possibly the presence of rectorectal lymph node involvement. In general it is accepted that the only treatment for the great majority of tumours which can be felt by the examining finger is an abdominoperineal resection. However, recently there has been a suggestion that small tumours palpable by the finger or in the lower third of the rectum which are mobile on the underlying rectal muscle and in whom no pararectal lymph nodes are palpable can be treated by local excision if multiple biopsies show that the tumour is well differentiated. This type of tumour with the characteristics described only account for about 10 per cent of all tumours in any series.

2 *Sigmoidoscopy and biopsy.* The former aids in establishing the level of the tumour and this enables the surgeon to decide on the type of resection required. However, it should be observed that in an intact patient the lower limit of the tumour may appear to be at 8 cm whereas when the rectum is fully mobilized and the lateral ligaments divided the tumour margin may lie as high as 11–12 cm above the anal margin. Whether it is now possible to perform a sphincter saving operation depends upon both the sex and the build of the patient. Biopsy, particularly if multiple biopsies of the tumour are taken, allow the surgeon to predict the downward submucosal spread. This is very important since it has been classically taught that the line of resection should

be some 5 cm below the lower margin of the tumour whereas in highly differentiated tumours it is now believed that 2 cm clearance is sufficient.

Carcinoembryonic antigen (CEA)

One of the most exciting developments relating to colorectal cancer has been the discovery of CEA. This antigen can now be estimated by radioimmunoassay techniques. It was named CEA because an apparently identical antigen can be detected in normal embryonic and fetal gut, pancreas, and liver during the first two trimesters. Thereafter it disappears only to reappear in appreciable quantities in patients suffering from carcinoma of these organs. CEA is a glycoprotein with a molecular weight between 200 000 and 370 000 daltons. Its appearance in malignant disease of the gastrointestinal tract is believed to be due to derepressive dedifferentiation, the antigen having been repressed during the course of differentiation of the normal bowel.

A positive CEA test with an absolute concentration of greater than 2.5 μg/ml is found in 70–80 per cent of patients suffering from carcinoma of the rectum and colon. The level tends to be higher with large tumours and higher still in the presence of hepatic secondaries. If the tumour is wholly removed, the CEA level falls to normal, only to rise if a recurrent tumour develops.

The estimation of CEA, therefore, is an extremely valuable diagnostic tool.

Among the various surgical manoeuvres which have been described to deal with rectal carcinoma, excluding local excision are the following:

1 *Anterior resection.* This operation is used when the tumour involves the upper end of rectum or rectosigmoid. Tumours in this situation can be resected without dividing the peritoneum of the pouch of Douglas or rectovaginal fold and without mobilizing the rectum from the hollow of the sacrum. The lateral ligaments are left intact and so a rectal stump some 10 cm in length remains viable.

2 *Low anterior resection.* This operation is indicated for tumours situated in the upper third of the rectum. The rectum must be mobilized from the hollow of the sacrum and the lateral ligaments divided. When the tumour lies in the upper third of the rectum there is relatively little difficulty in performing either a double or single layer anastomosis by hand.

3 When the tumour lies in the middle third of the rectum excision with preservation of the anal sphincters presents a problem which has been overcome in a number of ways, for example:

(*a*) by pull-through resection with delayed anastomosis, an operation developed in 1961 by Cutait and Figlioni and independently by Turnbull and Cuthberton. In one series reported the average distance of the lower margin of the tumour from the anal verge was 4.1 cm and the average distance of the tumour from the anus was 7.6 cm. The most troublesome complication of this operation is necrosis of the pulled through bowel which is resected some days after the initial operation. Whilst Kirwan reported an incidence of 2 per cent Goligher in a relatively small series reported this complication to be as high as 18 per cent.

(*b*) A modification of this technique was proposed by Parks (1972) who described an operation in which an immediate anastomosis was performed between the colon and the anorectal segment by sutures inserted from below after massive dilatation of the anal canal. This operation Parks called abdominotransanal resection. In order to perform the anastomosis a special anal retractor has to be used, and the sutures connecting the upper rectum to the anal canal have to be inserted by a modification of Turner-Warwick's urethroplasty needles, the needles having a round bodied tip rather than the cutting edge of the standard model. Because the needle is in the same axis as the handle of the instrument there is no problem with angulation such as exists using an ordinary needle holder and needle.

4   Many of the problems associated with reanastomosis following the resection of growths of the middle third of the rectum have, however, been overcome by the use of circular stapling guns. Two are in common usage, the Russian SPTU instrument and the American EEA stapler. Using either of these instruments an important technical step is the insertion of a purse string suture of 2/0 monofilament Prolene (polypropylene) into the cut edge of the rectal and colonic stumps. Following closure of the instrument and its withdrawal from the lumen of the gut this suture should be recovered intact and surrounding each should be a complete cuff of inverted bowel, the 'doughnuts'. If these criteria are not met the anastomosis will require reinforcement by hand inserted stitches. Using stapling techniques the postoperative anastomotic line may be as low as 4 cm.

Various incidences of leakage have been reported in different series using the stapling technique but if the above criteria are adhered to the radiological dehiscence rate appears to be about four times better than a hand sewn anastomosis at the same level when investigated radiologically and twice as good if measured in terms of clinical leakage.

Despite these various manoeuvres the mortality from carcinoma of the rectum has shown little improvement, the overall corrected 5-year survival for all rectal cancers is 30 per cent. The best prognosis is obviously obtained in Duke Class A tumours in which a 92 per cent 5-year survival can be expected. Of interest is the fact that tumours of the lower third of the rectum do less well than those of the middle and upper third.

5   *Hartmann's operation.* Essentially, this operation consists of leaving the rectal stump *in situ*, and in doing so the patient is saved from the additional trauma and blood loss of the perineal dissection.

6   *Transphincteric access to the rectum.* This type of rectal surgery was described in the earlier part of this century, abandoned, and then modified in the early 1970s by York Mason. The approach to the rectum is made by placing the patient on the operating table in the inverted V position, after which an incision is made extending from the anus just to the left of the midline posteriorly, passing obliquely upwards lateral to the coccyx and the lower part of the sacrum. The posterolateral aspect of the rectum is divided together with the sphincters and the puborectalis mass, all of which are carefully resutured when closing the lumen of the bowel. Primarily used for the excision of villous papillomas, York Mason has also used this method for the treatment of Duke Class A tumours on a highly selected basis.

Complications of surgical excision

Immediate. Shock, reactionary haemorrhage, ureteric injury.
Intermediate. Intestinal obstruction due to prolapse of a small gut loop through the pelvic peritoneum. Infection both in the perineal or abdominal wound. Necrosis of the colostomy.
Late. Persistent perineal sinus, sacral herniation, local recurrence. Metastatic disease. Stenosis of the colostomy, which is now rare due to direct mucosa-to-skin suture. Paracolostomy herniation appears to be much less common since the general adoption of the operative technique of extraperitoneal colostomy.

When an anterior resection or abdominoanal pull-through has been performed, a major cause of complications is the breakdown of the anastomosis. This is more likely when the resection is 'low', i.e. carried out below the level of the pelvic peritoneum.

Both abdominoperineal and anterior resection are followed by bladder disturbances. There can be a true neurogenic bladder only when the parasympathetic ganglia on both sides of the pelvis have been excised. This probably is more common in the 'easy' than the difficult case. Painless retention with incontinence develops.

Minor bladder disturbances are frequent (35 per cent) but are usually circumvented by leaving an indwelling catheter *in situ* for longer than the usual period of 4–5 days.

Ancillary methods of treatment

Because of the relatively poor results obtained by surgery alone various ancillary methods, none of which have led to striking improvement in the results, have been tried. These include:

1 *HER.* This has been given preoperatively or postoperatively and whilst there is some doubt as to its efficiacy as a form of adjuvant therapy there is little doubt that as a palliative treatment in the rare inoperable tumour it will cause relief of pain, if only temporarily in a proportion of cases.

2 *Chemotherapy.* Many trials proceed using a large number of drugs preoperatively to kill micrometastases and in inoperable growths. No positive results are yet available.

3 *Immunotherapy.* Many agents have been used to attempt to increase immunity to the tumour. These include BCG and its methanol extraction residue (BCG–MER), *Corynebacterium parvum* and lenamisole but none appears to delay recurrence or alter the ultimate prognosis.

6.19 Congenital deformities of the rectum and anal canal

Embryology
The rectum and anal canal are formed from the hindgut, cloaca, and proctodeal pit. The former contribute to the rectum from the level of the third

sacral vertebra to the junction of the proctodeal pit which lies at the level of the anal valves.

The term 'rectal agenesis' is used to describe malformations of the hindgut and cloaca. Anal anomalies, on the other hand, are due to abnormal development of the proctodeal pit and membrane and are nearly always associated with additional anomalies of the perineum and genital folds. The anatomical malformations associated with developmental rectal and anal anomalies are in large part determined by the sex of the embryo.

One of the most important differences between rectal agenesis and anal anomalies is that in the former the bowel terminates above the levator ani whereas in the latter the gut passes through this important portion of the sphincteric mechanism.

Rectal agenesis

1 *Male*
In approximately 50 per cent of children suffering from rectal agenesis a fistula is present into the urinary tract, this can be in either a rectovesical or rectourethral position.

2 *Female*
Rectal agenesis produces a variety of deformities. These include rectocloacal fistulae which may involve the bladder, vagina, and rectum, all of which open into a common cloaca. Lesser abnormalities leave the urethra opening in the normal position, but a fistulous hindgut tract commonly enters the vagina at the level of the vestibule in the fossa navicularis or, rarely, at a higher level on the posterior vaginal wall.

In both sexes communicating defects are commoner than non-communicating.

Associated abnormalities

Rectal agenesis is usually associated with one or all of the following defects:

1. Abnormalities of the bony skeleton. Varying degrees of sacral agenesis or spina bifida occur. The development of the levator ani and the associated pelvic diaphragm is related to sacral development. When less than three pieces of the sacrum have formed the whole of the levator ani complex is absent thus making adequate sphincteric action and, therefore, continence impossible to attain. Associated with lesser degrees of sacral agenesis a strong collar of muscle may form which represents the normal puborectalis. This results in a muscular sling being present which surrounds the lower part of the rectum and the fistulous tract.
2. Sphincter abnormalities. The internal sphincter is absent and if present the external sphincter is poorly developed.

3 Abnormalities of the cord and its coverings. A spina bifida associated with a meningocele or myelomeningocele may be present, the latter is attended by abnormal bladder innervation and thus a derangement of bladder function, i.e. a neurogenic bladder.
4 Abnormalities of the urinary tract. Nearly a third of the babies have a urological defect. In some patients this is limited to the bladder neck but in others there are malformations of the kidneys.
5 The major part of the rectum responsible for proprioceptive sensation is absent, this being a further factor leading to incontinence following attempted reconstruction.

Anal agenesis

Anal agenesis results from developmental defects of the proctodeal pit, anal membrane and, in the male, the inner genital folds. In most infants of both sexes the puborectalis and levator ani develop normally but the internal and external anal sphincters are usually incomplete.

1 *Male*
The following anomalies are seen:
(a) The anal membrane remains intact and bulges through the anal pit.
(b) Anal stenosis occurs due to incomplete breakdown of the membrane.
(c) A 'covered' anus is formed. This implies that the anus is, in part or completely, covered by an abnormal posterior fusion of the inner genital folds. Fusion may be so extensive that the fistulous tract opens on the undersurface of the shaft of the penis. In such infants the penile urethra is also improperly formed, with the result that the urethra and the fistula have a common opening on the penile shaft in association with a varying degree of hypospadias.
(d) Ectopic anus. This term is used to describe an anus that opens anterior to the normal position, but which in all other respects is normal. This condition is produced by the imperfect development of the tissues that later are defined as the perineal body.

2 *Female*
(a) An imperforate anus in which the anal pit fails to develop.
(b) The anal membrane remains intact and bulges through the anal pit.
(c) A vestibular anus in which the anus opens into the vestibule below the level of the hymen.
(d) Ectopic anus, in which the anus usually opens posterior to the vestibule.
(e) Covered anus, in which the anus opens in the perineum at any point between a normal postion and the vestibule. This anomaly is caused by the genital folds fusing posterior to the anus and continuing this fusion for a variable distance in an anterior direction.

Sacral, nervous and urinary tract abnormalities are rarely associated with anal agenesis.

Diagnosis
A clinical diagnosis of the type of congenital anomaly present can often be made by careful inspection and examination of the infant. An obvious sign, of course, is the complete absence of an anal pit. In the female, a tell-tale spot of meconium may be seen emerging from the vagina or, in the male, from the external urinary meatus.

A detailed clinical examination in good surroundings must be followed by a carefully performed 'inverted' plain radiograph. This is of greatest value when performed some 24–36 hours after birth because by this time the intestinal gas will have reached the lower reaches of the colon.

Radiographic position
The film should be a true lateral of the pelvis with complete overlapping of the ossification centres of the ischial bones. Before inversion the position of the underlying greater trochanter should be carefully identified on the skin and the film should be centred on this.

Interpretation of the film
The important radiological landmark is the pubococcygeal line extending from the upper border of the pubis to the ossification centre of the fifth piece of the sacrum. The importance of this line was described in 1953 by Stephens; prior to this date an estimate of the level of the atresia was made by measuring the distance between the gas column and an opaque body which was strapped to the perineal skin. This was the original method described by Wangensteen and Rice.

The resulting films may be difficult to interpret if rectal gas has escaped through a fistula or, alternatively, the puborectalis has contracted and so deformed the distal gut. In either event a false impression of the precise level of the atresia may be given.

Multiple films will overcome the problem of muscular contraction.

When rectal agenesis is present the lower boundary of the air shadow lies at or above the pubococcygeal line.

An alternative method of establishing the exact level of the lesion is the use of ultrasonography.

Neither method is of use if carried out after the performance of a colostomy because decompression is followed by the disappearance of gas from the distal bowel the detection of which is the all important feature of both investigations.

Treatment
Rectal or anal agenesis is associated with intestinal obstruction unless a large fistulous tract allows adequate decompression; therefore, the treatment is operative.

Rectal agenesis
Three alternative procedures have been described:
1 *Transverse colostomy.* Following the relief of obstruction the baby is allowed to grow for a period of one year or more before attempting a definitive

procedure. The protagonists of colostomy maintain that the enlargement of the pelvis and growth of the puborectalis sling makes subsequent surgery easier.

2 *Immediate abdominoanal pull-through.* In principle, the essence of such pull-through procedures is to divide the rectourethral or rectovaginal fistula and bring the bowel down anterior to the puborectalis sling as near to the prostate or cervix as possible in the hope that the nerve supply to the bowel, bladder and puborectalis will remain intact thus permitting the puborectalis to perform at least some part of the sphincteric action and thus preserve faecal continence.

3 *Sacrococcygeal reconstruction.* The protagonists of this approach argue that it enables the surgeon to preserve the whole of the puborectalis mass, particularly if the procedure is delayed for at least a year. The disadvantage of this method is that the preliminary colostomy may prolapse and the continued presence of the rectourethral fistula may lead to recurrent urinary tract infections.

Overall, the long term results of any procedure for rectal agenesis are poor. Long term follow-up suggests that only about 30 per cent of infants are continent by the age of 4, the majority suffering from recurrent faecal impaction due to lack of rectal sensation or persistent leakage requiring a perineal pad although the latter may be alleviated to some degree by regular bowel irrigation.

These clinical findings are reflected in manometric studies of the anorectal pressure profile. In a normal infant at about 4 years of age the anorectal reflex is firmly established, a fall in pressure in the anal canal occurring if the rectum is distended. However, in the incontinent child following reconstruction this reflex is absent and there is a decreased awareness of rectal sensation.

The mortality of both sacrococcygeal reconstruction and abdominoanal pull-through is between 10 and 15 per cent.

Other complications of reconstructive surgery include:

1 excessive protrusion of the rectal mucosa through the artificial anus which leads to leakage of mucus onto the perineum and, thus, perineal excoriation;
2 anal stenosis either at the level of the pelvic sling or, alternatively, at skin level;
3 recurrent urethral fistula;
4 disturbance of bladder function.

Anal agenesis
The treatment of anomalies associated with anal agenesis is accompanied by a low operative mortality and satisfactory functional results. The results are satisfactory because the puborectalis sling is usually perfectly developed.

The common 'covered' or ectopic anus is usually treated by a median episiotomy, the anal 'cut-back'. The orifice of the anus is enlarged to take the little finger end, and a direct mucosa-to-skin anastomosis is performed. The common complication of this operation is the development of a stricture but this can be prevented by dilatation with a Hegar's dilator. Because the cut-back operation in the female, performed for a rectovestibular or ectopic anus, leaves the female with a vagina 'stained' with faeces, attempts have been made to move the whole rectum and anal canal backwards. This operation is doomed to failure because of the improper development of the perineal body.

7 Urology

7.1 Causes and treatment of urinary tract infections
7.2 Diagnosis and treatment of carcinoma of the prostate
7.3 Benign prostatic enlargement: pathology, treatment and complications
7.4 Pathology, signs, symptoms, treatment and prognosis of renal tumours
7.5 Swellings of the scrotum, and the pathology and treatment of testicular tumours
7.6 Investigation and surgical management of stones in the renal tract
7.7 Causes and treatment of vesicoureteric reflux

7.1 Causes and treatment of urinary tract infections

Definition. A urinary tract infection exists when the bacterial count in 1 ml of a 'clean catch' specimen of urine is 10^5 or over, a count of this order indicating the presence of bacteria proximal to the internal urethral orifice. If it is impossible to obtain a clean catch specimen, an alternative diagnostic procedure is to puncture the distended bladder above the pubis.

Two major factors influence bacterial growth in the urine: pH and osmolality. The optimum pH for the growth of *Escherichia coli* lies between a pH of between 6 and 7. A pH of less than 5.5 delays growth and a pH of greater than 7.5 leads to total inhibition, but whereas a pH above 7.5 is physiologically unattainable, acidification to below 4.6 is possible. So far as osmolality is concerned, the usual physiological range is between 300 and 1200 mosmol/l; should the urine be diluted below 200 mosmol/l bacterial growth is reduced irrespective of the pH.

Urinary tract infection, apart from that in the first year of life and over the age of 60 years, is predominantly a problem of the female.

Classification
Infections of the urinary tract can be classified as follows:

(a) primary infections on which there is no previous history;
(b) secondary infections in which a primary infection has relapsed, or there has been an apparent reinfection.

It is also possible to divide urinary tract infections into those of childhood, those of adult life, and infections in the presence of a structural abnormality of the urinary tract. The structural abnormalities that may lead to infection of the urinary tract may be congenital or acquired, physiological or anatomical.

Congenital causes of urinary tract infection include:

1. urinary tract abnormalities associated with spina bifida and rectal agenesis. Both these conditions give rise to physiological disturbances due to interference with the nerve supply to the bladder and bladder neck.

    Spina bifida may be associated with gross anatomical and functional abnormalities of the whole urinary tract.

    Rectal agenesis itself gives rise to physiological disturbances because of its association with malformations of the pelvic plexuses, and, in addition, there are, also, anatomical abnormalities in the form of fistulae.
2. vesicoureteric reflux. This condition accounts for about 25 per cent of urinary tract infections in children, the dilated ureters serving as reservoirs of stagnant urine which form suitable breeding grounds for bacteria.
3. posterior urethral valves. In the male infant these lead to urinary tract infection due to chronic urinary retention.

Acquired abnormalities predisposing to infection include:

1. incomplete emptying of the bladder due to prostatic or urethral obstruction.
2. the presence of a tumour or calculus in the bladder or kidney.
3. the presence of a diverticulum of the bladder.
4. physiological disturbances due to spinal injury or acquired nervous diseases that produce retention.
5. retention treated by open catheter drainage.
6. vesicocolic fistulae. These are usually a complication of diverticulitis but they may be due to neoplastic disease of the colon or Crohn's disease.

In the majority of these acquired causes the treatment of the infection is secondary to the cure of the predisposing cause.

The significance of residual urine

The importance of residual urine, particularly in the lower urinary tract, has been extensively investigated in recent years. Apart from congenital anomalies leading to retention this factor is probably of greatest significance in prostatism and in the female suffering from recurrent infections. It is obvious, and it has been proven, that when infected urine is voided the total number of organisms in the urinary tract falls. However, as fresh urine is added to any residual infected urine the organisms multiply until once again they regain their original numbers. O'Grady showed that if the total bacterial population in the urine cannot be kept down by repeated micturition the response to antimicrobial therapy is poor.

Bacteriology of urinary tract infections

The majority of primary infections of the urinary tract are caused by *E. coli*, the strain usually corresponding to that found in the intestinal tract of the patient. This organism is a short Gram-negative rod which is usually motile. Grown on MacConkey's medium the colonies have a metallic sheen. In the primary attack these organisms are usually sensitive to a wide variety of antibiotics. In secondary or recurrent infections, although the *E. coli* remains the most common single dominant organism isolated, other coliforms also appear together with *Proteus, Pseudomonas aeruginosa, Streptococcus faecalis*, and even *Staphylococcus*.

Symptomatology and bacteriological investigation of urinary infection

Clinically, there is a considerable variation in the model of presentation of urinary infections. Catheter fever, with associated septicaemia and hypotension, represents one end of the scale. Merging with this syndrome is acute pyelonephritis associated with malaise, rigors, and pain. More restricted still is the development of prostatitis in the male, or the urethral syndrome of the female and, lastly, there is the totally asymptomatic, but infected, patient.

Recurrent urinary tract infection in the female appears most often in the absence of any overt anatomical abnormality, the common symptoms being urgency, frequency, and dysuria. Several factors predispose to infection in the female. First, her urethra is only 3.5–4 cm in length. Under normal circumstances it must withstand the trauma of sexual intercourse and, because of its anatomical position, it is exposed to contamination with faecal organisms. The importance of the former is suggested by the high frequency of urinary tract infection in sexually active women (prevalence rate 10 per cent) as compared to nuns in whom the incidence is of the order of 0.6 per cent. Furthermore, the wall of the female urethra is not a straight tube but, rather, an elongated cryptic prostate in which offending organisms once present can rapidly multiply.

When the female develops symptoms of an infected urinary tract the midstream specimen of urine is often clear and culture reveals no abnormality. The site of infection in such women can only be demonstrated by the use of differential urethrovesical urinary cell counts.

To perform these the external genitalia are first thoroughly cleansed, the first 50 ml of urine passed is then collected, and after this the midstream specimen. Every cell is counted except for squames and red cells. Normally the count does not exceed 5000 per ml, and the difference between the two specimens will be negligible. When infection is confined only to the urethral glands the first count is high and the second low. When infection, however, has reached the bladder both counts are high but in this situation the infecting organisms can usually be isolated by routine culture. In the male, a comparable method has also been described which involves the bacteriological examination of urine specimens obtained before and after prostatic massage. As would be expected, this method is only applicable to the male suffering from chronic prostatitis because differential growth does not take place in an overt acute infection in which the bladder is also involved.

Ascending infection

There is no clear explanation of the mechanism of ascending infection although it is known that there may be vesicoureteric reflux during and immediately after an acute attack of cystitis.

It has been suggested that infection reaches the upper urinary tract via the lumen of the ureter and *E. coli* is certainly motile.

In children suffering from persistent reflux, there is progressive renal damage but this is not necessarily due to infection but rather to the high pressure that occurs in the upper renal tract in this condition. When a bacteriuria is found in a child it should be fully investigated, and included in the investigations should be a micturating cystogram. In an adult the cause of repeated infections may be obvious, as for example, in the male suffering from prostatism. On the other hand, it may only become evident after investigation. Full investigations, including intravenous pyelography and cystoscopy, of both the male and female are justified in the presence of a relapsing infection.

Treatment of infection
When investigations have ruled out a lesion that requires surgical interference, the infection is treated by a combination of specific and general measures.

The common general measures include: in the female, scrupulous perineal hygiene, especially before and after sexual intercourse. Keeping the bladder empty and taking the last dose of the prescribed specific drug before retiring to bed and, possibly, rising in the middle of the night to micturate.

Specific measures relate to the drugs that may be used. A variety of sulphonamides, antiseptic agents, furan derivatives and antibiotics are now available. All these drugs are secreted in the urine in concentrations many times greater than the bacteriostatic or bactericidal level so that advantage can be taken of the dilution factor mentioned earlier. This not only reduces bacterial growth but also reduces the frequency of micturition.

The three questions, however, remain unanswered:

1. Do the drugs reach bacteriostatic or bactericidal levels in an area of kidney damaged by previous infection?
2. Irrespective of the growth of resistant mutants, are antibiotics of use in the elimination of altered bacterial forms?
3. For how long should treatment be continued and, if continued for long periods, does such therapy prevent damage to the urinary tract?

Miscellaneous
1. Mandelic acid 2–4 g four times a day using, simultaneously, ammonium chloride 2 g four times a day to acidify the urine.
2. Nitrofurantoin 5–10 mg/kg daily in divided doses. Active against *E. coli*.
3. Nalidixic acid 4 g daily in divided doses. Effective against *E. coli* and *Proteus*. Inactive against *Pseudomonas*.

Sulphonamides
1. Sulphafurazole, 6 g daily in divided doses active against *E. coli* and *Proteus*.

2 Co-trimoxazole. This is a combination of trimethoprim (one part) and sulphamethoxazole (five parts). The former drug inhibits the production of folinic acid by the organism and the latter the biosynthesis of folic acid. Extensive surveys have shown a high degree of sensitivity to this combination: 93 per cent of outpatients and 88 per cent of inpatients were found to be infected with organisms sensitive to this drug combination.

Antibiotics

Of the commonly used antibiotics, ampicillin and carbenicillin are both highly effective against *E. coli*. Carbenicillin is especially effective against *Ps. aeruginosa* which is an organism associated with recurrent rather than primary infections.

Gentamicin is also an effective drug but care must be taken in the presence of incipient or actual renal failure, because in these circumstances the concentration of the drug rises to ototoxic levels. Of the cephalosporins, cephradine, which can be administered orally is excreted at mean urine concentrations greatly in excess of the minimum inhibitory concentration necessary to kill all the organisms responsible for urinary tract infection.

In the male suffering from prostatitis, the antibiotic used should be basic and lipid-soluble so that it will be concentrated in the prostatic tissues; for these reasons erythromycin 1 g daily in divided doses is a useful agent but, unfortunately, it is predominantly active against Gram-positive organisms.

A patient treated with one of the above agents requires bacteriological follow-up. If there is a relapse within one week it can be safely assumed that the infecting organism has never been eliminated. When relapse occurs after many months it is a reasonable assumption that this is a reinfection and should be treated as such. A further unanswered question is, what is the correct treatment of an asymptomatic bacterial relapse, because there is little evidence that such an infection causes a deterioration of renal function.

7.2 Diagnosis and treatment of carcinoma of the prostate

Incidence
The incidence of carcinoma of the prostate varies from 3.1/100 000 of the male population over 35 years in Japan to 160/100 000 in Denmark. In part, the explanation for this low incidence in Japan is probably a reflection of lower recognition rates, but even in the most recently published figures, although the curves of age incidence are parallel with those of other countries, the overall incidence remains statistically lower. Post mortem, the incidence of prostatic cancer is much higher than the clinical incidence, being reported as high as 14 per cent in males over the age of 50.

The aetiology of the disease is unknown but since it is not found in eunuchs the changing hormonal patterns of advancing age must be of some significance. Of further interest is the finding that such tumours usually arise in the outer subcapsular glands which appear to be more sensitive to androgens than the inner group from which benign hypertrophy arises.

Clinical presentation
Many tumours are now being diagnosed at routine 'health checks' in completely symptomless males but when symptoms are present approximately two-thirds of the patients will have problems relating to the lower urinary tract and one-third symptoms due to disseminated disease. Lower urinary tract symptoms include frequency, difficulty, haematuria or retention. There may be diffuse perineal pain and eventually, as the tumour spreads across the pelvis, sciatic pain develops together with bilateral venous oedema due to obstruction of the external iliac veins. Blood stream dissemination may be associated with severe bone pain and leucoerythroblastic anaemia.

In the majority of patients the diagnosis can be made by digital examination of the prostate, although an infarct of the gland or, occasionally, a prostatic calculus may simulate a solitary nodule. When the tumour is more advanced the normal sharp palpable outline of the gland and the median sulcus are lost and once this stage has been reached the only *real* differential diagnosis is chronic prostatitis.

Pathology
Macroscopic appearance. In the early stages, nodules of prostatic cancer appear as butter yellow nodules in the gland, usually in the posterior lobe which lies below and behind the ejaculatory ducts. Such nodules must be at least 0.5 cm in diameter to be clinically recognizable.
Microscopic appearance. The majority of prostatic cancers are adenocarcinomata and are composed of small cells often arranged in microacinar or cribriform manner. Less commonly, squamous or transitional cell carcinoma occur and, very rarely, sarcoma.

Spread of prostatic cancer
As the tumour grows it involves the capsule, the base of the bladder and the seminal vesicles. Direct invasion of the rectum is rare because of the protection afforded by the fascia of Denonvilliers, although occasional reports appear in the literature of misguided abdominoperineal resections performed because a tumour has managed to breach this natural line of defence.

Lymphatic spread, often by permeation of the perineural lymphatics, begins relatively early. Venous spread via the vertebral venous plexus is responsible for secondary deposits in the lumbar spine, the pelvis and the femora. Death is normally from either uraemia, ascending infection, or cachexia due to widespread dissemination.

Diagnostic methods
Diagnosis of carcinoma of the prostate may be confirmed by the following methods.

1 *Prostatic massage*
Malignant cells may be found in the expressed secretion.

2 *Acid phosphatase*
Normal acid phosphatase is derived from both the prostate and the erythrocytes. The latter is inactivated by 0.5 per cent formaldehyde. The upper limit of normal is 3.5 KA units and this level is not usually exceeded until the tumour has extended beyond the capsule of the gland. A level of over 10 units indicates that metastases are definitely present, but in 40 per cent of patients suffering from metastatic disease the acid phosphatase may be normal. In the majority of patients with skeletal metastases the alkaline phosphatase is also raised.

3 *Radiology*
Intravenous pyelography may show evidence of bladder trabeculation, residual urine and/or a filling defect at the base of the bladder. When long-standing obstruction is present, there are also changes in the upper urinary tract.

In addition, skeletal X-rays may show the presence of bony metastases, these may be osteoblastic, appearing as areas of increased density within the bone, osteolytic when they appear as areas of rarefaction or they may be mixed. Skeletal metastases are present in a quarter of all patients at their initial attendance.

If a vertebra appears denser than the normal it is usually affected either by a secondary prostatic deposit, Paget's, or lymphoma. If Paget's is suspected the skull should be X-rayed, remembering that the precise radiological appearance depends upon whether resorption or deposition of bone is the predominant change.

4 *Prostatic biopsy*
This may be performed in various ways.
(a) By transurethral resection. If the tumour is limited to the posterior lobe such a resection is unhelpful but when the tumour is more extensive, particularly when it involves the bladder neck, it is simple to obtain worthwhile biopsy material.
(b) Transrectal biopsy. This type of biopsy is normally performed with a TruCut needle or a similar type of instrument. It is particularly valuable when a solitary nodule can be palpated in the gland per rectum. The major complication of this procedure is, however, the development of prostatic infection and for this reason tobramycin or gentamicin, dose 2 mg/kg should be given for 48 hours prior to the procedure. The former drug is possibly preferable since animal studies indicate that it is somewhat less ototoxic and nephrotoxic than the latter. Both drugs are active against Gram-negative organisms and some organisms resistant to gentamicin remain sensitive to tobramycin.
(c) By perineal biopsy. This method has a distinct advantage over transrectal biopsy in that it is a 'cleaner' procedure and can, therefore, be performed without any prior treatment with antibiotics. However, the disadvantage of

the method is that the operator may not locate the suspected nodule with the needle.

(*d*) *By aspiration cytology.* This may be performed using a narrow-bore needle introduced into the prostate via the perineum or rectum. If the latter method is used the procedure must be 'covered' by prophylactic antibiotic therapy.

5 Transrectal ultrasonography

This method which is non-invasive has achieved very satisfactory results when used in units in which the necessary apparatus is available. Basically a probe is passed through the anus and at various levels the prostate is scanned. The information gained from this type of investigation is as follows:

(*a*) the size of the prostate;
(*b*) variations in the texture of the gland, leading to the potential diagnosis of benign or malignant enlargement;
(*c*) the extent of extracapsular spread assuming the cause of the enlargement is malignant;
(*d*) the involvement or otherwise of the seminal vesicles.

6 CAT scan

Since lymphatic spread from the prostate takes place via the internal iliac nodes lymphograms give no indication of lymphatic spread. Computerized axial tomography allows:

(*a*) the size of the prostate and the extent of direct spread to be determined;
(*b*) the presence or absence of internal iliac node involvement to be established. In theory if not in practice this would obviate the necessity for a staging laparotomy.

7 Bone scan

If plain X-rays of the skeleton suggest the presence of metastases a bone scan may confirm or refute such a diagnosis. A bone-seeking nuclide is intravenously injected into the patient and is taken up in areas in which new bone is being laid down in an attempt to repair the destruction caused by tumour invasion. The discovery of compounds such as diphosphonate and pyrophosphate, both of which are bone seeking and can be labelled with ^{99m}Tc, has made available materials which are readily obtainable and which lead to a low radiation dose and a high photon yield.

When new bone is being formed the area is depicted as a zone of increased uptake.

Staging

T_0: no tumour palpable.
T_1: intracapsular tumour surrounded by normal gland.
T_2: tumour confined to the gland with a smooth nodule deforming the contour.
T_3: tumour extending beyond the capsule.
T_4: tumour fixed or invading neighbouring structures.

Treatment

In general terms the majority of patients suffering from prostatic cancer are treated by palliative means or not at all.

Indeed, Ferguson rightly pointed out that the overall merits of any particular form of treatment should be judged more by the relief of symptoms than by the survival time since in most patients the latter is in any case limited. It has indeed been estimated that the overall life expectancy of untreated cases from the onset of symptoms is 31 months, although 7 per cent may survive for 5 years. This demonstrates the great variability in biological activity of these tumours. If metastases are present when the patient is first seen two-thirds of the patients die within 9 months.

Surgical. Theoretically, prostatic cancer should be as radically treated as any other neoplasm but in only about 5 per cent of patients is this possible. The operation of radical perineal prostatectomy has gained little support in the UK. It involves the removal of the fascia of Denonvilliers, the prostatic capsule, vesical neck and trigone, seminal vesicles and the ampulla of the vas deferens. The major criticisms of this operation are the relatively high mortality, the frequency of postoperative incontinence and impotence, and the possibility of a retrovesical fistula.

Although retropubic or transvesical prostatectomy can be performed this results in only a limited excision of malignant tissue. Such operations are usually carried out when the correct preoperative diagnosis has not been made; the preferred method of dealing with obstructive symptoms is by transurethral resection.

Hormonal. Following the work of Huggins of Chicago in the 1940s and early 1950s it became a routine procedure to remove the testicular endocrine secretion by orchidectomy or enucleation or, alternatively, to inhibit the secretion of androgens by the administration of oestrogens.

Various studies have shown that a 5-year survival of 44 per cent can be obtained by the use of oestrogens and orchidectomy if the patient is seen and treated before metastases occur, and a 20 per cent 5-year survival thereafter.

However, oestrogen therapy is not without its problems. Nausea and vomiting are common, gynaecomastia and pigmentation of the nipples may occur. More serious are sodium retention leading to heart failure and the development of venous thrombosis. Indeed, the Veteran's Administration of America has published a series of papers that rejects the previous unqualified optimism that greeted the hormonal therapy of prostatic cancer and suggested that it should be administered only when definite indications exist such as bone pain.

About a third of patients respond to oestrogen therapy and gain relief from bone pain, the acid phosphatase falling and the alkaline phosphatase first rising and then falling as bone repair is completed. Both will rise again in the presence of any reactivity.

It is interesting to observe that following the administration of oestrogens the various clones of cancer cells which make up the whole tumour bulk may show differing response in different areas of dissemination. This feature is particularly noticeable in osseous metastases some of which may appear to respond totally whereas in other areas of the skeleton continuous progression can be observed. In general terms it would appear that small adenomatous-like foci respond whereas the anaplastic tumour areas remain unresponsive.

Irradiation. It has been shown that in T_3 tumours lymph node involvement is present in 60 per cent and that in 30 per cent this lymphatic extension will have reached the para-aortic nodes. In this type of case transurethral resection should be used to relieve urinary obstruction and the involved nodes should be treated by external irradiation using two large parallel opposed fields covering the prostate, internal iliac and common iliac nodes. A tumour dose of 35 Gy should be given in 15 fractions over 21 days.

Bony secondaries if causing pain, unrelieved by hormonal therapy, can be treated by external irradiation using a single field to deliver 24 Gy in five treatments over 7 days.

Cause of death
A common cause of death in sufferers from carcinoma of the prostate is chronic uraemia due to the eventual development of an obstructive nephropathy.

7.3 Benign prostatic enlargement: pathology, treatment and complications

Anatomy of the normal prostate
The prostate grows slowly from birth to puberty, then rapidly to about 30 years of age, after which it remains relatively static in size until the age of 45 after which it either atrophies or undergoes hypertrophy.

The apex of the normal prostate rests upon the external sphincter, its posterior surface is separated from the rectum by two layers of rectovesical fascia and has a depression towards its upper extremity through which the ejaculatory ducts enter the gland to open into the prostatic urethra on either side of the utriculus masculinus which itself lies on the crista urethralis. The plane of the ejaculatory ducts divides the gland into a number of lobes. Below the level of the ejaculatory ducts in the midline is the posterior lobe, above this level is the middle lobe. On each side of the middle and the much larger posterior lobe is situated the major portion of the gland, i.e. the lateral lobes which weigh between 6 and 7 g. The lateral lobes are joined anteriorly by the anterior lobe which contains few, if any, glands.

Two sets of glands are present in the normal prostate, an inner group which lie in the inner zone and directly surround the urethra and an outer group which lie in an outer zone which is separated from the true capsule of the prostate by a plexus of veins.

Pathology of prostatic hypertrophy
It must be appreciated that prostatic symptoms may develop in the absence of gross enlargement of the prostate and conversely a grossly enlarged prostate may be associated with minimal symptoms. The hyperplastic gland may be large and

soft, or small and hard, depending on the relative contribution made by the glandular elements and the fibromuscular ground substance.

When the gland is large and soft histological examination shows that the number of glands in the stroma has increased, 'adenosis' and that the number of cells forming these new glands has also multiplied, 'epitheliosis', although there may be little or no increase in the stromal elements. Approximately 25 per cent of all large adenomatous glands show evidence of secondary change such as infarction and in about 10 per cent an unsuspected carcinoma will be found. In addition if secretions are retained within the new glands cyst formation will occur. Such changes most commonly occur in the lateral lobes so that rectal examination readily reveals the enlargement, if they occur only in the middle lobe the prostate may feel normal in size even though middle lobe enlargement can produce severe obstructive symptoms. A further pertinent point is that prostatic hypertrophy begins in the inner zone of the prostate producing compression of the outer zone which then forms the false capsule from which the 'adenomatous gland' is enucleated.

When the gland is small and hard a minimal degree of epithelial proliferation is present accompanied by a considerable overgrowth of the fibromuscular components of the gland. Such a gland may feel almost normal on rectal examination but cystourethrography may reveal a so-called median bar seen best with a fore-oblique lens with the urethroscope situated just proximal to the veru so that the prostatic urethra above this level can be viewed as a whole. Normally the bladder neck forms a circle but in the presence of a median bar the circle is interrupted inferiorly by a ridge which appears to stretch across and interrupt the inferior boundary of the circle.

Aetiology
The cause of prostatic enlargement is unknown. The condition increases in frequency with advancing age and it is well documented that about the male menopause the production of androgens diminishes and there is a relative increase in oestrogens. It is known, however, that testicular activity is necessary for prostatic hypertrophy since castrates never develop prostatism. One hypothesis is that the oestrogens produce an increase in the fibromuscular stroma whereas androgens act upon the epithelial elements.

Clinical presentation
The common symptoms of prostatic hypertrophy include:

(a) difficulty of micturition associated with hesitancy;
(b) repeated attack of retention;
(c) persistent frequency;
(d) recurrent infection leading to frequency and dysuria;
(e) nocturnal waking associated with hesitancy;
(f) haematuria;
(g) chronic retention with overflow incontinence.

Clinical examination of a patient suffering from prostatism may reveal little. If the patient has developed acute retention the bladder may be visible and will certainly be palpable and tender. In chronic retention the bladder wall may be so thin and atonic that the bladder, though grossly enlarged, may be impalpable.

Rectal examination may reveal an apparently normal-sized prostate or, alternatively, if there is hypertrophy the lateral lobes bulge these backwards into the rectum. When benign, however, the prostate is clearly delineated and the median sulcus is palpable.

Special investigations

1 *Measurement of residual urine.* This investigation is rarely performed because of the more sophisticated techniques available. However, a residual urine exceeding 60 ml can be regarded as pathological.

2 *Blood urea and more complex tests of renal function.* A blood urea estimation is simple to perform and exceedingly valuable because marked elevation indicates that there is no purpose in performing an intravenous pyelogram. More complex tests seldom need to be performed.

3 *Intravenous pyelography.* This investigation may show a variety of physical changes in the urinary tract including:

(a) non-function;
(b) dilatation of the pelvicalyceal system;
(c) hydroureter;
(d) bladder trabeculation;
(e) diverticulum formation;
(f) filling defect at the bladder base, indicating the degree of prostatic enlargement;
(g) measurable quantities of residual urine.

4 *Acid phosphatase* (see section 7.2).

5 *MSU.* In the majority of patients suffering from prostatism the urine will not be infected but in the presence of long-standing obstructive symptoms and a large residual urine infection is almost inevitable. This feature is important to establish since urological procedures are one of the commonest precipitating causes of bacteraemic shock.

6 *Measurement of peak flow.* This investigation, particularly if repetitive results are obtained, now plays an important role in the investigation of lower urinary tract disease. When the peak flow of urine falls to below 10 ml/sec following the intake of 2 litres of fluid not only does it indicate that operation is required it also indicates that if surgery is not undertaken in the relatively near future acute or acute on chronic retention is almost bound to occur sooner rather than later.

7 *Cystourethroscopy.* This examination establishes:

(a) prostatic size;
(b) the degree of bladder trabeculation, which is an anatomical indication of the physiological difficulty;
(c) the presence or absence of bladder diverticuli;
(d) whether the urinary obstruction is due to prostatic hypertrophy or some other cause such as urethral stricture, hypertrophy of the bladder neck or carcinoma of the bladder.

Differential diagnosis
The other common causes of 'prostatism' include:
1 *Carcinoma of the prostate.* An identical history may be obtained but rectal examination often reveals a hard irregular gland lacking the normally palpable median sulcus and lateral borders.
2 *Urethral stricture.* Infective strictures due to untreated or improperly treated gonorrhoea are now rare in Western society. The common site for such strictures was in the bulbous urethra distal to the triangular ligament. More common are strictures due to trauma, usually instrumental but occasionally traumatic.
3 *Chronic prostatitis.* This condition is normally associated with a history of recurrent urinary tract infection and deep perineal pain.
4 *Bladder neck obstruction.* Palpation reveals little but the cystourethroscopic findings as already described are typical.
5 *Bladder tumour.* A bladder tumour, especially of the undifferentiated variety arising in the region of the bladder neck may produce urinary obstruction but this will normally be accompanied by intermittent haematuria.

Complications of prostatism
The major complications associated with enlargement of the prostate are:

1 acute retention;
2 chronic retention with overflow incontinence;
3 urinary tract infection;
4 back pressure effects leading to bilateral hydronephrosis and eventually a reduction in renal function.

Indications for prostatectomy
1 The most frequent indication for prostatectomy is to relieve the various symptoms of urinary obstruction. However, when considering surgical treatment the age and general condition of the patient, as well as the severity of the symptoms, must be taken into account. This is important because if the effects of back pressure are limited to the bladder there may be long asymptomatic intervals.
2 Eradication of an infected area, e.g. a chronic prostatic abscess.
3 Correction of physiological imbalance, i.e. in the neurogenic bladder.
4 Diagnostic measure when prostatic cancer is suspected. Prostatectomy in these circumstances is nearly always performed by transurethral resection.

Prostatectomy

This operation may be performed by closed techniques, i.e. transurethral resection, or by open methods. In general, a prostate weighing 30 g or less is nearly always treated by transurethral resection whereas a prostate weighing 40 g or more is usually removed by open operation. Between these two extremes either method can be employed.

The recorded series suggest that the retropubic or transvesical route will be used in just over half the patients, and transurethral resection in the remainder. Commonly, as the age of the patient group rises, there is a decreasing incidence of operations for prostatism and an increase in the number of operations performed for retention. This, not unnaturally, contributes to an increasing mortality since an average 'acceptable' mortality is about 2 per cent for prostatism alone, 6 per cent for patients suffering from acute retention, and 9 per cent in patients suffering from chronic retention. The most frequent causes of death following prostatic surgery are cardiovascular, respiratory, and renal complications.

Complications of retropubic prostatectomy

1 *Immediate*
(*a*) *Clot retention*. This can usually be dealt with by perurethral means using some form of evacuator but, occasionally, the prostatic capsule has to be reopened. This complication is avoided by:

 (i) carefully controlling the bleeding prior to closure of the capsule;
 (ii) the use of diuretics to flush out the bloody urine in the early postoperative period;
 (iii) continuous bladder irrigation.

(*b*) *Shock*. This is due to excessive blood loss after enucleating the adenoma and should not occur if the blood loss is corrected by immediate transfusion.
(*c*) *Uncontrollable haemorrhage*. Rarely, bleeding from the prostatic bed continues despite all efforts to stop it. One method of dealing with this is to insert a Foley catheter through the urethra, pack the prostatic bed, inflate the catheter bulb and bring it down under tension in order to squeeze the pack against the prostatic cavity. A cystotomy is then performed high on the anterior wall of the bladder. Through this, the end of the pack is brought to the surface and by its side another Foley catheter is inserted into the bladder. The capsule is then closed, followed by the abdominal parietes. The pack can be removed by gentle traction after 48 hours, the suprapubic catheter after 6 days, and the perurethral catheter after 12 days.

2 *Intermediate*
(*a*) *Fistula formation*. This complication usually arises when the capsule has been difficult to close or excessive coagulation has led to extensive necrosis. A fistula usually closes if the bladder is drained by a urethral catheter for several days.
(*b*) *Epididymitis*. It was once considered that epididymitis could be prevented by ligation and division of the vas, and this was originally a routine procedure following retropubic prostatectomy.
(*c*) *Secondary haemorrhage*. This is fortunately rare. It is more common if the bladder is infected at the time of operation.

3 *Late*
(*a*) *Incontinence*. This is nearly always temporary and is usually better within 3 months.

(b) *Osteitis pubis.* This should be suspected when the patient complains within a few weeks of operation of pain in the pubis and down the inner aspect of the thigh. Spasm of the adductors forces the patient to take small shuffling steps. The condition spontaneously improves and is nearly always better within a year. Occasionally there is pus formation which may track within the tissue planes.

(c) *Stricture formation.* Strictures can develop at the external urethral meatus, in the urethra, or at the bladder neck. The latter tend to develop when there has been a too limited resection of the bladder neck. Strictures of the urethra and external meatus are due to irritation by the indwelling urethral catheter which should be small in diameter and removed as soon as possible.

Complications of transurethral resection

The common complications of this type of prostatectomy include the following.

1 *Early*
Haemorrhage

2 *Intermediate*
(a) *Stricture.* Strictures following transurethral resection usually form in the penile urethra at the point where it is supported by the suspensory ligament. This type of stricture can be avoided by using a small sheath and preventing undue trauma to the urethra by excessive angulation and movement of the instrument.

(b) *Incontinence.* Incontinence following transurethral prostatic resection is nearly always permanent and is due to damage to the external sphincter. It can be avoided only by restricting the lower limit of prostatic resection to the level of the verumontanum.

3 *Late*
The continued complaint of prostatism, indicating that the initial resection was too conservative.

Conservative treatment of prostatic symptoms

In the presence of a median bar, as opposed to median lobe enlargement, it may be possible to improve the symptoms by the administration of the α-blocking agent, phenoxybenzamine. Since this drug may cause faintness in the erect posture it is best given in a dose of 10 mg at night when the patient is already in bed.

However, in the majority of patients in whom this drug is potentially of value the condition may be simply ameliorated by dividing the bladder neck at the two lateral angles between the median bar and the lateral lobes using a Colling's knife via a resectoscope.

7.4 Pathology, signs, symptoms, treatment and prognosis of renal tumours

Tumours of the kidney may be benign or malignant. The former, except when arising from the urothelium of the renal pelvis are of little importance.

Malignant tumours are classified into the following three groups:

1. nephroblastoma; this tumour arises in the fetal or infant kidney and is eponymously known as a Wilm's tumour;
2. carcinoma of the renal parenchyma, eponymously known as the Grawitz tumour;
3. carcinoma of the urothelium of the renal pelvis.

Nephroblastoma

This tumour accounts for approximately 6 per cent of all paediatric neoplasms.

Pathology
This is an embryonic tumour belonging to the same category as the medulloblastoma of the brain, neuroblastoma of the sympathetic nervous system and the hepatoblastoma of the liver. Many pathologists believe that this tumour develops before birth and develops rapidly thereafter.

This tumour causes gross enlargement of the affected kidney. The cut surface is white or whitish grey and it may be homogeneous or contain cystic spaces, areas of haemorrhage and gelatinous 'degeneration'. Whilst the tumour may spread into the renal vein in keeping with the paucity of renal symptoms the renal pelvis is only rarely penetrated.

Microscopic examination reveals a stroma chiefly consisting of spindle cells which possess hyperchromatic nuclei. Within this mass of cells are collections of somewhat more differentiated tissue so that tubules, primitive glomeruli and areas of cartilage and bone together with both smooth and striated muscle can be recognized.

Nephroblastomata spread chiefly by the blood stream to the lungs, bones and liver and also by direct invasion of the surrounding tissues and by the lymphatics to the lumbar lymph nodes.

Clinical presentation

The peak incidence of Wilm's tumour is between 3 and 4 years and this tumour rarely presents after the age of 6 years. Occasionally the tumour is clinically apparent at birth. In 10 per cent of affected children the tumour is bilateral and interestingly bilateral tumours do not tend to metastasize.

The common presenting symptoms of a nephroblastoma include:

1. a mass. This is frequently first noted when the parent is dressing the child. If nothing is done the mass tends to enlarge rapidly and the general health of the child deteriorates.
2. abdominal pain.
3. vomiting.
4. fever, approximately 50 per cent of affected children are pyrexial when first seen.
5. occasionally haematuria.
6. rarely hypertension develops due to compression of the renal tissue inducing activation of the renin–angiotensin mechanism.
7. polycythaemia, due to the excessive production of erythropoietin.

The following investigations should be performed:
1. *Intravenous pyelography.* This may reveal the following:

(a) enlargement of the renal outline.
(b) a non-functioning kidney.
(c) distortion of the calyceal system.
(d) calcification; this is rare in nephroblastoma and its presence suggests a diagnosis of neuroblastoma.

2. *Cavography.* An inferior cavogram may demonstrate the presence of renal vein involvement.
3. *Chest X-ray.* Whole lung tomography is required to exclude small pulmonary metastases.
4. *Skeletal survey or skeletal scan.* The investigation of both the pulmonary and skeletal systems is mandatory because at the time of the initial consultation metastases will be present in 10 per cent of the infants.

Apart from a congenital hydronephrosis the only swelling from which a Wilm's tumour must be distinguished is a retroperitoneal neuroblastoma.

Treatment
There are three possible methods of treatment.
1. *Surgery.* The kidney is removed either by a transabdominal or thoracoabdominal approach. If possible the hilum is tied early and every effort should be made to remove the kidney without tearing the capsule. As soon as the surgeon has satisfied himself by examining the tumour that it is a nephroblastoma an injection of vincristine should be given.
2. *Irradiation.* Except in Stage I tumours, i.e. T_1 and T_2 on the TNM classification radiotherapy will be administered in the first postoperative week. T_1 and T_2 tumours in which the tumour has not breached the renal capsule do not require such treatment. Radiation is given by parallel opposed anterior and posterior fields in a dose between 1800 and 3000 rads.
3. *Chemotherapy.* Children suffering from early disease, i.e. in Stage 1, are normally given vincristine as a single agent therapy for a few months. Vincristine is a *Vinca* alkaloid which interferes with mitotic spindle formation, ribosomal RNA and protein synthesis, it is classified as a phase-specific drug and its chief toxic effects are the development of alopecia, peripheral

neuropathy and gastrointestinal disturbance. The dose of vincristine is 1.5 mg/m^2 twice a week for approximately one month in Stage 1 tumours. When tumour is present outside the confines of the renal capsule radiotherapy should be followed by an initial course of vincristine after which actinomycin D 2.4 mg/m^2 over 7 days should be given every 6 weeks.

Prognosis

The majority of metastases occur early. Note Colin's rule, which states: 'diagnosis is preceded by a period of silent growth which at a maximum is equal to the nine months gestation period, plus the age of the child at the time of diagnosis. Diagnosis is followed by a period of risk equal to the maximum period of silent growth. A patient living beyond the period of risk without recurrence should be beyond the risk of recurrence.'

Before the introduction of radiotherapy only 27 per cent of children survived for 5 years if the tumour could be removed. This was increased to 50 per cent 5-year survival following treatment with radiotherapy and with the addition of chemotherapy the 5-year survival of resectable tumours has risen to 80 per cent. Even if distant metastases are present at the time of diagnosis survival can be remarkably prolonged in approximately 50 per cent of children.

Adenocarcinoma of the kidney

Pathology

This relatively rare tumour is approximately one-third as common as carcinoma of the bronchus.

On cross-section the tumour may be lobulated or surrounded by a pseudocapsule. The cut surface is usually yellow in colour, old areas of haemorrhage may be seen together with areas of necrosis.

Microscopically the cells of a renal adenocarcinoma are polygonal or oval and may be arranged in tubules, a papillary formation or a solid trabecular pattern. They possess either a clear cytoplasm which contains glycogen and neutral fat or a granular cytoplasm which contains large numbers of mitochondria.

Renal adenocarcinomta spread by direct invasion of the surrounding tissues, by the lymphatics and by the blood stream.

Clinical presentation

These tumours commonly present with a classic triad of symptoms which includes haematuria 60 per cent, pain 30 per cent, and a palpable mass 10 per cent. Alternatively, the tumour may be small and produce systemic rather than local signs, presenting with pyrexia or polycythaemia. Lastly, a solitary metastasis in bone or lung may be the presenting symptom, although one of the characteristic features of hypernephroma is the possibility of considerable growth without any evidence of metastases.

One classical but rare symptom is the rapid development of a left-sided varicocele due to obstruction of the left testicular vein by tumour permeating the renal vein. Occasionally also, metastases in the left ovary or testes may be produced by retrograde venous embolization. Bony metastases are common, as also are secondaries in the lung and brain.

Investigations
Confirmatory investigations include:
1 *Straight X-ray of the abdomen and intravenous pyelography.* This may demonstrate:

(a) distortion of the renal outline and spicules of calcification.
(b) displacement, elongation, compression or obliteration of one or more calyces, the classical calyceal deformity is known as the spider calyx.
(c) displacement, distortion or a filling defect in the renal pelvis.

2 *Selective renal angiography.* Lesions as small as 2 cm in diameter can be identified by this means. The classic changes include:

(a) displacement of the arterial aborizations.
(b) a 'snow storm' appearance in the later films due to the presence of abnormal vessels in the tumour.

3 *Cavography.* In some centres this diagnostic method is used to detect involvement of the renal veins.
4 *Ultrasound.* This may be used to ascertain the size of the lesion, extracapsular spread and distinguish the mass from a renal cyst.
5 *Plain X-ray and tomography of the lungs.* Using a complex system which must involve the use of computerized axial tomography a renal carcinoma can be staged by the TNM classification.

Treatment
This tumour is one in which excision of the primary tumour and an apparently solitary metastasis appears to be worthwhile.
1 *Surgery.* The treatment of choice is surgical excision. Very extensive exposure of the involved kidney can be obtained by the use of a combined thoracoabdominal approach at the level of the tenth rib. If the tumour is small a simple upper transverse incision will suffice. Blockage of the renal vein can be assumed if large numbers of thin walled friable collateral veins are found within the perinephric fat. In theory an attempt should be made to expose and ligate the renal vein and artery before mobilizing the kidney itself in order to minimize the risk of disseminating metastases during renal mobilization. In the author's experience this is extremely difficult to achieve in the presence of a large tumour.
2 *Radiotherapy.* This is indicated when:

(a) extracapsular spread has been found.
(b) involved adjacent hilar and para-aortic nodes are present.

   Two parallel opposed fields are applied and a tumour dose of 35–40 Gy is given in equal fractions spread over 15 days.
3 *Hormone therapy.* In a small proportion of cases the tumour regresses following the administration of progesterone, medroxyprogesterone acetate 100 mg three times a day. This is never used as a primary procedure but for palliation in advanced disease.

Prognosis
Widely divergent figures for survival have been reported in different series. Prognosis is made difficult by the fact that metastases already present may regress following the removal of the primary tumour.

Approximately 50 per cent of all patients survive for 3 years, between 20 and 40 per cent for 5 years and 15 per cent for 10 years if there are no obvious metastases present at the time of the original operation. When metastases are present few patients survive for longer than 2 years.

When bony metastases occur, confirmed by X-ray or an isotope bone scan, pain relief can be achieved in a high proportion of patients by the use of 20–24 Gy in five fractions delivered by a single field.

Carcinoma of the urothelium of the renal pelvis

Pathology
Macroscopically these tumours vary in appearance according to the degree of malignancy. The more benign the tumour the longer and slimmer are the papillary fronds. With more malignant tumours the fronds become shorter and fatter and when the tumour is highly malignant from its inception it may present as a solid plaque associated with central ulceration.

Microscopically these tumours may be classified as:

1. transitional cell carcinoma—
   (*a*) well differentiated,
   (*b*) differentiated,
   (*c*) undifferentiated;

2. squamous carcinoma; this type of tumour is associated with calculi in the renal pelvis.

All types of tumour spread by direct invasion, by the lymphatics and by the blood stream.

Clinical presentation
The commonest presenting symptom of urothelial tumour of the renal pelvis is haematuria. This may be painless or painful if clot colic occurs.

1. In any patient complaining of haematuria a specimen of urine should be examined for the presence of exfoliated cells.
2. Intravenous pyelography. This may show:
   (*a*) a non-functioning kidney on the affected side;
   (*b*) a papilliferous type of tumour filling the renal pelvis, the precise appearance of which depends upon the tumour type and the degree of anaplasia.
3. Cystoscopy. This is an essential investigation because transitional cell tumours metastasize by direct spread, and tumour implantation along the ureter to the bladder is not infrequent.

Treatment
The treatment of a transitional cell tumour of the renal pelvis is nephrouretectomy, removing at the same operation a cuff of bladder mucosa surrounding the ureteric orifice.

The kidney and the upper half of the ureter are first mobilized through a loin incision after which the patient is placed supine on the operating table, and, through a lower paramedian or midline subumbilical incision, the lower half of the ureter together with a cuff of bladder are dissected free. The bladder is repaired and the kidney and ureter removed.

Radiotherapy is not indicated unless there has been spread through the wall of the pelvis or involved para-aortic nodes are present.

Prognosis
Few long term survivors were reported until the operation briefly described above was generally adopted. However, using this technique, 50 per cent of patients survive for 5 years, so long as there has not been extrapelvic extension. The histological grading has considerable influence on the prognosis. When the tumour is histologically in Grade 1 or 2 a 5-year survival approaching 60 per cent can be expected, whereas if the tumour is Grade 3 or 4 the 5-year survival falls to as low as 10 per cent.

7.5 Swellings of the scrotum, and the pathology and treatment of testicular tumours

Swellings of the scrotum may be divided into the following groups:

I *Cystic*
A Unilateral:

1 Hydrocele
(a) Congenital
(b) Infantile
(c) Encysted hydrocele of the cord

2 Spermatocele
3 Cystic collections in embryonic remnants

B Bilateral:

1 Epididymal cysts
2 Hydrocele

II *Solid*
A Of the epididymis:

Inflammatory conditions
(*a*) Acute epididymitis
(*b*) Chronic tuberculous epididymitis

B Of the testes:

1 Inflammatory conditions
(*a*) Mumps
(*b*) Gumma
(*c*) Granulomatous orchitis

2 Neoplastic
(*a*) Tumours that may be benign or malignant
   (i) Interstitial cell tumours
   (ii) Sertoli cell tumours

(*b*) Malignant tumours
   (i) Seminoma
   (ii) Teratoma
   (iii) Mixed seminoma and teratoma
   (iv) Lymphoma
   (v) Yolk sac tumour

C Of the tunica vaginalis

Haematocele

Only testicular tumours will be the subject of further discussion here.

Testicular tumours are relatively uncommon. Their incidence is about 3 per 100000 of the population, or approximately 1 per cent of all male cancer patients.

Clinical presentation
The majority of testicular tumours are brought to the attention of the patient by observing the one testis is larger in size, or possibly heavier, than the other. The tumour usually retains the overall shape of the testes because it is confined within the thick tunica albuginea. Once it has reached a certain size two classical physical signs develop: the total insensitiveness of the body of testes invaded by tumour and a relative heaviness of the affected organ.

Occasionally, metastatic deposits, either in the retroperitoneal lymph nodes or lungs, draw attention to hitherto unsuspected testicular swelling, and very occasionally a tumour may produce a hormonal derangement. The infrequent choriocarcinoma, which is a rare variety of teratoma, may manufacture sufficient gonadotrophins to cause gynaecomastia. Similarly, Sertoli cell tumours and Leydig cell tumours may both secrete oestrogens and the latter may also secrete sufficient androgens to produce sexual precocity in affected children.

Diagnosis
There are only three other important causes of swelling of the body of the testes. They are mumps, in which the history should be typical, the swelling usually being painful and exquisitely tender; gumma, which usually affects a much older age group and is now rare and granulomatous orchitis which is also relatively rare. Seminomata are most common in the fifth decade whereas teratomata are found at all ages.

Tumour markers

When the clinician anticipates that the correct diagnosis will be one of a malignant testicular tumour a search should be made for the presence of tumour markers before attacking the testicular swelling itself. The two markers produced by testicular tumours which bear a good correlation with the body's tumour burden are the glycoprotein, alphafetoprotein and the β-subunit of human chorionic gonadotrophin. The former is a normal serum protein of the human fetus and is synthesized from the tenth week onwards by fetal liver cells, the cells of the gastrointestinal tract and the yolk sac. The neosynthesis of this protein after the age of 3 months indicates the presence of increased hepatocyte turnover or neoplasia of tissues originally capable of synthesizing this protein in embryonic life. The latter, i.e. HCG, is produced by syncytial trophoblastic and non-gestational trophoblastic elements in gonadal and extragonadal tissues.

Not all germ cell tumours produce markers. They are much more commonly found in teratomata than seminomata and when present their concentration is related to tumour burden, overall prognosis, response to therapy and following therapy their reappearance is indicative of relapse.

Pathology
Ninety per cent of testicular tumours are either derived from epithelial tissue, i.e. the seminoma, or are tumours of embryonic origin, teratoma. In addition a further group of tumours principally occurring before the age of 3 has also been recognized, the yolk sac tumour, formerly referred to as the orchioblastoma. It must also be pointed out that even in a seminoma teratomatous elements may be found.

The classification of these tumours has always represented a considerable problem since so many factors may be taken into consideration including the microscopic appearance of the tumour, its histogenesis, its morphological, immunological and biochemical characteristics and in addition its immunochemical and serological features.

So far as testicular tumours are concerned consideration of these various factors has led to an increasing subdivision of the various tumour types.

The recognized WHO classification of Testicular Germ Cell Tumours drawn up in 1977 is given below and contrasted with the somewhat earlier classification of the Testicular Tumour Panel which was chiefly based on the work of Pugh, 1976.

WHO classification	Testicular Tumour Panel classification

Seminoma:
  typical
  spermacytic
  anaplastic
	Seminoma

Teratoma:
  mature
  immature
	Previous classification—teratoma differentiated (TD)

Embryonal carcinoma with teratoma: teratocarcinoma	Previous classification—malignant teratoma intermediate (MTI)
Embryonal carcinoma	(MT undifferentiated)
Choriocarcinoma	(MT trophoblastic)
Yolk sac tumour	Yolk sac tumour
Tumours of more than one histological type	Combined seminoma and teratoma

Seminoma accounts for some 40 per cent of all malignant testicular tumours. They are usually soft greyish white tumours with obvious areas of haemorrhage and necrosis. Enlarged distended veins can be seen beneath the thickened tunica albuginea, and bisection of the testes shows that the normal testicular tissue is squashed to one side. Microscopically the tumour is composed of uniform polyhedral cells which are occasionally arranged in tubular fashion.

Direct spread may involve the epididymis and the spermatic cord and, in addition, lymphatic and blood stream metastases also occurs. The lymphatics carry the tumour to the retroperitoneal lymph nodes while blood stream spread results in secondary deposits in the lungs and liver. Two aetiological factors have been described: trauma and maldescent of the testes.

In many cases of established testicular tumour a preceding history of trauma is elicited but it is more probable that the incident draws attention to an already pathological organ. So far as maldescent is concerned the weight of evidence leads to the conclusion that there is an increased incidence of malignancy in the maldescended testis but whether this is due to a direct effect of maldescent, the increased environmental temperature associated with this condition or some unknown agency remains an enigma. The risk of developing a tumour in a maldescended testes is approximately 30 times higher than in a normally descended testes, a risk much lower than was originally postulated when the association was first recognized.

Teratomata account for most of the remaining neoplasms. They are derived from all three germ layers but, unlike the ovarian teratoma, they are usually extremely active and behave in a malignant fashion. Less than 1 per cent of teratomata are differentiated to such a degree that a dermoid cyst is produced. In approximately 14 per cent of teratomata typical seminoma tumour tissue is to be found.

On section, teratomata have a varied appearance. The tumour mass contains cystic spaces, cartilage and areas of solid or degenerate tumour tissue. Microscopically a well-differentiated tumour may show areas of mature bone, cartilage, or numerous epithelial layers, whereas anaplastic tumours are composed of masses of pleomorphic cells.

Hormonal disturbances

Gynaecomastia may be associated with any testicular tumour. Leydig or interstitial cell tumours, which comprise only between 1 and 2 per cent of all testicular tumours can secrete either androgens or oestrogens. In general Leydig cell tumours produce a virilizing effect particularly in childhood whereas interstitial cell tumours produce gynaecomastia.

Treatment of testicular tumours

Assuming that obvious metastases are not present at the time of the initial clinical diagnosis the first step is orchidectomy. The inguinal canal is first exposed by dividing the external oblique aponeurosis to the level of the internal ring after which the cord is clamped with vascular clamps and the testes dislocated from the scrotum so that it can be examined. If the diagnosis is confirmed either by the external appearance of the testes or by inspection of the bulk of the enlarged testes by dividing the tunica albuginea the cord is immediately divided, the testis and cord removed and the wound closed.

Further investigations are now required to establish the stage of the disease which, in turn, determines the subsequent regimen.

1 *Plain chest X-ray.* If this is negative in the presence of a proven testicular tumour whole lung tomography should be performed.
2 *Intravenous pyelography.* This investigation may establish the presence of enlarged para-aortic nodes due to the distortion of the ureter on the affected side.
3 *Bipedal lymphography.* This investigation is of greatest use in detecting the presence of involved iliac glands but much less acurate in determining the state of the para-aortic lymph nodes in the area of the coeliac axis artery. However, if positive lymphographic evidence of nodal involvement is established the field of irradiation will be widened but not more than one-third of a kidney should be irradiated, otherwise an irradiation nephritis may develop.
4 *CAT scan.* This investigation will only be available in some centres but, if available, it allows the easy detection of involved nodes in the coeliac axis region and the mediastinum.
5 *Repeated estimation of the tumour markers if initially present.*

As a result of the above investigations the Stage of the tumour can be assessed. A staging classification commonly used in the UK and Europe is that proposed by Peckham and his co-workers in 1980 in which four stages with further subdivisions of Stages II, III and IV are proposed.
Stage I. The tumour is limited to the testicle.
Stage II. Infradiaphragmatic nodal disease is present, this stage is subdivided into three depending upon the size of the nodes. In Stage IIA the metastases are less than 2 cm and in Stage IIC greater than 5 cm in diameter.

Stage III. Supradiaphragmatic, i.e. mediastinal and/or supraclavicular, nodes are involved. This stage is subdivided into six subsets depending upon the position of the involved nodes and their size.

Stage IV. Extranodal disease is present. This is commonly in the lungs, liver, bone or brain.

Further treatment

1 At various times, particularly in the USA, pelvic and para-aortic lymph node dissection has been advocated following a positive diagnosis. This has never found favour in the UK and elsewhere.

2 *Radiotherapy.* In all types of tumour, even when nodal involvement is not proven, postoperative X-ray therapy should be applied to a field including the homolateral inguinal, pelvic and para-aortic lymph nodes up to the xiphisternum. The lower margin of the field should include the seminal vesicles and if unfortunately a trans-scrotal biopsy has been performed on the scrotum, a tumour dose of 35 Gy is delivered.

If it is also demonstrated by CAT scan that the mediastinal lymph nodes are also involved or the supraclavicular nodes are palpable this field should also be irradiated.

In general terms seminomata are relatively radiosensitive, Smithers reporting a 5-year survival in this group of tumours of 94 per cent even when the abdominal lymph nodes were involved. Teratomata are not so radiosensitive particularly those in which a yolk sac element is present.

If a teratoma is well differentiated, i.e. mature, and histological examination of the cord shows that no local spread has occurred no irradiation is given at the time of the initial diagnosis since in approximately 20 per cent of patients dissemination will eventually occur and since irradiation causes some bone marrow damage aggressive chemotherapy cannot then be used in the treatment of such a recurrence.

3 *Further surgery.* If after several months a CAT scan shows that a nodal mass is remaining it is appropriate to remove or debulk the tumour mass. Due, however, to the natural lymphatic drainage of the testicle to the higher para-aortic nodes this may prove difficult because of the danger to the renal vessels. This form of attack has been encouraged by the finding by some workers that undoubtedly undifferentiated teratomata may become benign following irradiation.

4 *Chemotherapy.* A drug in common use in the treatment of disseminated testicular tumours of the teratomatous, mixed or pure yolk sac type is *cis*-platinum. This is a Class III chemotherapeutic agent as defined by Bruce and his colleagues which means that although the drug is markedly selective against malignant stem cells it also promotes, unfortunately, a marked bone marrow stem cell kill and, therefore, a careful watch must be kept on the peripheral white cell count. Renal function should be good if this drug is used. It is given by intermittent intravenous injection after which the patient is hydrated with isotonic saline in order to eliminate the nephrotoxic effects of the drug.

Other regimens which have been applied to the treatment of disseminated testicular tumours are combinations of cis-diamine-dechloro-platinum (CDDP) combined with vinblastine (VBL) and bleomycin (BLM) or combinations of vinblastine with methotrexate, actinomycin D and folinic acid. Long term remission in Stage III tumours is claimed by the protagonists of combination chemotherapy in a large proportion of cases. It would appear from the results obtained that if a complete remission occurs over a period of 2 years then the life expectancy of the treated patients is almost comparable to that of age matched controls.

When combinations of CDDP, VBL and BLM are administered the chief danger is the development of agranulocytosis leading to sepsis.

Prognosis
Due to the advancing science of chemotherapy the prognosis of testicular tumours is constantly changing. However, the prognosis in patients suffering from a seminoma at whatever stage is considerably better than for teratoma. So far as the latter are concerned mature teratomata, previously classified as Teratoma Differentiated (TD) have the best prognosis, with some 80 per cent of patients surviving for 5 years whereas embryonal carcinoma (MTV) and combined tumours have the poorest prognosis, about 40 per cent surviving for 5 years.

7.6 Investigation and surgical management of stones in the renal tract

Formation of renal stones

All stones in the renal tract, with the exception of primary bladder stones, develop in the kidneys. In 1937, Randall suggested that they formed from nuclei of crystalline material deposited in the interstitial tissues at the tips of the renal papillae, the Randall's plaque. This theory was later modified by Carr when he found that microliths were commonplace in the region of the papillae and calyces. Because of this finding, Carr felt that there must exist a mechanism for their removal, and he suggested that this involved the lymphatic system. Carr postulated that if this clearance mechanism was overloaded, as in hyperparathyroidism which produces nephrocalcinosis, or renal infection which produces obliteration of the lymphatic channels, the microliths might remain *in situ* and enlarge.

Eventually, whatever the primary site of microlith formation, the mucosa over the affected calyx or calyces ulcerates and then the accumulation of crystals on the surface begins and finally leads to the formation of a plaque. Such a plaque may remain fixed, growing slowly to the size of a calculus, or it may fall off and be passed, possibly unnoticed, by the patient. Once the plaque separates, there may be further crystal deposits on the ulcerated surface unless rapid healing takes place.

Chemical composition

From the clinical point of view, urinary stones may be classified into four main groups according to their chemical composition:

1 triple phosphate stones containing varying mixtures of calcium phosphate, magnesium ammonium phosphate, and calcium carbonate. Such stones usually form in an alkaline infected urine.
2 calcium oxalate calculi forming, usually, in an acid, often uninfected, urine.
3 mixed stones which are composed of calcium oxalate together with one or other of the insoluble salts listed above.
4 organic stones formed of uric acid, cystine or xanthine. These are rare.

X-ray diffraction studies of renal calculi show that calcium oxalate and calcium phosphate are the most abundant and frequently occurring crystalline constituents, and that the most common variety of stones are those composed of pure calcium oxalate or a mixture of calcium oxalate and phosphate.

A patient suffering from stone in the renal tract should have the following investigations performed:

1 radiological examination of the urinary tract;
2 bacteriological examination of the urine;
3 serum calcium estimation;
4 blood uric acid;
5 measurement of the urinary calcium and oxalate excretion.

Radiological investigations

These include:

(a) acute intravenous pyelography, if the patients is suffering from renal colic;
(b) intravenous pyelography in the quiescent stage (interval pyelography);
(c) retrograde pyelography.

The dyes in common use for intravenous pyelography include sodium diatrizoate (Hypaque) and meglumine iothalamate (Conray 280). If the examination is carried out when the patient is actually suffering from renal colic no preparation and no compression are used. If the procedure is elective, the patient is usually deprived of water overnight and a vegetable laxative is administered on the evening before the examination in order to remove intestinal gas and faeces. The commonest contraindication to pyelography is iodine sensitivity.

1 *Acute pyelography*
This is now an accepted procedure in a patient complaining of suspected renal colic. The percentage of positive results obviously varies with the accuracy of the clinical diagnosis that indicates the need for the investigation. In any examination an opaque stone must be differentiated from other causes of

calcification including: calcified costal cartilages, gall-stones, calcified iliac vessels, phleboliths, and fibroids. The common radiological signs indicating obstruction due to stones include:

(a) the presence of an opaque calculus;
(b) delayed excretion;
(c) enlargement of the renal shadow on the affected side;
(d) the appearance of a nephrogram;
(e) films taken up to 24 hours after injection showing dilatation of the collecting system proximal to the point of the obstruction.

2 *Elective or interval pyelography*
This examination is usually performed after preparation of the patient and with preliminary compression. The findings include:

(a) the presence of an obvious calculus on the preliminary film;
(b) delayed or absent renal excretion;
(c) dilation of the calyces, pelvis and/or ureter to the point of obstruction;
(d) enlargement of the renal shadow.

The appearance of the opacity gives some indication of its chemical composition. Uric acid and xanthine stones are radiolucent. Calcium oxalate calculi are frequently laminated and form 'jack stones' with a central nucleus, or have projecting thorn-like processes. Phosphate stones grow rapidly, attain a larger size, and may form a cast of the renal pelvis and calyces, the 'staghorn'. Stones within the ureter are often small and elongated.

3 *Retrograde pyelography*
When the only question is to decide whether an observed opacity is within the ureter, an AP and oblique film with the catheter *in situ* are usually all that is needed. If, however, a catheter cannot be passed beyond the point of obstruction a bulb catheter may be inserted into the ureteric orifice and retrograde filling performed.

Bacteriological investigations of urine

The commonest organisms found in the urine are *Escherichia coli* and other coliform organisms including *Proteus* and *Pseudomonas*. *Streptococcus faecalis* and *Staphylococcus* may also be found.

The importance of infection in the urinary tract lies in the fact that urea-splitting organisms produce a high urine ammonia and an alkaline urine which reduces the relative solubility of triple phosphate, i.e. calcium magnesium ammonium phosphate and, hence, leads to its precipitation.

Serum calcium estimation

In the vast majority of patients serum calcium is normal. Any elevation above the normal range of 2.25–2.60 mmol/l should lead to investigation of the patient for hyperparathyroidism which is probably responsible for stone formation in approximately 2–10 per cent of stone formers.

Blood uric acid estimation

The normal blood uric acid level lies between 0.20 and 0.45 mmol/l in males. Elevation suggests gout, which is complicated by stone formation in approximately 10 per cent of patients. Although the level of uric acid secretion may be normal the important abnormality is an excessively acid urine which leads to a lowered uric acid solubility.

Urinary calcium and oxalate excretion

Hypercalciuria is met with in specific conditions such as a hyperparathyroidism, sarcoidosis, and secondary bone metastases, but in the majority of patients the cause is unknown, when the condition is termed idiopathic hypercalciuria. Normal calcium excretion on a normal diet varies between 50 and 250 mg (1.25–6.25 mmol) over a 24-hour period. A figure in excess of the latter demands investigation.

Primary oxaluria. In a small number of recurrent stone formers, abnormal amounts of oxalate in excess of the normal average urinary secretion of 33 mg (0.27 mmol) a day are excreted. The underlying cause of this condition is believed to be an abnormality of glycoxylic acid metabolism.

Surgical treatment of renal stones

Common indications for surgical removal of renal stones are:

1. severe recurrent symptoms;
2. increasing renal destruction;
3. associated infection.

Progressive renal damage may be caused by a number of factors including direct pressure of the stone on the renal tissues, indirect pressure by blockage of the neck of a calyx or the pelviureteric junction and, lastly, associated infection. Slow deterioration of renal function may eventually lead to the secretion of a hypotonic urine of low specific gravity. Rarely, a renal stone leads to metaplasia of the urothelium followed by the development of a squamous cell cancer of the renal pelvis.

Recurrence following operation

Any operation for renal calculus is followed by a high recurrence rate, the frequency of which is related to the length of the follow-up. Thus, after 10 years the recurrence rate following nephrolithotomy is 24 per cent as compared to a recurrence rate of 37 per cent following pyelolithotomy, but after 20 years both operations are followed by a recurrence rate of approximately 80 per cent.

Such high recurrence rates suggest that stones should be conservatively treated wherever possible, that nephrectomy should be avoided, and that any underlying cause should, if possible, be treated.

True and false recurrence
It has become apparent that recurrence may be true or false. The latter are due to particles of stone being left *in situ* at the time of the original operation, and in order to avoid them radiological facilities should, if possible, be available at the time of operation in order to take plain X-rays of the exposed kidney.

Operations performed
1 *Pelvic stones.* Calculi lying in the pelvis are treated by pyelolithotomy, incising the pelvis in its long axis. The incision is normally closed by fine sutures of plain catgut.
2 *Stones in the lower calyx.* These are commonly treated by lower polar partial nephrectomy, an operation first described by Czerny in 1887. The operation is performed using meticulous haemostasis rather than large mattress sutures through all layers of the renal tissue. The opened calyx should be closed by catgut sutures. True recurrence rates, after partial nephrectomy, as low as 12 per cent were reported by earlier writers after 5 years, although the same degree of success that led to this operation becoming popular have not been substantiated.

Staghorn calculi
The treatment of these stones has always been a problem. Staghorn calculi usually present with pain, haematuria or infection and many series have shown that if they are ignored the patient dies of renal failure when the condition is bilateral or if the condition is unilateral a nephrectomy is ultimately required because of the development of intolerable symptoms or a pyonephrosis. They must rarely be symptomless since they are an infrequent incidental finding at post mortem. Whilst some surgeons would argue that there is no need for surgical interference the overwhelming majority argue in favour of surgical treatment since operative removal of a staghorn calculus will relieve the patient of pain, may relieve renal infection, prevents deterioration of renal function occurring as a result of infection and obstructive nephropathy and avoids the possible danger of a pyonephrosis with its attendant complications and dangers.

Of the various methods described for dealing with staghorn calculi that of Gil Vernet, which is based on the following surgical procedures, deserves special mention.

1 Posterior vertical lumbotomy replaces the more commonly used oblique approach to the kidney. Using this approach no muscle fibres are divided, only the lumbar aponeurosis, and no nerves are usually damaged, both factors helping to diminish the possibility of a postoperative lumbar hernia.

2 The pelvis and upper ureter are reached posteriorly, thus avoiding the necessity of mobilizing the entire kidney.

Once the upper end of the ureter and the kidney have been identified the pelvis of the kidney is approached in an extracapsular plane. The surgeon must maintain contact with the adventitia of the renal pelvis since this keeps him in a bloodless plane. At one point a bunch of fibres will be encountered which form a capsular diaphragm between the pelvis itself and the renal capsule. This must be divided before access to the renal sinus can be gained. Once divided, however, a retractor can be placed on the mass of peripelvic adipose tissue, the internal lip of the posterior edge of the kidney and the retropelvic artery, the whole of this being reflected without any danger of tearing the renal parenchyma. Gauze dissection is now used to expose more and more of the renal pelvis and as this dissection proceeds larger retractors are necessary and as these are lifted posterolaterally so the organ rotates and the sinusal space becomes perpendicular to the surgeon, offering, when the dissection is completed, a complete view of the posterior surface of the pelvis and the major calyces. Difficulty will only be encountered in performing such a dissection if inflammatory changes have led to thickening and adherence of the adipose tissue.

Once adequate exposure has been obtained the pelvis is incised and if the whole of the staghorn cannot be removed through this single incision intrasinusal calicotomy incisions are made into each affected calyx. The latter step is unnecessary, however, when large ball-shaped calyceal cysts are present which are covered only by a thin layer of renal parenchyma. In such cases the offending stone is removed through a nephrotomy incision, the section being virtually bloodless due to atrophy of the overlying parenchyma.

It is essential when dealing with a staghorn calculus to have, if possible, radiological facilities available to make certain that all the calculus has been removed. If complete removal is achieved the incidence of recurrence and residual infection appears to be considerably reduced, although a relatively high incidence of recurrence occurs if the urine remains infected by *B. proteus*.

Another method, recently described, but as yet of limited use is to attempt to label the stone with ^{99m}Tc-methylene diphosphate before operation and then at the completion of its removal attempt to identify residual fragments, if any, with a gamma scintillation probe. As, however, one might expect, the success of this method depends on the chemical composition of the stone.

Management of ureteric calculus

A ureteric stone may be treated in any of the following ways:

1 conservative;
2 manipulative;
3 operative.

Radiological investigations will establish the site, size, shape and degree of obstruction. Bacteriological examination establishes the presence or absence of infection. With these facts a decision about management can be made.

According to different reported series, between 20 and 70 per cent of ureteric calculi are passed spontaneously. If the stone is less than 5 mm in size a high proportion, probably 80 per cent, will pass spontaneously. Holmlund investigating the passage of experimental renal calculi in rabbits found that the traditional regimen of forced fluids and muscle relaxants was of little use.

When a stone reaches the lower third of the ureter and then makes no further progress, especially if a progressive hydronephrosis develops, endoscopic removal can be attempted. The success obtained by using a Councillor's or Dormia's basket again varies according to the series examined. Some urologists claim successful removal of a calculus in as many as 90 per cent of patients, whereas others find the method of little use.

The contraindications to the use of this method include:

1 a stone lodged above the junction of the lower and middle thirds;
2 a stone known to have been present for a long time, because such stones are normally associated with inflammation of the ureter and periureteric tissues;
3 the presence of a gross hydroureter.

The complications of this method include perforation of the ureteric wall and avulsion of the ureter.

When the stone is impacted in the intramural portion of the ureter a transvesical ureteral meatotomy may be successful, but this operation is open to the criticism that partial destruction of the vesicoureteric junction may be followed by vesicoureteric reflux.

Stones situated in the middle and upper third of the ureter associated with obstructive symptoms or obstruction can be removed by ureterolithotomy. Operation should always be preceded by a plain radiograph to detect any change in the position of the calculus. The upper third of the ureter is usually approached through a loin incision and the lower ureter through a midline subumbilical incision, in both instances the approach is normally extraperitoneal. If possible, the stone is milked from the position of impaction before incising the ureteric wall.

The rate of stone recurrence following ureterolithotomy is approximately 20 per cent at 5 years, 35 per cent at 10 years, and 70 per cent at 20 years.

7.7 Causes and treatment of vesicoureteric reflux

Aetiology
Vesicoureteric reflux may be classified as primary or secondary. In adults, reflux is always secondary to one or other of the following causes.
1 *Bladder neck obstruction.* Bumpus showed that approximately 5 per cent of males suffering from prostatic hypertrophy suffer from reflux, and reflux should always be suspected when a Gram-negative septicaemia develops after prostatectomy.

2 *Neurogenic bladder*. Reflux occurs because of recurrent infection, hypertonicity of the bladder, and bladder neck obstruction.
3 *Cystitis*. Transient reflux may come about during an acute attack of cystitis in the female, temporarily disturbing the competence of the ureterovesical junction.
4 *Operations*. Interference with the ureteric orifice, e.g. meatotomy for the removal of stone, is not infrequently followed by reflux.
5 *Chronic inflammation*. Tuberculosis may result in a rigid ureteric orifice and a spastic bladder.

In childhood, the secondary causes of reflux include such simple factors as phimosis in the male, or distal urethral obstruction in the female. Less common causes are:

(*a*) posterior urethral valves producing bladder outlet obstruction;
(*b*) the neurological complications of spina bifida;
(*c*) postoperative reflux as a complication of ureteric implantation.

These are relatively rare, and the most frequent and important cause of infantile reflux is associated with no abnormality other than ureterovesical incompetence, the basic cause of which is believed to be failure of maturation of muscles at the ureterovesical junction.

Normally, the ureter penetrates the bladder wall in an oblique fashion, losing in its passage all muscular layers with the exception of the longitudinal coat. Expressed in absolute terms, the average intramural length of the ureter in the newborn infant is 5 mm, and in the adult 13 mm. In a normal infant the ratio of the intramural length to the ureteric diameter is 6 or 7 to 1 as compared to 0.75 to 1 in an infant suffering from reflux. This oblique entry of the ureter into the bladder is believed to produce a flap valvular mechanism whereby, as the intravesical hydrostatic pressure rises, so the submucosal portion of the ureter is compressed, thus preventing reflux. Sometimes the intramural length may appear normal but when the intravesical pressure rises, as in micturition, the ureter recedes through the ureteric hiatus. In this situation the basic fault is believed to be caused by lax fixation of the ureter due to deficient tone in the muscles of the trigone.

Presentation
In all series the incidence of 'primary' reflux is higher in girls than boys, in some series the incidence in females being three times greater than the incidence in boys. However, ureterovesical reflux tends to be more severe in boys possibly because of the higher urethral resistance in the male.

Primary reflux is not associated with any specific symptoms other than repeated attacks of urinary infection. These may produce one or all of the following—fever, vomiting, diarrhoea, irritability, meningism and convulsions. When any of these symptoms repeatedly occur in a child a search should be made for a urinary tract infection and its underlying cause. A minority of children present with enuresis.

Age of presentation
Approximately 50 per cent of children present before the age of 4 years but the

diagnosis is frequently delayed so that in nearly one-half the affected infants' symptoms have been present for over one-half of their lives before the diagnosis is made.

Diagnosis
Diagnosis of reflux depends upon clinical suspicion and a series of special investigations including:

1. bacteriological examination of the urine.
2. excretion pyelography which will give some indication of renal function and renal scarring.
3. micturating cystography, paying particular attention to the degree of reflux and the urethral voiding image particularly in girls. The incidence of unilateral and bilateral reflux can be shown to be approximately equal by this means.
   Furthermore, if there is duplication of the upper urinary tract, micturating cystography shows that reflux occurs in the majority of infants into the ureter from the lower component.
4. urethral profile pressures, especially in girls, which enable a diagnosis of distal urethral obstruction to be made.
5. biochemical tests of renal function.
6. cystourethroscopy. Not all surgeons would perform this investigation if the previous investigations indicate that surgical interference is necessary. However, should it be performed a cause of urethral obstruction may be found and within the bladder in infants suffering from primary reflux the ureteric orifices may be found to be more widely separated than normal.

On the basis of the findings on micturating cystography the severity of the reflux can be graded in a variety of ways.

One such classification is as follows:

(*a*) the mild case. The ureters and calyces fill with dye.
(*b*) the moderate case. The calyces are dilated during micturation.
(*c*) the severe case. The calyces are markedly dilated and renal scarring, otherwise known as reflux nephropathy, may be evident.
(*d*) the extremely severe case. In this, the ureters are tortuous, profoundly dilated, and probably asystolic. In this condition the bladder may also be grossly enlarged, the syndrome of megaureter megacystica. However, despite a similarity to Hirschsprung's disease no deficit of ganglion cells in the walls of either bladder or ureters can be demonstrated.

Complications of untreated reflux
Reflux, particularly if severe, leads to progressive dilatation of the ureters, dilatation of the renal pelvis and the destruction of the renal parenchyma, these effects being due to the intermittently increased hydrostatic pressure in the upper urinary tract combined with an ever increasing severity of infection.

Management
Once the primary causes, such as phimosis in the male or distal urethral

obstruction in girls, have been eliminated there are two ways of managing the condition.

By a conservative regimen. When the degree of reflux is mild and there is little if any demonstrable change in the renal pelvis or kidney the condition should be treated conservatively using the antibiotics appropriate to the urinary tract infection which is present. Reports indicate that long term treatment in this fashion in this group of infants is followed by a cessation of reflux in approximately 50 per cent of children and in these infants the urine will usually remain sterile. However, all such infants should be reinvestigated, say one year later, and if this reveals that the reflux is persistent, a urinary tract infection is present and that changes are taking place in the renal tissue itself, there is a strong argument in favour of surgical intervention.

Surgical intervention. The indications for surgical intervention are:

1   the presence of reflux nephropathy at the time of the original diagnosis;
2   rapidly repeated severe urinary tract infection despite adequate treatment.

Approximately one-half of the infants when first diagnosed will present with these indications for early operation and the majority will be boys rather than girls.

Technique

Many techniques for the reimplantation of the ureter or ureters have been described. One in common usage is based on the Politano–Leadbetter technique which is carried out in the following way.

The ureteric orifices are identified by a transvesical approach after which the ureters are divided at their point of entry into the bladder and wounds in the vesical wall are repaired. Each ureter is then brought through the bladder wall in such a fashion that their intramural length is some four to five times their diameter.

Following surgery appropriate antibiotic therapy should be continued for some months.

Complications of reflux surgery

The major complications following reimplantation of the ureters are:

1   failure of the operation and continued reflux with persistent infections;
2   ureteric obstruction;
3   diverticulum formation.

Results

The overall results reported indicate that total relief from both reflux and infection is obtained in between 70 and 90 per cent of children according to the series examined. It is obvious, however, from the literature that reimplantation gives the most satisfactory results when the ureter is not too dilated. Since this type of operation has now been performed for more than two decades long term results are now available. These show that some degree of hypertension develops in about 12 per cent of affected individuals usually within 15–20 years, at which point the infants are young adults. In about 50 per cent of these patients the hypertension is sufficiently severe to warrant treatment. Although the development of hypertension may be associated with visible renal scarring on the intravenous pyelogram this is not necessarily so. Recurrent urinary tract infection may also occur in approximately 10 per cent of children even though on micturating cystography the reflux appears to have been adequately controlled.

8 Vascular Diseases

8.1 Anatomy of the sympathetic system, and the place of sympathectomy in surgery
8.2 Embolism and the treatment of arterial embolus
8.3 Pathology, symptoms, signs, and investigations of atherosclerosis in the lower limb
8.4 Arterial reconstruction in the lower limb
8.5 Diagnosis and management of the postphlebitic syndrome

8.1 Anatomy of the sympathetic system, and the place of sympathectomy in surgery

Anatomy of the sympathetic system
Origin. The cell bodies of the first order neurones that form the sympathetic outflow lie in the intermediolateral column (visceral efferent column) of the spinal cord between the first thoracic and the second or third lumbar segments.

Distribution. The thinly myelinated preganglionic axons leave the spinal cord via the anterior ventral spinal roots and then pass via the white rami communicantes to the paravertebral ganglionic trunks which extend on either side of the vertebral column from the base of the skull to the coccyx. Once the first order neurone has reached the sympathetic chain it may end locally in the corresponding ganglion or turn up or down the trunk. In either event, the fibres synapse with the postganglionic (second order) neurones which then send their axons directly back into the corresponding spinal nerve via a grey ramus communicans, or through the sympathetic trunk, to enter another spinal nerve. Since first order neurones arise only between T1 and L2, white rami communicantes are found associated only with these segments, but grey rami communicantes reach every spinal nerve.

The second order axons reach the organs innervated by:

1 passing via the spinal nerves until they end in the effector organs;
2 forming nerves or plexuses around blood vessels and following their course. In general, the arterial side of the circulation is more richly endowed than the venous.

Source of the sympathetic innervation of the upper and lower limbs. The preganglionic fibres supplying the upper limb arise from the second to the ninth thoracic segments. The majority of the postganglionic fibres leave the sympathetic chain via the grey rami at the level of the first thoracic and inferior cervical ganglia, which are often fused to form the cervicothoracic 'stellate' ganglion. Some fibres are also derived from the second and third thoracic ganglia. The vasomotor supply is distributed via the fifth and sixth cervical nerves from the middle cervical ganglion and via the lower components of the brachial plexus, from the stellate ganglion.

The preganglionic fibres of the lower limb arise from the fourth thoracic to the second lumbar segments and synapse in the lower lumbar and upper sacral ganglia. The majority of the vasomotor fibres supplying the leg and foot are carried in the sciatic nerve and its branches.

Although the anatomical pattern of innervation of the upper and lower limbs is similar there are significant physiological differences; for example, the lower limb circulation appears to be under greater sympathetic control than the upper because a sympathetic block of the lower limb produces a far greater rise in the skin temperature of the foot than a similar procedure in the upper limb. Furthermore, indirect methods of inducing vasodilatation, such as body heating, have a much greater effect on the lower than the upper limb.

SYMPATHECTOMY: SURGICAL TECHNIQUES

1 Upper limb

The most commonly used approach is the anterior cervical. A transverse incision is made above the clavicle, the clavicular head of the sternomastoid is divided, the carotid sheath is retracted medially, the scalenus anterior is divided, and the subclavian artery is retracted downwards and forwards. The fascia strengthening the cervical pleura is divided to allow the apex of the lung to be retracted and, thus, the inferior cervical ganglion, the first and second thoracic ganglia and the sympathetic chain are exposed. Sympathetic denervation of the upper limb can be achieved by resecting the second and third thoracic ganglia and the intervening chain, although some surgeons suggest that the cervicothoracic 'stellate' ganglion, together with the upper three thoracic ganglia, should be removed.

A second technique for approaching the lower cervical and upper thoracic chain is the transaxillary transpleural approach. This method was popularized in the UK by Hedley Atkins in 1954 although it has been previously described by Schultze and Goetz. The patient is placed in the lateral or semilateral position; if the latter, the patient is propped up by sandbags beneath the buttock and shoulder. The arm is flexed, and abducted to lie vertically, the elbow is fixed to 90 degrees and the forearm supported horizontally in an arm rest.

The skin incision, made with the surgeon sitting, may be made in the line of the third rib or a more vertical oblique incision immediately behind and parallel to the posterior border of the pectoralis major muscle. Following exposure of the third rib a section is resected. The pleura is usually torn during this procedure after which a Tudor Edwards retractor is inserted between the second and fourth rib and the lung retracted. Using a fibreoptic light source the interior of the wound is illuminated and the sympathetic ganglia can either be seen or palpated. Having identified the ganglia the pleura is divided and the second, third and fourth ganglia together with the intervening chain are removed. If the operation is being performed for severe axillary hyperhidrosis the fifth ganglia will also be removed. A chest drain is inserted which is connected to an underwater drain, normally this is removed on the following day when full expansion of the lung has been established by plain radiographs of the chest.

The complications of the anterior cervical approach include:

(a) accidental and unrecognized perforation of the pleura leading to a pneumothorax;
(b) bleeding from a torn intercostal vein or less commonly, artery leading to a large retropleural haematoma;
(c) Horner's syndrome;
(d) on the left side the thoracic duct may be injured. This leads to a troublesome lymph fistula which, fortunately, will close spontaneously although it may take many weeks.

The chief complications of the transaxillary transpleural approach are:

(a) chest pain, usually temporary;
(b) pleural effusion;
(c) chest infection, normally due to segmental collapse.

2 Lower limb

Three anatomical approaches to the lumbar sympathectomy chain have been described: the transperitoneal anterior, the extraperitoneal anterior, and lastly, the posterior extraperitoneal approach. Whichever approach is made, the sympathetic chain is found more easily on the right, lying on the bodies of the lumbar vertebrae just medial to the psoas origin; on the left side the chain is somewhat hidden by the inferior vena cava.

To denervate the lower limb, the second, third and fourth lumbar ganglia and the intervening chain are removed. If the first lumbar ganglion is excised the area of anhidrosis extends proximally almost to the level of the inguinal ligament. In the treatment of peripheral vascular disease this is a useless extension, and furthermore, such an operation will be complicated by impotence in the male.

Complications of lumbar sympathectomy
These include haemorrhage, which is nearly always caused by injury to the lumbar veins which are tributaries of the inferior vena cava. The bleeding may be severe enough to warrant early interference, or much later when the patient presents with a mass in the affected loin together with fever if there has been infection.

Another significant complication is postsympathetic neuralgia, which usually affects the proximal part of the limb and begins some 10 days after operation, lasting for several months.

Furthermore, lumbar sympathectomy is not an innocuous surgical procedure. The majority of patients upon whom this operation is performed are old, suffering not only from ischaemic changes in the lower limbs but also accompanying cardiac and pulmonary disease. A mortality rate in excess of 5 per cent must be expected.

This operation has, therefore, been virtually supplanted particularly in the UK by phenol sympathectomy, destroying the sympathetic ganglia by the paravertebral injection of 5 ml of 1:15 solution of phenol, the injection site being controlled in many centres by radiographic positioning of the needle point.

Physiological response to sympathectomy
1   The only apparently beneficial effect of sympathectomy in a limb suffering from occlusive vascular disease is to decrease the distal resistance to blood flow by causing maximal dilatation of the arteriovenous anastomoses. This occurs because the arteriovenous anastomoses are not already dilated in an ischaemic limb in contrast to the afferent arterioles. As a result of the latter change a transient increase in collateral blood flow occurs in ischaemic limbs.

There appears to be no effect on the skin or muscle arterioles despite the oxygen debt in an ischaemic limb.

2   Although skeletal muscle is diffusely innervated by sympathetic nerves the response to sympathetic stimulation is limited to resting muscle blood flow. Whilst a maximal sympathetic discharge lowers the resting muscle blood flow by approximately 85 per cent of its normal value the abolition of sympathetic activity increases the muscle blood flow approximately 3 times as compared to a 15 times increase on active exercise, a finding which shows that the afferent arterioles in skeletal muscle have a high intrinsic myogenic tone which compensates for sympathetic ablation.

3   So far as the skin is concerned, changes in skin temperature, i.e. a rise in skin temperature, occurs in response to sympathectomy. However, it would appear that this change is due to changes in the flow of blood through the arteriovenous anastomoses rather than the skin capillaries which have a high myogenic tone and which are primarily responsible for the nutrition of the skin.

4   Sweating is abolished.

Indication for cervical sympathectomy

1   *Raynaud's disease*
This is a primary condition, first described by Raynaud in 1862, seen mostly in young women who suffer episodes of digital ischaemia due to an excessive reaction to cold or emotional stress. On exposure to cold the fingers become pale due to acute ischaemia as the digital vessels shut down. As the attack ends the affected fingers become cyanotic due to the rapid deoxygenation of the blood which stagnates, after which there is a period of reactive hyperaemia associated with redness. In severe cases there are skin and nail changes, including ulceration and dry gangrene.

Initially because it was thought that the disease was wholly due to sympathetic overactivity sympathectomy was commonly practised for the treatment of this disease. It is now appreciated that at least three-quarters of all patients can be treated conservatively.

The most important single factor is to avoid exposure to cold, less important is to stop smoking and avoid emotional upset. The many individual treatments described include the use of tolazoline hydrochloride, reserpine, griseofulvin and methyldopa. None of these regimens carries any guarantee of success.

Sympathectomy is reserved for those patients in whom the disease progresses. Varying results have been reported and it appears that only about 20 per cent of patients are permanently cured, the remainder relapsing within 1 year. A number of theories have been advanced to explain this, including:

(*a*) incompleteness of the original operation;
(*b*) regeneration and relinking of fibres;
(*c*) increased sensitivity of the denervated limb to circulating catecholamines;
(*d*) the development of some previously undiagnosed predisposing cause such as scleroderma.

2 Raynaud's phenomenon

This is a descriptive term describing a symptom based on a wide variety of underlying diseases which include:

(*a*) the 'collagen diseases' among which are systemic sclerosis, dermatomyositis and rheumatoid arthritis. The first of these conditions is the commonest cause of Raynaud's syndrome in women.
(*b*) atherosclerosis. This is the commonest cause of Raynaud's phenomenon in males and may develop in the presence of minimal proximal disease. In affected individuals a single digit or the whole hand may be affected and digital arteries involved in the disease may undergo sudden thrombosis leading to digital gangrene.
(*c*) thoracic outlet compression due to a cervical rib or the scalenus anterior muscle.
(*d*) trauma particularly in workers whose hands are exposed to vibrating tools such as pneumatic road drills, pneumatic chisels or the chain saws used by forestry workers. The symptoms develop after a latent period which may be several years in duration and the actual fingers affected depend not only upon the particular tool which is being used but also on the manner in which a particular workman holds his specific tool. It has been shown that the blood flow in the digital vessels is reduced to the greatest degree when the frequency of vibration is between 70 and 120 Hz and that the reduction in digital flow is directly related to the amplitude of vibration.

Among the rarer causes of Raynaud's phenomenon can be listed:

(*a*) underlying malignancy, usually of the gastrointestinal tract;
(*b*) exposure to the manufacturing processes involved in the production of vinyl chloride;
(*c*) ergot poisoning;
(*d*) chemotherapeutic agents, notably bleomycin.

A cervical sympathectomy is of doubtful value in the majority of the conditions described. It is of little use in scleroderma. In thoracic outlet compression attention should be devoted to excising the cervical rib particularly if embolic phenomena are occurring. In vibration-induced disease further exposure to the causative agent should be avoided.

In cases of Raynaud's phenomenon due to atherosclerosis cervical sympathectomy may be useful in securing healing after excision of necrotic tissue and the same applies if digital gangrene complicates rheumatoid arthritis although it should be appreciated that in neither case will further episodes of Raynaud's phenomenon be abolished. All the surgeon is seeking to achieve is rapid and successful healing of remaining tissue.

It should be noted that in Raynaud's due to scleroderma a variety of medical treatments have been examined. These include the administration of reserpine, guanethidine, the anabolic steroid, stanozolol and prostaglandin E. None of these drugs appear to exert anything other than a negligible or transient beneficial effect. One further treatment in vogue some years ago was plasma exchange but the beneficial effects of this treatment, if any, also appear to be transient.

In summary, therefore, it can be stated that cervical sympathectomy is a rarely performed operation.

8.2 Embolism and the treatment of arterial embolus

Definition. The word embolus is derived from the Greek word that means peg or stopper, and the generally accepted definition of an embolus is an abnormal mass of undissolved material that is transported from one part of the circulation to another.

Types. Emboli may travel in arterial, venous or lymphatic vessels and they may be solid, liquid or gaseous. The common emboli are composed of tumour cells, thrombus or clot, atheromatous plaques, fat or oil, bacteria, air or nitrogen.

Effects. These depend upon the composition, size and the tissue in which they become impacted. Thus, a solid embolus of even small dimensions produces considerable disturbance when there is impaction in the cerebral or coronary vessels, whereas the same embolus carried to the pulmonary circulation may cause neither symptoms nor signs.

Specific emboli

Gas emboli
Gas emboli that result from surgical misadventure during operations on the head and neck, mismanaged blood transfusion, or insufflation of the Fallopian tubes, may be fatal. In man, approximately 200 ml of air may be lethal due to the heart being unable to deal with the frothy mixture of blood and air that forms in the

right ventricle and pulmonary artery. The sudden introduction of air into the right side of the heart leads to loss of the peripheral pulses, pallor, cyanosis, peripheral circulatory failure, hyperpnoea, and death. Treatment is to turn the patient onto the left side so that the outflow tract is no longer at the highest point at which air collects.

Another form of air embolus is caisson disease. This is an occupational hazard of divers and others working in air under pressure. In this situation air goes into solution, the oxygen and carbon dioxide are removed but nitrogen remains in solution. When the pressure is reduced the nitrogen comes out of solution and forms small bubbles which may lodge in the cerebral, myocardial, pulmonary, or osseous vessels. Emboli in the nervous system give rise to the painful condition known as the bends, and respiratory and nervous effects may develop with great rapidity.

Solid emboli
The effect of solid emboli impacting in an artery supplying solid tissue depends in part on the blood supply of the organ. Thus the lungs are supplied not only by the main pulmonary artery but also by the bronchial arteries and the liver whilst receiving its major supply of blood via the portal vein is also supplied by the hepatic artery. If a solid embolism impacts in a major artery supplying an extremity, depending largely on the site and the possibility of an alternative route around the block the result is a variable degree of ischaemia which at its worst will end in gangrene.

Infected emboli
These are normally associated with a pyaemia and are normally carried in the venous circulation. Impacting in the branches of the portal vein within the liver they produce not only infarction but also local infection. This is the origin of the multiple liver abscesses which occur in a portal pyaemia caused most commonly by appendicitis or diverticulitis.

Fat emboli
This condition, following major trauma accompanied by fractures of the long bones, was first described by Zenker in 1862 who not unnaturally assumed that the fat globules entered the circulation from the torn veins of the marrow in the bones fractured by trauma. However, in 1965 Evarts put forward an alternative hypothesis suggesting that the fat emboli were not simply due to mechanical factors but rather to a physicochemical alteration in the solubility of the lipid emulsion in the blood stream. On the basis of this hypothesis Evarts suggested that all severely injured individuals should be given clofibrate (Atromid-S) which has been shown to be effective in Types IIb, III and IV hyperlipoproteinaemias.

Once in the systemic venous circulation the fat particles block the microcirculation of various regions including the lungs, brain, kidney, skin and retinal circulation.

In the lungs, if a sufficient number of emboli are present, AV shunting, alveolar hypoperfusion and an increased resistance to pulmonary blood flow occurs. These changes lead to the development of symptoms within 24–48 hours and are associated with dyspnoea, cyanosis, tachypnoea, cough, a fever of around 38.5 °C, a marked tachycardia and haemoptysis. Auscultation of the lung fields reveals crepitations and râles and cyanosis of the lips and nail beds may be obvious.

Plain radiographs of the chest show bilateral opacities that are particularly marked at the periphery. The absence of a pleural effusion or hepatomegaly virtually rules out the possibility of pulmonary oedema due to heart failure. Fat appears in the sputum and urine and may even be observed in the retinal arteries.

When the main feature of fat embolism falls on the microcirculation of the brain the patient may become disorientated, drowsy, uncooperative and confused and less often delirium, coma and decerebrate rigidity develop. The basis for the symptoms and signs of cerebral fat embolus is, in part, the inadequate oxygenation of the blood following pulmonary involvement and the local hypoxia which follows occlusion of the cerebral arterioles by emboli.

Involvement of the kidneys may lead to the finding of fat in the urine but there are seldom signs of renal failure.

Involvement of the skin vessels leads to a petechial rash, commonly 2–3 days after injury. The rash is brownish in colour and may be mistaken for normal skin pigmentation if not carefully examined. Its location is chiefly across the root of the neck, the axillae, and the anterior chest wall. The rash is transient, fading in one area as it appears in another.

Diagnosis
1. In approximately 50 per cent of patients free fat can be demonstrated in the urine using the stain Sudan 3.
2. Fat globules may be seen in the retinal vessels.
3. The serum lipase rises about the fourth day.
4. The Po_2 falls if there is major lung involvement.
5. X-ray changes as described appear in the lung fields.

Arterial emboli
Arterial emboli arise from many sources and vary considerably in size. In more than 80 per cent the origin of the embolus is the heart. Less common sources include aneurysms of the aorta, thrombi forming on atherosclerotic plaques in peripheral vessels or mural thrombi forming in peripheral arteries which are the site of continual trauma, e.g. from the subclavian artery in the thoracic outlet syndrome when mural thrombus forms which may discharge microemboli which impact in the digital arteries causing digital gangrene.

Larger emboli usually originate in the heart, the initial cause of thrombus formation being:

1. rheumatic heart disease associated with mitral stenosis. The causative thrombus tends to form on the atrial septum. At first, it is mushroom-shaped, but ultimately it may lie free in the lumen as a ball thrombus. In the presence of auricular fibrillation, thrombus tends to develop in the auricular appendages and may suddenly pass into the general circulation when a normal cardiac rhythm is restored. The chance of an embolus is

seven times greater in a fibrillating heart than in a heart in normal sinus rhythm.
2 atrial fibrillation. In this condition clots form in the left atrium due to incomplete emptying of the chamber due to the feeble contractions of the atrial wall. The resulting stasis predisposes to the development of thrombi which then enter the left ventricle to be propelled into the blood stream by the force of ventricular contraction. Atrial fibrillation may arise from many causes including rheumatic heart disease associated with mitral valve disease, arteriosclerotic heart disease, hypertension and occasionally hyperthyroidism.
3 myocardial infarction. In at least one-half of fresh infarcts which have extended to the endocardium mural thrombosis occurs. In some 10–20 per cent of affected individuals pieces of the thrombus break loose and enter the peripheral blood stream. In the majority of patients embolization occurs within three weeks of the initial infarct. In some patients suffering from a severe myocardial infarct an aneurysm of the left ventricle develops which eventually becomes the site of thrombosis and clot formation.
4 cardiac emboli also complicate cardiac surgery or endocarditis. The last named condition was always rare but in recent years a new cause has developed, i.e. staphylococcal endocarditis in patients who have undergone valve replacement. Approximately one in every hundred valves is lost per year due to infective complications. In classical subacute endocarditis emboli frequently occur in the cerebral, peripheral and visceral vessels.
5 emboli from great vessels such as the aorta are nearly always the result of atherosclerosis and/or aneurysm.

Sites of infarction
Peripheral emboli generally occlude arteries at their bifurcation at which point there is usually a sudden narrowing in the luminal size. When the aorta is occluded this event always occurs at the bifurcation, the so-called 'saddle' embolus.

In order of descending frequency the site of impaction is in the common femoral artery just proximal to the origin of the profunda femoris, 40 per cent; superficial femoral, 30 per cent; iliac bifurcation 10 per cent; aortic bifurcation 10 per cent; and popliteal artery 10 per cent.

Symptoms
When the blood supply to a limb is suddenly cut off, 90 per cent of patients suffer immediate severe pain. This may initially be felt over the site of impaction, and so, in the presence of an embolus impacted at the aortic bifurcation there may be at first pain in the back and suprapubic region whereas an embolus impacting in the common femoral artery causes pain and tenderness in the thigh. Apart from these local signs there is an abrupt and rapid onset of severe ischaemic pain in the muscles distal to the site of impaction associated with paraesthesia, numbness and coldness which begin distally and spread centripetally. As the duration of anoxia increases so the

symptoms usually increase in intensity until the peripheral nerves become non-functioning, at which point a sense of numbness replaces the pain. Loss of function almost immediately follows the occlusive episode.

Physical signs
Examination usually reveals marked pallor of the limb distal to the block. Palpation reveals tenderness along the course of the artery at the site of the occluding embolus. There are no pulses present distal to the point of obstruction, and at some point on the skin surface there is an abrupt change in temperature. Cutaneous sensation usually disappears as far as the midthigh following an aortic embolus, as far as the knee in the common femoral artery, and to above the ankle when the superficial femoral or popliteal arteries are blocked. The muscles below the block are often tender and slightly swollen. As time progresses, the skin pallor changes to cyanosis and mottling and within 24–36 hours the limb is usually brownish blackish in colour as gangrene develops.

Differential diagnosis
An arterial embolus of the lower limb must be distinguished from:

1 *arterial thrombosis*. This is commoner in the femoral and popliteal arteries. The patient is usually over 40 and there may be a long history of arterial disease before the onset of sudden pain without any history of cardiac disease.
2 *phlegmasia caerulea dolens*. This condition is an extensive deep venous thrombosis associated with arterial spasm. Unlike arterial occlusion, a massive deep venous thrombosis is usually associated with severe swelling.
3 *dissecting aneurysm*. This may be difficult to distinguish. There is usually no obvious site of origin of an embolus and the femoral pulses are of different magnitudes on the two sides.

Treatment
The first duty of the surgeon is to relieve pain, after which treatment of the limb can be considered. It is now appreciated that the more proximal the embolus the less chance there is of limb survival. Thus, when aortic, iliac, and common femoral emboli are treated conservatively, gangrene develops in approximately 50 per cent of limbs. Below the common femoral artery, gangrene develops in about 30 per cent of cases. However, when a distal embolus is conservatively treated the limb often suffers from chronic ischaemia, causing claudication, thereafter. In general terms, therefore, the treatment of emboli above the level of the popliteal trifurcation is operative.

The development of the balloon catheter described by Fogarty has considerably reduced the operative hazards for, if necessary, the affected artery can be explored using a local anaesthetic only. The Fogarty catheter is used in the following manner: the catheter is inserted into the arterial lumen up to a known length with the balloon deflated; at the desired point the balloon is then inflated with saline until a slight resistance is felt as the balloon reaches the diameter of the vessel. The catheter is then slowly withdrawn, keeping a gentle and gradually decreasing or increasing pressure on the balloon so that it remains in contact with the inner surface of the vessel.

If there has been a saddle embolus lying across the aortic bifurcation, both femoral arteries must be controlled before using the catheter in order to prevent distal embolization, after which both arteries can then be explored from below. It is essential that clot distal to the thrombus is also removed by passing the catheter distally. Following embolectomy the arteriotomy wound is sutured and the patient anticoagulated with heparin.

Postoperative course
In some patients in whom the immediate relief of the occlusion is delayed oedema of the muscles, haemoconcentration, hypovolaemic shock, acidosis, myoglobinaemia and myoglobinuria may develop. If the affected muscles are enclosed in a rigid compartment, e.g. the anterior tibial compartment, extensive fasciotomies may be required to relieve the intracompartmental pressure and hence the secondary ischaemia which may lead, if severe, to the onset of gangrene. The metabolic disturbance accompanying this syndrome is related to the muscle mass involved in the initial episode.

In patients in whom embolectomy is unsuccessful in re-establishing the blood flow through the involved artery the viability of the limb depends on the previous role of the vessel in supplying the limb with blood and the functional state of the collateral circulation.

8.3 Pathology, symptoms, signs, and investigations of atherosclerosis in the lower limb

Definition. Atherosclerosis was defined by the World Health Organization study group as a variable combination of changes in the intima and media of arteries consisting of focal accumulations of lipids, complex carbohydrates, blood products, fibrous tissue and calcium deposits.

Pathology
Stage I. The first visible evidence of atherosclerosis is the development of fatty streaks on the inner walls of the arteries. To the naked eye these appear as slightly raised yellowish thickenings of the intima which are microscopically seen to be produced by the deposition of lipid material within the intima. The major portion of the lipid, which consists of a mixture of cholesterol and its esters, phospholipids and triglycerides, is deposited within the 'myogenic foam' cells.
Stage II. This stage is the beginning of irreversible disease. The plaques, either scattered in isolated patches or, alternatively, forming large coalescent areas, are still confined to the intima but, in addition to the chemical components, histological examination shows many additional changes. These include:

1 the invasion of the lesion and the surrounding area by macrophages and fibrous tissue;
2 fragmentation of the internal elastic lamina;
3 degeneration of the media and the replacement of elastic and muscle fibres by fibrous tissue;
4 calcification;
5 invasion of the plaque by small vessels derived from the vasa vasorum.

Even when this stage has been reached the intimal lesion may still remain covered by endothelium but the affected vessel may well appear abnormal to the naked eye. Internal inspection reveals thickening of the vessel wall, and the progressive changes in the media lead to dilatation.

Stage III. The final stage is reached when there is ulceration of the overlying endothelium followed by surface thrombosis. Ulceration may allow discharge of atheromatous material into the blood stream, resulting in the appearance of embolic phenomena, or surface thrombosis may be sufficient to occlude the artery, either partially or totally, and produce ischaemic changes in the parts distal to the disease. There may also be occlusion because of bleeding into the deeper layers of the plaque. Advancing calcification at this stage leads to the characteristic stone-hard shell in the arterial wall.

Mechanism of lipid accumulation
The precise mechanism by which lipids accumulate in the arterial wall is unknown. Three opposing theories deserve mention:

1 *The thrombogenic theory.* This was first proposed in 1842 by Rokitansky, who suggested that the lipids were deposited on the vessel wall from the blood stream; this theory has recently received support from Duguid.
2 *The filtration theory.* This theory postulates that the lipids reach the deeper layers of the intima after being deposited on, and filtered through, the endothelium.
3 *The haemodynamic theory.* This was proposed by Texon. He suggests that intimal proliferation is due to a suction effect on the arterial wall, an effect brought about because the lateral pressure in the arterial system falls as the velocity of the blood increases, due to the arteries becoming smaller. This theory offers a possible explanation of the increasing incidence of atherosclerosis in the lower abdominal aorta and the common iliac vessels and also of the manner in which the lesions progress once they have begun.

Possible aetiological factors
The various factors that have been incriminated in this disease include:

1. mechanical factors, e.g. haemodynamic stress. Atherosclerosis does not develop in the low pressure pulmonary arterial system except in the presence of pulmonary hypertension. The rate of development of atherosclerotic lesions probably increases in hypertensives.
2. diabetes mellitus. Atherosclerosis is two to three times commoner in the diabetic than normal controls.

3 cigarette smoking. Statistical evidence shows that atherosclerosis is more common in cigarette smokers.
4 oestrogens. These hormones are known to depress the serum β-lipoproteins and, in keeping with this, women are relatively unaffected by arterial disease until they are postmenopausal.

Symptoms of atherosclerosis

The symptoms of atherosclerosis are due to the decrease in blood supply to the tissues supplied by the affected blood vessels. This is usually gradual, but may be sudden if there is subintimal haemorrhage or thrombosis. In the majority of people, atherosclerosis must be symptomless, because it is a common post mortem finding in asymptomatic patients. In others, the onset of symptoms is not necessarily associated with progression, indeed, only 14 per cent of patients presenting with intermittent claudication eventually require an amputation. The main symptoms of atherosclerosis are as follows.

1 *Intermittent claudication*
This indicates a reduction, usually by more than 60 per cent, in the blood flow to muscle groups undergoing exercise. Although it is most often a symptom of arterial occlusion it may also be apparent when there is a deficient oxygen supply to muscle, as can happen at a high altitude or in severe anaemia. The pain of claudication is usually typical; it is produced by muscular effort and it is relieved by stopping the exercise even when the limb remains dependent. This distinguishes claudication from the pain of venous stasis which may be felt on exercise but which can only be relieved by elevating the affected limb.

The precise algogen responsible for the pain of claudication is unknown. Lewis, in his original papers in the 1930s concluded that the factor responsible, the P factor, was a product of muscle metabolism.

If a patient continues to walk after the pain of claudication begins, the muscles gradually stiffen and tighten so that, regardless of the patient's pain threshold, he or she must eventually stop. Variations in the amount of exercise required to produce pain, 'the claudication distance', gives an approximate measure of the progress of obliterative arterial disease, and the site of the pain is an indication of the site of the block, which is always proximal to the area of complaint. Thus, claudication in the foot, often interpreted as 'foot strain' indicates occlusion at or above the ankle. Claudication in the calf indicates femoropopliteal disease whereas pain in the buttocks and thighs indicates occlusion of the aorta or iliac vessels (Lériche's syndrome).

Claudication is nearly always associated with absent peripheral pulses. If this happens not to be so, the usual explanation is the presence of an aortic block, in which condition the femoral pulses are absent but the popliteal and posterior tibial pulses are palpable. However, if clinical examination reveals that all the pulses are present, the patient should be asked to walk until claudication develops. Re-examination at this time often reveals that the previously palpable pulses have vanished, but as the pain disappears the pulses slowly return. The explanation of this phenomenon is the shift of the blood flow into the muscle bed.

Differential diagnosis. Symptoms superficially resembling claudication may be produced by many conditions including orthopaedic, muscular and neurological pathologies. In nearly all cases, however, the minutiae of the history, together with the obvious physical signs allow the diagnosis of occlusive vascular disease to be made with comparative ease.

A very similar pain, known as pseudoclaudication, may be experienced due to compression of the cauda equina. However, in this condition the distress may also be brought on by standing or bending, and it is usually associated with numbness or muscle weakness, which is relieved by sitting or lying down.

2 Constant limb pain

This is nearly always due to ischaemic neuritis which may be felt after either a sudden or gradual occlusion of the arterial supply to the limb.

In this condition the pain is usually severe, diffuse, and bears no relationship to dermatomes. Typically, it is worse in bed at night. It may be associated with paraesthesiae, formication, and a sense of numbness and coldness in the affected extremity. At some point in time the patient usually observes that putting the foot out of bed into a dependent position brings relief. Still later, the patient may begin to sleep sitting upright in a chair.

Because the pain of ischaemic neuritis is nervous in origin, physical examination may reveal reduced sensation to touch, pain and/or vibration. A similar pain, known as rest pain, which cannot be differentiated on clinical grounds from ischaemic neuritis, is sometimes experienced before the onset of gangrene. Both conditions indicate a serious deterioration of the peripheral circulation.

Occasionally, severe rest pain is felt in a limb that seems completely normal but in which the pulses are absent. In such a limb gangrene is inevitable.

Differential diagnosis. Once again in the presence of physical signs the diagnosis of ischaemic neuritis or rest pain is simple. However, it must occasionally be distinguished from causalgia which follows injury to peripheral nerves and any type of peripheral neuropathy.

In aged people, even in the highly developed countries, there is a syndrome known as the burning feet syndrome. This is probably caused by dietary deficiencies since the majority of people are cured if given a good diet with vitamin supplements. The major symptoms of this disease are intense burning in the foot associated, often, with shooting pains. Some patients obtain relief by sitting out of bed with their feet in cold water.

Diabetic neuropathy, which is relatively common in older people, often gives rise to gross sensory changes together with pain in the presence of relatively normal motor function.

Physical signs of arterial occlusion

The major physical signs associated with the *gradual* occlusion of a limb artery are those associated with atrophy. The affected limb or limbs are wasted, the toe pads disappear, and the hair vanishes.

In addition, there are always significant colour and temperature changes in any limb in which the arterial supply is in danger. In general, the skin becomes cyanotic when the limb is dependent because the rate of blood flow is so slow that it allows longer for the reduction of oxyhaemoglobin. When the limb is elevated it usually becomes pallid because the blood pressure in the diseased limb cannot overcome gravity. Because the skin temperature is determined by both blood flow and heat loss, the affected limb nearly always feels cooler to the examining hand and coldness may, indeed, be a cause of bitter complaint by the patient.

Following inspection of the limb a search is made for arterial pulsations.

Absent pulsations
The pulses normally palpable in the lower limb include those of the common femoral artery, the popliteal artery, the posterior tibial artery, and the dorsalis pedis. If it appears that there is an element of vasospasm associated with absent pulses, a sublingual tablet of glyceryl trinitrate will release the spasm and the pulses will become palpable within 2–5 minutes. Pulses in vessels permanently occluded by organic disease remain impalpable. When the lower femoral and popliteal arteries are blocked, pulsation may be felt in the medial or lateral geniculate arteries.

Bruits
Arterial murmurs develop in partially occluded arteries due to the turbulence of the blood flow. Bruits can be made more obvious by exercising the limb because this increases the rate of proximal blood flow and dilates the artery distal to the block so increasing the rate of 'run off'. This increases the velocity of blood flow across the stenotic segment and a louder systolic bruit is heard. As an affected segment narrows, the bruit may be apparent even under resting conditions. Any bruit is usually conducted peripherally so that a partial occlusion at the bifurcation of the common iliac artery may be heard in the thigh.

Venous changes
As arterial occlusion progresses and the blood flow to the affected limb diminishes, so the veins lie empty and collapsed, forming grooves rather than elevations under the skin.

In the clinical disease known as thromboangiitis obliterans, or Buerger's disease, the veins may be involved in a segmental thrombophlebitis. This leads to acutely, red, raised and slightly indurated tender cords along the course of the vein, usually a few centimetres in length. This acute stage lasts for a few weeks after which the pain disappears but the occlusion persists. This condition must be distinguished from thrombophlebitis in a varicosity and from thrombophlebitis migrans. This differentiation is again not usually difficult because of the associated symptoms and signs of arterial insufficiency.

Ulceration
Ischaemic ulcers most commonly develop on the heel and digits but may be

found elsewhere on the leg following injury. Such ulcers may penetrate the deep fascia and expose both muscles and tendons. They are usually locally painful and nearly always associated with the generalized pain of ischaemic neuritis. Other symptoms of vascular impairment appear and the distal pulses are usually absent. These ulcers have, of course, to be distinguished from other causes of limb ulceration of which there are many. Some of the commoner causes are as follows.

1 *Stasis ulcers*. These are commonest on the medial aspect of the leg and they are usually associated with severe venous insufficiency.

2 *Hypertensive ulcers* (Martorelli's syndrome). These lesions are commoner in women than men and are usually bilateral, and located on the lower third of the leg posterolateral to the medial malleolus. They are painful, superficial, and often associated with satellite infarctive lesions in the immediate vicinity. They have a necrotic central eschar which is surrounded by rather indolent granulation tissue. Whereas ischaemic ulcers tend to progress slowly, hypertensive ulcers usually heal spontaneously over a long period. This type of ulcer is due to an obliterative lesion of the small arterioles of the cutaneous arterial plexus.

3 *Neurotropic ulcers*. These appear in peripheral neuritis, usually on the soles of the feet, and often under the first metatarsophalangeal joint. They are indolent, painless, and penetrating.

Other less common causes of leg ulceration include the blood dyscrasias, especially sickle-cell anaemia and chronic haemolytic anaemia, and specific ulcers such as the gumma of syphilis and ulcers found in the presence of a general disease such as pyoderma gangrenosum complicating hypogammaglobulinaemia and ulcerative colitis.

Gangrene

When gangrene is due to atherosclerosis it is really an advancing ischaemic ulceration. It commonly begins on the digits themselves or in the interdigital clefts. It is often precipitated by injury or interdigital fungal infections which macerate the affected skin. The gangrene of atherosclerosis is usually dry; the tissues involved are at first purple, later black, and in the absence of infection the affected part becomes dry and shrunken with a line of demarcation developing between the affected part and viable tissues.

Acute occlusion

When the limb vessels are suddenly occluded ischaemic pain usually develops with great rapidity. The generalized pain in the affected portion of the limb is associated with a feeling of coldness, numbness, and tingling. When the artery is blocked by an embolus, for example at the bifurcation of the common femoral, the artery is very often tender to pressure at the point of impaction.

Distal to the block the muscles of the limb are at first tender on pressure and there is usually total paresis. There are marked temperature changes in the affected limb and the position of the block can be judged in time by finding a line of demarcation between warm and cold and the progress of the condition can be assessed by the gradual shift of the temperature gradient in a distal direction.

Acute occlusion is nearly always associated with instant pallor.

According to the level of the acute occlusion the limb behaves in different ways. A block at the common femoral bifurcation which is unrelieved leads to gangrene, a more distal block in which the popliteal artery continues pulsating may be followed by a persistent cold foot and, possibly, some weakness of the small muscles, but gangrene is rare.

Special investigations

1 Non-invasive techniques

Oscillometry. An oscillometer consists of a pneumatic cuff connected to an aeronoid capsule which measures the pulsatile variations with each cardiac systole in the volume of the limb segment under examination. The use of an oscillometer confirms the presence of a palpable pulse and may establish the presence of a pulse which an examiner has failed to palpate.

Ultrasound echography. This is a very useful, rapid and accurate non-invasive method for identifying the contour, lumen size, and wall thickness of an aneurysm and since it can be repeated as often as is required it is very helpful in establishing whether such a lesion is expanding.

Doppler ultrasonic flowmeter. This is a useful technique for measuring the flow velocities in major arteries. The principle on which the method is based is the Doppler phenomenon whereby sound reflected from a moving object undergoes a shift in frequency which is proportional to the velocity of the object. The commercially available instruments consist of a probe housing two piezometer electric crystals. One of these, driven by an oscillator, projects a 2- to 10-megacycle continuous ultrasound beam which is directed transcutaneously through the tissue overlying the artery under study. The reflected beam is detected by the second crystal in the probe and converted to an electric signal. By sensing and amplifying the phase shifts that occur when the ultrasound waves are scattered by the moving cells in the blood stream, the instrument is able to detect changes in the velocity of flow, either visually or audibly.

Normally the sound heard over arteries is multiphasic with a high-pitched hissing noise present during systole, followed in diastole by one or two short medium-pitched sounds of lower intensity. An increase in velocity, as after a period of exercise on a treadmill, causes all the sounds to be higher pitched.

When a partial or a complete block exists in the local arterial tree causing damping of the systolic peak and loss of retrograde flow a monophasic low-pitched sound can be heard which lasts through most of the cardiac cycle, the discrete diastolic sounds being lost. Partial obstruction of distal vessels produces a 'waterhammer' effect which consists of a short, sharp, higher-pitched sound. As the probe is passed over the skin along the course of the stenosed artery under study the intensity of the sound tends to become greater until the point of total occlusion is reached after which and immediately beyond it all sound disappears.

The Doppler ultrasonic flow meter can be used to measure the blood pressure in the tibial arteries at the ankle and the anterior tibial and dorsal pedal arteries in the ankle and foot. The probe is positioned over the artery, e.g. the posterior tibial artery, a blood pressure cuff is wrapped around the middle or upper part of the leg and the pressure is raised to above the systolic level and then dropped until sounds reappear over the artery. The level at which this occurs is considered to be the systolic pressure in the vessel.

In a normal individual the resting ankle pressure is approximately the same as that in the brachial artery, proximal blocks causing considerable reduction both at rest or following exercise.

2 Invasive techniques

Arteriography. This is not necessarily an essential investigation but it is always performed if direct arterial surgery is contemplated. The lower aorta and iliac vessels may be visualized either by translumbar aortography or by the introduction of a flexible catheter into the aorta via the femoral artery. The distal blood vessels are usually visualized by an injection of contrast medium into the common femoral artery or a small catheter can be introduced from the groin and passed into the distal segment of the popliteal artery, the contrast medium being delivered from this point. As soon as large quantities of contrast medium are injected the patient may experience an unpleasant burning sensation which may be particularly noticeable in the perineal region.

The dangers of arteriography include:

(a) anaphylactic shock. The intra-arterial injection of a large quantity of contrast medium should be preceded by the intravenous administration of a small test dose.

   Medication should also be available to combat an allergic response including adrenaline 1:1000.

(b) transfixion of an atheromatous plaque, when there may be either local dissection, dislodgement and embolization, dissection or failure to cease bleeding on withdrawal of the catheter.

(c) severe vasospasm. This produces severe pain and blanching of the affected limb and after several hours the appearance of scattered violaceous plaques in the skin below the point of injection which represent cutaneous and subcutaneous haemorrhages. Motor paralysis may be present but this, together with any loss of sensation normally recovers within a week to 10 days.

The radiological physical signs of atherosclerosis include:

(a) diffuse narrowing of vessels;
(b) irregularity of the vascular contour;
(c) variations in the density of the opaque column. If there are variations they give a clue to the presence of plaques and mural thrombi. Unfortunately,

there can be large plaques even in the absence of any radiological appearance;
(d) tortuous vessels which indicate fragmentation of the internal elastic lamina;
(e) aneurysm formation;
(f) frank occlusion;
(g) decrease in the magnitude of the 'run off' following a narrow segment.

The surgeon nearly always finds a greater degree of luminal compromise, intimal disease, mural thrombosis and calcification than is apparent from the aortograms or arteriograms.

3 *Electrocardiography*
Since atherosclerosis is a generalized disease it is frequently associated with disease of the coronary arteries. Between 10 and 20 per cent of patients with peripheral arterial disease have suffered from a myocardial infarction.

4 *Biochemical changes in peripheral atherosclerosis*
Investigations have shown that the mean serum total cholesterol and triglyceride levels are higher in patients of both sexes suffering from peripheral vascular disease than in control subjects although the only significant difference is in respect of the triglyceride level in males. This difference is not, however, associated with a significant reduction in the high density lipoprotein cholesterol concentration although there is some difference in the levels of this fraction between the sexes.

In ischaemic heart disease due to coronary artery disease there is an increase in the very light density lipoproteins (VLDL) and light density lipoproteins (LDL) and this is thought to promote atherosclerosis by enhancing the rate of deposition of cholesterol in the arterial wall.

In contrast it has been suggested that increased levels of high density lipoproteins (HDL) which are known to be associated with a decreased risk of coronary artery disease counteract the accumulation of cholesterol either by promoting its removal from the arterial wall or by preventing the uptake of low density lipoprotein.

One way of expressing these contrasting effects of serum lipoproteins is to calculate the ratio of 'protective' HDL cholesterol to the sum of atherogenic VLDL and LDL cholesterol. The HDL ratios are reduced in both male and female with peripheral vascular disease but in males this is partly due to an increase in VLDL and LDL whereas in females a decrease in HDL is probably more important.

Unfortunately there is as yet no 'hard' evidence that any treatment of these biochemical abnormalities delays or stops the progression of peripheral atherosclerosis once it has become a clinical entity.

8.4 Arterial reconstruction in the lower limb

Only about 25 per cent of patients presenting with symptoms of arterial occlusion in the lower limb due to arterial disease require direct arterial surgery, 15 per cent eventually undergo amputation, and about 10 per cent die within a year from involvement of arteries elsewhere, usually the heart.

The common sites of occlusion producing lower limb symptoms are:

1. adductor region of the femoral artery in 70 per cent;
2. aortoiliac area, 50–60 per cent;
3. popliteal artery, 12 per cent;
4. popliteal bifurcation, 12 per cent.

The proximal parts of the superficial femoral artery, and the popliteal artery below the level of the knee joint are relatively uncommon sites of occlusion. In recent years it has also been realized that the artery of supply in the thigh, the profunda femoris or deep femoral artery, is seldom involved along its length but only at its junction with the common femoral and along its first few centimetres.

It is also important to recognize that a considerable proportion of patients suffering from aortoiliac disease also have disease in the femoropopliteal segment and that this can dramatically alter the results of surgical interference if this is deemed necessary, about 25 per cent of such patients presenting with intermittent claudication progressing to severe ischaemia.

Indications for direct arterial surgery

1 Claudication
This is a relative indication for direct arterial surgery because the degree of disablement with similar claudication distances will be different in each individual owing to various factors such as work, hobbies, and age. The individual degree of disablement is, therefore, important.

2 Rest pain
This may be regarded as an absolute indication since it always leads to general deterioration in the patient's general condition, because of interference with sleep and the depressive effect of chronic pain. Furthermore, this type of pain is difficult to control with non-addictive analgesics of low or intermediate potency.

3 Ischaemic ulceration of the leg, incipient or actual gangrene
Ischaemic ulceration, incipient or actual gangrene are an indication for arterial surgery assuming that the radiological findings indicate that some benefit will be achieved. If, however, investigation shows only small vessel disease or occlusion below the trifurcation it is unlikely that any benefit will accrue from

direct arterial surgery. However, an operative or chemical sympathectomy will sometimes prevent incipient gangrene from becoming a true necrosis of tissue.

Investigations

1 *Non-invasive techniques*
Doppler ultrasonic probe measuring the ankle pressure, known as the ankle pressure test. The ankle pressure is measured at rest and then after standard exercise on a treadmill, the patients walking at a fixed speed, up a fixed incline for a fixed period or until stopped by the severity of their claudication. In patients with significant ischaemia the ankle systolic pressure falls after exercise, occasionally to zero and may take 20 minutes or more to recover to pre-exercise levels.

2 *Invasive*
When contemplating direct arterial surgery in the presence of the indications listed above, angiography is the most essential of the preoperative investigations. By this means the distribution and the severity of the disease can be established together with the presence of adequate 'run off' in vessels distal to the block.

Neither aortography, used when the common femoral pulse is absent or weak, or femoral arteriography, used when the most proximal absent pulse is in the popliteal segment, are free from complications.

Retrograde transfemoral aortography using a Seldinger catheter may, for example, be complicated by local thrombosis, embolism due to dislodgement of an atherosclerotic plaque, and local damage to the arterial wall resulting in either immediate haemorrhage or later aneurysm formation.

Translumbar aortography may be complicated by a dissection if the dye is injected into the wall of the vessel rather than the lumen and this may produce ischaemic changes in the viscera.

HISTORICAL DEVELOPMENTS OF ARTERIAL SURGERY

Homologous arterial grafts

The first surgical operations on the arteries consisted of excision of the diseased portion of the artery and replacement by arterial homografts. This method was derived from the work of Gross (1949) who used both fresh and preserved aortic homografts for the treatment of children suffering from coarctation of the aorta. The use of arterial homografts continued until the late 1950s, by which time synthetic substitutes were being introduced. At the same time, autologous vein grafts, first introduced by Kunlin (1949) were being extensively used. It is interesting to note however, that Martin wrote in 1956 that the latter were generally unsuccessful.

Synthetic grafts

Homologous arterial grafts, difficult to procure, were gradually abandoned when their tendency to thrombose or become aneurysmal became generally recognized. Synthetic grafts were at first made of a large number of different artificial fibres, many of which were eventually discarded for a variety of different reasons; nylon, for example, was found to lose its tensile strength, others kinked. The latter difficulty was partially overcome by crimping. Currently, the most popular synthetic grafts are made of knitted Dacron which possesses sufficient porosity to ensure that the neointimal lining is firmly fixed in place by fibroblasts growing though the interstices of the material from the host tissues. This degree of porosity, however, means that a new graft, exposed immediately to a normal arterial flow, leaks in an alarming manner. To overcome this difficulty such grafts are 'preclotted' before insertion by allowing them to lie in the recipient's blood, and then flushing them free of clots.

Two more recently introduced graft materials which have been introduced are:

1. polytetrafluoroethylene (PTFE) otherwise known as the Gore-Tex graft. This was introduced into the UK in 1976 and is a prosthetic graft made of fibrillated PTFE. It is of low thrombogenicity and the thin flexible fibres allow tissue ingrowth and hence the formation of a satisfactory neointima. The grafts are 6 mm in diameter and are anastomosed to the recipient vessel with a continuous polypropylene suture. The graft has the advantage of flexing without kinking. Unlike Dacron it requires no preclotting and does not bleed. It does not tend to become aneurysmal and the short term patency rates are equal to those of a reversed saphenous graft.
2. glutaraldehyde-stabilized umbilical vein grafts. These were introduced by Darlik *et al.* in 1979. This type of graft is said by its protagonists to be useful in replacing small vessels such as the peroneal and tibial arteries. However, the thick wall of the graft makes it difficult to sew and the Dacron mesh with which it is surrounded makes it more difficult to pull through tissue tunnels.

Endarterectomy

In the latter part of the 1940s Dos Santos described the operation of thromboendarterectomy. The technical efficiency of this operation depends on the presence of a plane of cleavage between the adventitia and the media in the diseased artery. This plane is between the external elastic lamina and the media, so that in performing an endarterectomy the entire intima and media are removed. Endarterectomy is only technically possible because calcification rarely extends into the external layer of the artery. The dissection can be accomplished under direct vision by using multiple arteriotomies, removing the disease between arteriotomies, or by dissecting instruments such as the Cannon loop or by the injection of gas.

The precise form of arterial surgery used, assuming that reconstruction is possible, appears to depend on the individual surgeon's preference and the technical expertise he has developed. It is doubtful whether the results reported in the literature, using any one of the three major techniques, are statistically different. Furthermore, an individual surgeon's indications for surgery may differ slightly from his colleagues, making the end result difficult to assess. The important aspects of each operation will now be briefly discussed.

1 Aortoiliac disease

In many, but not all, surgical centres endarterectomy has replaced the use of synthetic grafts for atherosclerosis of the aortoiliac region although Dacron grafts are still mandatory in the management of aortic aneurysms. Following exposure of the diseased area, the patient is heparinized immediately before arterial clamps are placed on the aorta and iliac arteries, the distal vessels then being flushed with a dilute solution of heparin, 150 mg/500 ml. The disobliteration is then performed through incisions along the axis of the major vessels. Care must be taken not to leave a ragged edge of diseased intima and media protruding into the lumen of the vessel in case this forms a focal point for dissection or thrombosis.

Results. The 5-year patency rate for aortoiliac disobliteration, as reported in various series, is between 50 and 75 per cent. In about 10 per cent of patients further arterial surgery is needed in the legs. Although the aorta frequently becomes larger than normal after endarterectomy, it does not lead to progressive dilatation and aneurysm formation is rarely seen.

2 Femoral artery disease

(a) Femoropopliteal disease. The initial site of occlusion of the superficial femoral artery is in the femoral canal, the occlusion starting at the adductor magnus hiatus and then extending proximally to the origin of the profunda femoris. This type of block is eminently suitable for direct arterial surgery and although endarterectomy can be used the published results in the literature suggest that in the long term a reversed saphenous vein graft, or if this is impossible a Gore-Tex graft will yield superior results.

Endarterectomy is successful in approximately two-thirds of all patients in whom investigation proves the operation to be feasible. Early failure is nearly always due to bleeding, infection, or both, either of which may lead to a secondary haemorrhage. This must be treated by immediate proximal and distal ligation of the main vessel, an operation usually followed by amputation. Late failures are nearly always due to rethrombosis of the endarterectomized segment or deterioration of proximal disease.

(b) Profunda femoris artery. The importance of this artery was first recognized by Morris *et al.* (1961) but it was not until 1968 that Martin and others described the operation of endarterectomy of its origin. A number of separate studies have shown that the profunda arteries, which supply the large muscles of the thigh, communicate via the geniculate arteries with the arteries of the leg. Thus, if the superficial femoral artery is blocked by disease the profunda forms an alternative pathway by which blood may reach the periphery. It has also been shown that if the profunda is involved in atherosclerosis the disease tends to be limited to the orifice and the first few centimetres of the artery. Thus, disobliteration of the profunda would appear to be a reasonable alternative to surgery involving the superficial femoral artery.

The first operation of this type described was that of endarterectomy of the orifice. This was later succeeded by extended endarterectomy carried out over approximately 15 cm of the main trunk of the profunda. Recently, Cotton (1971) has described the operation of extended deep femoral angioplasty. The artery is exposed throughout the proximal 15–18 cm, after which it is opened and a long autogenous vein patch graft is inserted so that the cross-sectional area of the vessel is doubled. In the original operation, an endarterectomy was also performed at the same time, but Cotton later omitted this step in order to avoid the possibility of intimal flap dissection. Cotton has reported that extended angioplasty is immediately successful in approximately 70 per cent of claudicants, these clinical results being parallel to the results of objective testing. The long term results in patients followed for between 10 and 40 months are also encouraging, some 75 per cent of the limbs remaining satisfactory. In the majority of patients, both claudication and rest pain are relieved but the results in patients whose legs were already gangrenous were disappointing. His enthusiasm for this operation is such that he suggests femoropopliteal bypass operations should be limited to cases of gangrene in which angiography has shown that a bypass is possible, or limbs in which this alternative operation has failed.

Autogenous vein grafts

This operation is performed using a reversed segment of the patient's own long saphenous vein which must be dissected from the thigh with great care. The vein used must be free from disease and at least 5 mm in diameter.

Following exposure of the diseased vessel, the graft is inserted between the superficial femoral and popliteal arteries. One major limiting factor in the performance of this operation is the state of the popliteal artery. When it is severely diseased the distal anastomosis must be performed in the post-tibial segment, which is technically a more difficult manoeuvre but does not necessarily alter the result, although various investigations have shown that the flow rates are significantly higher when the inferior anastomosis is performed above the level of the knee joint. Fortunately, in the great majority of patients the anastomosis can be performed at the higher level.

Balloon angioplasty

This technique consists of dilating strictures in the peripheral vessels by means of a balloon under direct vision in the X-ray department. Initially used for short occlusive lesions this method is being applied by the Swiss to strictures several centimetres in length.

Factors governing the success of direct arterial surgery
There is little doubt that the major factor governing the result of any of the surgical procedures described above is the run-off resistance. When this is high, the incidence of both early and late failures is increased whereas when all

vessels at the popliteal trifurcation are patent an initial success rate of about 90 per cent can be achieved.

In general, the long term results using vein grafts appear to be somewhat better than endarterectomy but the interpretation of an individual surgeon's results is always difficult because of slight differences in the type of patient upon whom the operation is performed. A typical large series reported in the literature claimed a success rate of 90 per cent in patients complaining of severe claudication, 80 per cent in patients complaining of rest pain, and 75 per cent in patients with threatened gangrene.

Long term results. Long term graft patency at 5 years is reported to be as high as 60 per cent. The late bad results are nearly always due to advance in proximal disease.

General remarks

The general consensus of opinion is that at least three-quarters of lower limbs endangered by occlusive vascular disease can be salvaged by direct arterial surgery using one of the methods described. Less common methods of restoring blood flow include crossover grafts between the iliac vessels. When the saphenous vein is unsatisfactory an endarterectomy *must* be performed, although a substitute for a vein graft has been described: this is bovine carotid artery treated with proteolytic enzymes to remove antigenicity and then tanned so that the final product is an inert collagenous tube.

After reconstructive surgery has been performed it is essential that the patient's general health is improved. Nearly all observers maintain that the cessation of smoking is essential and indeed many surgeons will not operate until the patient has abstained from this habit. Interestingly some large series have shown that age at the time of arterial reconstruction, the presence of diabetes, the graft diameter and the site of the distal anastomosis on lower limb surgery have little influence on the results of surgery.

8.5 Diagnosis and management of the postphlebitic syndrome

Anatomy of venous drainage of lower limb
It was not until the work of Cockett in the early part of the 1950s that the total anatomy of the venous drainage of the lower limb was fully appreciated. Until his work the veins of the leg had been divided into superficial and deep systems which, it was recognized, were joined at intervals by the communicating veins, the largest of which being the junction of the long saphenous with the femoral vein at the saphenous opening. Cockett's contribution was to describe a third group of veins known as the perforating system, which was composed of

vessels draining the skin on the medial and lateral aspects of the lower part of the leg directly into the vena comites surrounding the posterior tibial artery.

Thus, any alteration in pressure in the deep system can be, and is, immediately transmitted to the skin and subcutaneous tissues in the area drained by the perforators. Normally, all three systems are protected from undue increases in pressure by a series of valves that also impose the following pattern of venous return.

Blood in the deep system normally flows upwards, pumped by the compression caused by the contracting calf muscles acting within the ensheathing layer of deep fascia; this system has been called the peripheral 'venous heart'. Blood from the skin on the medial and lateral aspects of the leg flows inwards to the deep system, and blood in the superficial system can move either upwards or centripetally; in all, about 85 per cent of the blood from the legs is returned to the vena cava via the deep veins.

Venous pressures in the lower limb
The venous pressure in the lower limb has been investigated under different conditions by many workers. The normal pressure in the foot in a standing person is equal to the pressure of a column of blood extending from the heart to the point in the venous system at which the vein has been cannulated. If the venous system is normal, this pressure falls by 30–40 per cent during walking.

When uncomplicated varicose veins are present, although the pressure falls it does not do so to the same degree. However, if the varicose long saphenous vein is occluded by extrinsic pressure at the level of the knee, there is an additional fall in venous pressure so long as the communicating veins are functioning normally. This physiological measurement parallels the clinical test attributed to Perthes who described how the superficial varicosities below the knee emptied on walking if the superficial veins were occluded at the level of the knee joint by a tourniquet. When the deep venous system is blocked or incompetent, there is little or no reduction in venous pressure on walking, and occlusion of the long saphenous vein makes no difference, a state of affairs called by Linton 'ambulatory venous hypertension'.

Aetiology of the postphlebitic limb
The postphlebitic syndrome follows defects in the venous circulation in the deep venous system, usually the result of thrombosis. In general, the more proximal and extensive the original thrombosis the greater the chance of developing the symptoms and signs of venous insufficiency at a later date.

Thus, a previous history of phlegmasia caerulea dolens, the painful blue leg indicates that a high and extensive iliofemoral block has taken place and such an episode will nearly always be followed by venous incompetence and stasis. When, however, a venous thrombosis is limited to the intramuscular sinuses of the soleal muscle, producing minimal pain and tenderness in the calf, together with little sign of clinical disease, there is no evidence of venous incompetence unless proximal spread involving the posterior tibial and popliteal veins takes place. However, even a limited thrombosis may rapidly be followed by consecutive and propagated clot so that the deep vein is temporarily occluded. Such occlusion, however, is seldom long lasting; the clot shrinks and is invaded by granulation tissue so that eventually the vein is, at least in part, recannalized. However, there is gross physiological disturbance in the venous circulation because once the venous valves are destroyed persistent high pressure is exerted in the deep venous system, a pressure that increases on exercise.

Symptoms and signs

1 *Pain*. One of the major symptoms may be pain, although it is remarkable how painless the postphlebitic limb can be. The pain of severe venous insufficiency develops with exercise and is felt as a bursting sensation in the calf. Unlike intermittent claudication, cessation of activity does not produce relief, which can be obtained only by lying in a recumbent position with the leg elevated. Such pain can be disabling and may occasionally follow walking as little as 100 metres.

2 *Dermal changes*. In the course of time, dermal changes appear in the skin areas drained by the perforating veins, the incidence of such changes increasing with the passage of time. The first change is usually the development of multiple small tortuous veins under the skin in the ankle region in the absence of any demonstrable abnormality in the superficial veins. At the same time, the patient may note that the foot and leg are oedematous, particularly after standing. As time passes, the pitting oedema gives way to an indurated pigmented area. The induration is produced by a low-grade inflammatory reaction which is probably chemical in origin, possibly stimulated by the haemosiderin liberated into the subcutaneous tissues from red blood cells escaping by diapedesis from the dilated venules. Eventually, the indurated area forms a large plaque which involves nearly the whole circumference of the lower leg. Once in this condition the leg itches and the subsequent scratching may lead to an extensive eczema involving the whole area. If there should now be a bacterial infection cellulitis follows, and many patients give a history of repetitive attacks controlled by intermittent bed rest and an appropriate antibiotic.

3 *Ulceration*. Local trauma, infection or thrombosis may all lead eventually to ulceration and even when the ulcer heals in response to treatment the scar is usually atrophic and so easily breaks down.

Typical postphlebitic ulceration is situated in the region of the ankle joint above or below the malleoli. Ulceration may be so extensive as to be circumferential. It must be distinguished from other causes of ulceration on the leg, e.g. ulceration due to atherosclerosis, gumma, hereditary spherocytosis, ulcerative colitis, or tuberculosis.

Treatment

1 *Conservative*. The treatment of the postphlebitic leg is support and rest; many of the patients are overweight and a reducing diet may be helpful. The most efficient support for the ambulant patient is an elastic bandage some 10 cm in width extending from the toes to the level of the tibial tubercle. This can often be applied by younger patients without any help, but older patients need assistance.

Ulceration will nearly always heal with prolonged bed rest, elevation of the limb, and compression bandaging, although ambulant treatment should be tried first, using some non-irritant local application to the ulcerated area itself.

2 *Surgical treatment.* Surgical treatment is usually reserved for severe intractable ulceration or for patients who are unable to comply with the rigid conservative regime necessary to achieve healing.

Special investigation before surgery
Before operation, venography can be helpful in defining the deep system and demonstrating the incompetence of both the communicating and perforating veins. It is performed either by the injection of 30 ml of opaque water-soluble medium into a superficial vein on the dorsum of the foot, or by an intraosseous injection into the calcaneum. In the former method, which is less hazardous, the superficial veins are occluded prior to the injection by a tourniquet at the ankle. The presence of tortuous leashes of veins which have no valves in the deep circulation, or trunks with irregular outlines demonstrates that the deep system is abnormal.

Surgical techniques
The surgery of varicose ulcer owes much to Linton and Cockett. Linton originally described an operation that consisted of the following steps:

1 excision of the ulcer and the underlying deep fascia; this, he stated, severed the communications between the deep and superficial veins;
2 removal of all large superficial varicosities, especially in the lower leg;
3 ligation of the superficial femoral vein at its junction with the profunda, the latter being preserved.

Once Cockett had demonstrated the existence of the perforating veins, Linton's operation was placed on a sounder physiological basis although Cockett modified the operation by leaving the femoral vein untouched. Cockett's operation involves removing the incompetent perforators, the subcutaneous plaque of thrombosed venules and fibrofatty tissue and the ulcerated area. The latter is then allowed to granulate, and when the base of the ulcer is clean and healthy in appearance a split thickness skin graft is used to close the defect. The patient should be kept in bed with the leg elevated until the first dressing at 6 days. After this, the graft can be supported by a foam dressing and elastic bandages, although there is always a little separation at the line of junction with the abnormal skin.

Management following surgery
Even when the graft has firmly healed, continuous support is usually required and, if possible, the patient should avoid long periods of standing.

Treatment of venous pain
Deep bursting pain in the limb represents an almost insoluble problem. One operation described in the literature is to divide the deep fascia from the level of the knee to the ankle. The author has used this with complete lack of success and little has appeared in the literature following the initial reports, which again suggests that the operation carries little hope of success.